*Activity Measurement
in Psychology
and Medicine*

APPLIED CLINICAL PSYCHOLOGY

Series Editors:
Alan S. Bellack, *Medical College of Pennsylvania at EPPI, Philadelphia, Pennsylvania,*
and Michel Hersen, *University of Pittsburgh, Pittsburgh, Pennsylvania*

A Continuation Order Plan is available for this series. A continuation order will bring delivery of each new volume immediately upon publication. Volumes are billed only upon actual shipment. For further information please contact the publisher.

Activity Measurement in Psychology and Medicine

Warren W. Tryon
Fordham University
Bronx, New York

Plenum Press • *New York and London*

Library of Congress Cataloging-in-Publication Data

Tryon, Warren W.
    Activity measurement in psychology and medicine / Warren W.
Tryon.
        p.   cm. -- (Applied clinical psychology)
    Includes bibliographical references and index.
    ISBN 0-306-43786-4
    1. Behavioral assessment. 2. Exercise tests. I. Title.
II. Series.
        [DNLM: 1. Activities of Daily Living. 2. Behavior. 3. Mental
Disorders. 4. Monitoring, Physiologic.   WB 142 T875a]
    RC473.B43T79 1991
    616.07'5--dc20
    DNLM/DLC
    for Library of Congress   91-3683
                                                                  CIP

Material from DSM-II, DSM-III, and DSM-III-R (American Psychiatric Association: *Diagnostic and Statistical Manual of Mental Disorders, Third Edition, Revised,* Washington, DC, American Psychiatric Association, 1987) reprinted with permission of the American Psychiatric Association.

ISBN 0-306-43786-4

© 1991 Plenum Press, New York
A Division of Plenum Publishing Corporation
233 Spring Street, New York, N.Y. 10013

Printed in the United States of America

To my parents, who would be proud,
To Georgiana, my wife, and
To Elizabeth, for being herself

Foreword

In his treatment of activity measurement in the fields of medicine and psychology, Tryon gives us a book that clearly accomplishes the three purposes set out in its preface. The reader is definitely encouraged to wrestle with the concepts of behavior and activity in terms of "dynamic physical quantities." Moreover, the reader cannot help but become familiarized with the technology available for performing activity measurements. Motivation to use some of this technology is enhanced by the very extensive summary of other people's uses of it provided throughout the book.

Readers may find the book provocative on a number of levels. It is conceptually provocative to those of us struggling with understanding basic issues in the assessment and measurement of behavior. It is practically provocative to those of us working with various forms of behavioral difference, especially in clinical populations. The book provokes because it is essentially an unfinished exploration, opening us to numerous pathways that, when traveled, reveal still more paths to explore. In this sense the book should be heuristically useful both in the more traditional empirical sense, and in terms of its stimulation of conceptual discussion.

For me, the more interesting of these provocations is found in the conceptual challenges. Tryon nicely drives home the importance of measurement in science, reminding us that measurement may drive as well as be driven by theory. In reading the book and reflecting on it afterward I was struck with how clearly behavior can be seen on a continuum, ranging from chemical actions in the molecular biologic substrate through neural activity, to minute muscle twitches and aggregates of these at specific bodily locations sufficient to enable detection, to larger movements of particular body parts, to combinations of these propelling the organism through space. Tryon makes the very telling argument that assessing the stability of behavior requires aggregation to permit adequate detection at the individual-person level. As he notes, the logic of the Spearman-Brown prophecy formula provides tacit support for the relationship between consistency and aggregation. Consistency can be achieved if one is willing to increase the number of units of behavior observed to adequate levels of aggregation. Using this logic one might expect that specific activities detected by the actometers, pedometers, stabilimeters, accelerometers, and other devices reviewed by Tryon would evince a minimal amount of consistency. This is because, as very small aggregations (VSAs), they are difficult to detect. At the other end of the continuum, the behavioral dispositions referred to by trait labels should be relatively stable, as indeed they are, because traits, being very large aggregations (VLAs), are easy to detect (or at least their manifestations are).

Pursuing the question of temporal consistency raises further conceptual and methodological issues. As Tryon points out, the usual establishment of temporal generalizability with humans confounds instability in the human repertoire with that of the instrument being evaluated. Thus, the denominator in the classic reliability formula contains error due to both the person and the measure. The result is a conservative estimate of the reliability of the measure. As solutions to this problem, Tryon offers simultaneous measurement (with another identical instrument), aggregation (à la Epstein, 1980), or the use of a mechanical behavior generator (à la McGowan, Bulik, Epstein, Kupfer, & Robertson, 1984; Tryon, 1985). It seems that only the first two of these really treat reliability as we generally conceive of it. The simultaneous measurement solution, using two or more identical measures, seems conceptually akin to the process of alternate form reliability analysis. When the two measures are not identical and there is some reason to place one in criterion status (e.g., our operations reliably and completely define it), it is probably safest to regard the process as involving an analysis of the measure's accuracy.

The book could have benefited from clarifying the differences among terms such as these. Not that this would be desirable in a truly definitive way, since years of the best work of some preeminent measurement specialists have not completely settled our conceptual arguments in this area. Tryon's presentation of the psychometric issues concerning activity measurement forced me to reevaluate my own views. As a result, it seems clearer to me that accuracy and validity (and perhaps even reliability) are really waypoints along the same continuum. When scores on an instrument are totally controlled by objective features of the phenomenon being measured, we say the instrument is accurate. This total control can be known when we deliberately construct the phenomenon being measured to have objective features of a certain type. If our instrument detects these objective features, we say it is accurate.

Tryon refers to the process just described as studying validity. For example, he suggests that the validity of pedometers could be established by oscillating or vibrating them varying numbers of times. Correlations between pedometer readings and the number of oscillations or vibrations would provide evidence of the validity of the measure. He then goes on to note that there is a more important question to be asked of the measure's adequacy. This has to do with how small a difference in activity the actometer could detect a certain percentage of the time, e.g., 95% or 99%. Tryon suggests that this be referred to as the sensitivity of the measure. If we restrict our definition of accuracy to the extent to which an instrument detects objective, independently establishable features of the behavior, however, then

Tryon's concepts of validity and sensitivity are subsumed therein. Within such a framework, validity can be viewed as the process of relating scores on the instrument to those on measures that have nothing to do with operationally defining the phenomenon being assessed in any absolute sense. Correlating actometer readings with heartrate would be one example. When scores on the measure are related to scores on the same or identical measures (as in the simultaneous measurement example), the characteristic being examined is reliability. And when the measure is being related to the output of a mechanical behavior generator or some other instrument the output of which is completely defined, the characteristic being examined is accuracy.

It is quite clear from Tryon's exposition, though he does not address it directly, that as behavioral scientists, we need to consider behavior in the broadest sense. If we think of it as that which an organism does, involving action on and reaction to stimulus (environmental) conditions, we have a suitably broad—if not particularly precise—definition that encompasses both the very small aggregations dealt with in this book, and the very large aggregations typically seen as the province of psychology. But what of the terms "action" and "reaction"? The book deals with the measurement of activity, and it does so remarkably well considering that the term lacks precise definition anywhere therein. Activity appears to be defined solely operationally, thereby being relative. Wrist counters result in "activity units," which used to be defined as the amount of movement necessary to produce a complete revolution in the minute hand of a suitably modified self-winding watch. Pedometers result in units representing distance traveled. Tryon disputes the common calibration of pedometers in terms of distance traveled by pointing to the topographic differences in street crossing of adults on the one hand and children on the other. As Tryon describes it, the adult walks comfortably, taking relatively few steps to accomplish the crossing. The child, being less motorically efficient, takes many steps and perhaps engages in arm swinging, head turning, and other movements not directly relevant to crossing the street. Because of the conversion and calibration processes customarily used, most pedometers will give the same score to both. Tryon would regard the child as more active. Another interesting question is, How do we deal with the problems posed by different readings from the same device attached to different parts of the same person's body?

We need attention to these basic definitional issues. If we resort to physics for help, we might use energy or energy expended as our anchors for activity. Thus, activity might be equated with energy in the well-known $e = mc^2$ equation. Such a definition would give the edge in our above example to the adult. Skinner (1938, p. 6) saw behavior as "the movement of an organism or of its parts in a frame of reference provided by the organism itself or by various external objects or fields." He also noted that it "is often desirable to deal with an effect [of the behavior on its environment] rather than with the movement itself." If we use Skinner's definition of behavior as our definition of activity we might see the adult and the child in the above example as engaging in the same amount of activity. That is, topography aside, the effect of the movement of both was to reach the other side of the street. This strictly functional definition does not appear entirely satisfactory, however. What if the adult had been a paraplegic and navigated the crossing in a wheelchair? What if the child used a skateboard? In contrast to the functional approach, equating activity with mc^2 would give the edge to the adult, since m would be greater. Perhaps energy expended would be a better approach to defining activity. What, if any, difficulties would be encountered by relying on kilocalories (Kcal) as the basic unit? Of course, such a measure would be derivative in that the behavior or activity that caused the heat to be generated is not being assessed directly. However, given suitable control over the temporal relations between the activity and the kcal generated, one would be hard pressed to defend an alternative explanation for the energy expended.

Qualitative aspects of VSAs (or activity) are not dealt with by activity sensors as currently conceived. Tryon suggests the possibility of establishing a "physical signature" characterizing organized and disorganized behavior as one attempt to distinguish qualitatively different repertoires in diagnosing attention deficit–hyperactivity disorder in children. To accomplish this, persons with "organized" and "disorganized" behavior would be assessed using multisite actometry. Presumably some sort of norm or "physical signature" would be produced thereby, allowing a reference point for similar measures made on children for whom the diagnosis was in question. Confirming our definition of activity to kcal would appear to circumvent this requirement, however. Surely the organized repertoire would result in fewer kcal than the disorganized one. It is intriguing to speculate on the practical utility of such objectification.

The practical provocations in the book are as interesting as the conceptual. I will not go into these in detail, preferring to leave something to the reader's own discovery. A few ideas are too exciting to ignore, however, such as the notion of a physical signature mentioned above. While Tryon was thinking of it in a more nomothetic sense, it seems to have some potential value at the idiographic level as well. For example, it is now possible to determine a person's unique genetic signature and to identify people on this basis. Fingerprints provided the structural precursor to genetic signatures or genetiprints, and to behavioral signatures as represented in voice prints. The physical signature suggested by Tryon might be thought of as a more comprehensive type of behavioral or activity signature (actiprint?). While it would not be used for the same identification purposes as voice, finger, and genetiprints, it could serve the very useful purpose of establishing baselines representing the organizational level or quality of one's activity. Extent of loss and the success of rehabilitation efforts following injury could then be gauged more objectively, for example. It might be reasonable to obtain activity signatures along with the usual biochemical and physical assays collected during routine physical examinations. Studies showing changes in signature following other types of event (e.g., golf lessons, piano lessons, aging) would also benefit from the increased objectivity offered by such technology, especially if activity were defined in some absolute terms such as kcal.

While I have concentrated on the conceptual provocations that I have experienced in reading this book, others will no doubt find it stimulating in other ways. What Tryon has done for me, and will perhaps do for others, is to set the occasion for challenging the barriers between behavior and physiology. It will be interesting to see if this form of psychological "glasnost" is experienced by the scientific community at large.

John D. Cone

United States International University
San Diego, California

REFERENCES

Epstein, S. (1980). The stability of behavior. II: Implications for psychological research. *American Psychologist, 35,* 790–806.

McGowan, C. R., Bulik, C. M., Epstein, L. H., Kupfer, D. J., & Robertson, R. J. (1986). The effect of exercise on nonrestricted caloric intake in male joggers. *Appetite, 7,* 97–105.

Skinner, B. F. (1938). *The behavior of organisms.* New York: Appleton-Century-Crofts.

Tryon, W. W. (1985). Measurement of human activity. In W. W. Tryon (Ed.), *Behavioral assessment in behavioral medicine* (pp. 200–256). New York: Springer.

Preface

Activity is integral to behavior regarding both its presence and absence. The emission of behavior requires moving in space and time while the omission of behavior is characterized by no, or greatly reduced, movement in space and time. Therefore, all motor behavior can be placed somewhere on a movement (activity) spectrum ranging from zero to very high.

Given that all motor behavior involves movement, it follows that behavior disorder involves abnormal activity that psychologists and physicians can measure to describe these disorders, diagnose their presence in particular cases, and assess the impact of treatment on.

In addition to its central theoretical importance, activity has the desirable property of being physically measurable in natural science units, i.e., the centimeter, gram, second (cgs) or meter, kilogram, second (mks) system. This property immediately brings the study of activity within the scope of natural science while preserving many important social science implications. Physical measurement of activity enables objective longitudinal transduction and recording of motor behavior, thereby making possible extensive naturalistic studies as well as prolonged controlled clinical trials, feats that have previously not been feasible. For example, a review of activity studies of hyperactive children quickly reveals that very limited behavioral samples have typically been used both with respect to time (20–30 minutes) and situations (office or laboratory). Chapter 4 discusses this literature and recent encouraging actigraphic exceptions. Technological developments in recent years have greatly expanded our ability to obtain longitudinal activity measurements without artificial restriction to enable data collection. The advent of ambulatory activity monitoring has allowed more rigorous and extensive study of existing research questions, such as whether children diagnosed as hyperactive are measurably more active, and allowed new questions to be addressed, such as changes in circadian activity as a function of affective disorder.

This book has three major purposes: one, to encourage the reader to think of behavior (activity) in terms of dynamic physical quantities found at various sites of attachment rather than as a uniform trait such as eye color (a corollary of this perspective is that one should obtain representative behavioral samples prior to drawing activity inferences); two, to familiarize the reader with the full spectrum of technology available for obtaining activity measurements; and three, to summarize as much of what is currently known through activity measurements as is possible within available space and time constraints. Hence, topics of adult mood disorders, schizophrenia, hyperactivity in children, eating and sleep disorders, drugs and substance use, and effects of chronic diseases are restricted to findings obtained by behavioral measurements with instruments. While every effort has been made to be thorough, no doubt some studies within the above-stipulated scope of this book have been omitted. I therefore invite anyone with knowledge of such omissions to send me a reprint of the omitted article.

Warren W. Tryon

Bronx, New York

Acknowledgments

I am especially grateful to Michel Hersen for his confidence in me and invitation to write this book and for his intellectual support during its formative stages. I also wish to thank the many people who graciously sent me reprints and preprints of their work, hardware specifications, photographs, and references to published articles I would have otherwise likely missed. On the basis that citation and coverage are the most sincere forms of acknowledgment that science offers, I refer the reader to the text.

Contents

Introduction to Behavioral Physics: Activity

The history of science is largely coextensive with the history of measurement. Theory existed from the time humans first began to reason, but knowledge accumulated very slowly. The supremacy of theory often led to static dogma. Subordinating theory to experience was the critical epistemological development giving rise to science and the resulting explosive increase in new knowledge. Experience is gained through the senses; we learn by observing, listening, touching, tasting, and smelling. Instruments often quantify experience into standard units of measure. Instruments can extend the senses into new domains. The telescope allows us to see farther than possible with the naked eye. The microscope allows us to visit the world of the exceedingly small. High speed cameras and lasers allow us to slow down time so that we can study sequences of events that appear instantaneous to the unaided eye and ear. Time lapse photography allows us to better appreciate dynamic changes that take place very slowly. X-ray, computed axial tomography (CAT), magnetic resonance imaging (MRI), and positron emission tomography (PET) scans allow us to visualize the insides of live beings without surgery. Chemical analysis of blood and other specimens has greatly advanced our understanding of disease to the modern point where disease is thought of in terms of laboratory measurements and the results of physical examination. Examples could be continued at greater length but by now the point should be crystal clear; our present scientific understanding of many phenomena is critically dependent upon instrumented measurements. Consider what the state of contemporary science education would look like if all knowledge based upon instruments were stricken from existing textbooks.

An equally important feature of instruments is that they correct for sensory limitations. The Weber-Fechner Law indicates that where humans perceive linear increases, exponential changes are occurring. Instruments standardize experience. The amount of physical change in temperature, weight, or any other physical event necessary for one person to perceive a just noticeable difference (JND) is not the same amount as is required for another person to perceive a JND. Said concisely, individual differences in perception clearly exist. Properly calibrated instruments provide a common experience which facilitates arriving at a common understanding of the events under study. Of special importance to the social sciences is that instruments are not influenced by sex, race, personality, and other characteristics that can prejudice observations.

The major purpose of this book is to seriously embrace a *natural science* orientation to the study of behavior by emphasizing knowledge obtained through instrumentation. The term *behavioral physics* is used to emphasize the premise that behavior, activity, involves motion in time and space which has historically been the province of physics. Hence, obtaining data about behavior from a physical perspective constitutes the natural science approach to the study of behavior exemplified by this book.

Adopting the behavioral measurement perspective requires a major theoretical adjustment. The basic challenge is to forgo generic global behavioral referents, such as activity, for the perspective of a sensor transducing the physical events in question. This philosophical move requires that we thoroughly understand both the operational characteristics of the sensor and its associated recording mechanism, and also where the sensor has been placed on the individual. The first issue pertains to *construction validity*; the second to *site of attachment*. Current questions and uncertainties will be reviewed and recommendations will be made regarding desirable future lines of research. In sum, the purposes of this book are as much or more toward theoretical as toward temporal empirical ends.

UNITS OF MEASURE AND THEIR THEORETICAL IMPORTANCE

Most investigators in the natural and social sciences give little thought to the units of measurement entailed in their discipline. In the natural sciences, this inattention is partly because the centimeter, gram, second (CGS) and meter, kilogram, second (MKS) measurement systems have been well-established international standards for some time now. While the exact value of these basic defining quantities may still be in transition as one or other atomic standard is considered, current textbook values serve the scientific and engineering communities quite well. Future modifications will likely be in terms of referents such as the number of wavelengths of a particular atom rather than in either final numerical value or theoretical nature. Currently, one meter equals 1,650,763.73 wavelengths of orange-red light emitted from krypton-86. One second equals 9,192,631,770 transitions between two energy levels of the cesium-133 atom.

Units of measurement have theoretical implications that are rarely considered despite their substantial importance. Consider the meaning of the term "velocity." Its definition is in terms of distance per unit time; a ratio of two fundamental units of measurement (meters/second). Continuing such division further yields the concept of acceleration (meters/second/second). A new basic unit is then constructed relative to the natural phenomenon of how rapidly things fall at sea level at 45 degrees latitude (9.80616 meters/second/second). This development sets the occasion to conceptualize force in terms of accelerating mass. The force necessary to accelerate a mass of one kg to an acceleration of one meter per second was defined as one newton consistent with the equation: $F = MA$. We should remember that the equals sign means "is conceptually equal to" in addition to "is numerically equal to." The term "equation" indicates that both sides mean the same thing. The term "formula" means that we have formulated a theoretical relationship between quantities of interest.

It was intended that one gram be equal to one cubic centimeter of water at its maximum density in a vacuum. Problems of measurement caused the resulting platinum-iridium cylinder taken today as defining one kilogram to depart from the intended standard of 1000 cubic centimeters of water by a small amount. The point here is that mass was conceptualized in terms of a volume of a very common substance—water. Dividing the weight of an object in grams by its volume in cubic centimeters formulates its density.

The above examples can be extended until we have reconstructed essentially all of the *ideas* of modern natural (physical) science since they all are expressed in some unit(s) of measure. Conceptualizing and defining *concepts in terms of measurements* has set the occasion for the considerable hierarchically integrated achievements of the physical sciences.

Operational definitions are related to but not coextensive with the developments just described. It is true that all of the above conceptual definitions constitute operational definitions because they specify the procedures necessary to obtain the indicated quantities. To obtain density values, one divides weight measurements in grams by volume measurements in cubic centimeters. Changing the measurement procedures changes the meaning of the concept in question. I could have defined density to equal the time it takes for a penny to drop one foot—but now we are talking about something altogether different than weight per unit volume. While this example may seem absurd, we shall shortly see that activity has been measured in distinctly different ways while thinking that essentially the same thing has been measured. Sensors that respond to a 5° deflection from vertical are not equivalent to sensors that measure acceleration. Nor are the conceptualizations of activity equivalent.

No Units Equal Limited Understanding

The first major problem of not having basic units of measurement is that one lacks a fundamental definition of the phenomenon under study. Consider the measurement of intelligence. We lack a meaningful unit of intelligence which, given the above discussion, indicates that we have yet to concisely conceptualize what the essence of intelligence is. We have yet to formulate the concept "intelligence" in an explicit manner. To say that intelligence is what an intelligence test measures both begs the question and is a correct evaluation of the current conceptualization of intelligence. It begs the question only because intelligence tests lack a theoretical unit of measurement, the IQ and related scores being but convenient statistical conventions. We indirectly refer to the nature of intelligence by specifying the various tasks used to quantify it.

It may well be that intelligence can only be adequately evaluated by obtaining many measurements and combining them in a complex *formula*. The point here is that each contributing measurement should be based upon a specific unit of measurement in order to have rigorous meaning. Consider the following two approaches to the facet of intelligence called information processing. We might measure the number of bits of information correctly processed in a fixed time period and calculate a processing rate of bits per second. Or, we could measure the time necessary to correctly process a fixed number of bits of information and calculate seconds per bit. While these two approaches are probably positively correlated, they represent different formulations. Bits per second emphasizes the importance of dividing the task into temporal units of one second each and studying the time-series and aggregate distribution of amount of information (bits) processed by a single individual during the task and over individuals presented with the same task. The interest is in how the amount of information processed varies with each uniform temporal interval.

Seconds per bit emphasizes the importance of dividing the task into single bits of information and studying the time series and aggregate distribution of time measurements obtained from a single individual during the task and over individuals presented with the same task. The size of the "chunk" to be processed is held constant, controlled, at one bit and the duration of its processing is measured.

An entirely different example regarding manipulations to study the effects of crowding may make the contrast even greater. If one hypothesizes that crowding, population density, is related to aggression, one might experimentally study this hypothesis in one of two ways. We might take three 2 ft × 2 ft cages and put 2 rats in the first, 4 in the second, and 8 in the third. Here we control for living space but increase the number of occupants, which dramatically increases the total number of pairwise relationships present. Alternately, we might select three groups of 4 subjects placing one group in a 1 ft × 1 ft cage, another group in a 2 ft × 2 ft cage, and the last group in a 3 ft × 3 ft cage. Here we control for group size and consequent social interactions while changing the amount of space they have to live in. Both manipulations are valid aspects of crowding, may yield correlated findings, but are conceptually different.

No Units: Reliable, Valid, but Probably Inaccurate

A second problem associated with not having fundamental units of measurement is that one can have reliable and valid measuring devices that are also inaccurate, as illustrated by the following thought experiment.

Consider a situation where five persons wish to measure temperature. They are all aware of the mercury-in-a-glass-tube sensor and therefore partially fill a glass tube with mercury. They each test their thermometers by repeatedly placing them in a one-liter beaker of ice water and recording the height of the mercury on the tube each time with a millimeter rule. The thermometers are left out of the ice water for 10 minutes in between trials to bring them to a new higher level. Assume that nearly the same result is repeatedly observed such that no question exists as to the high reliability of each of the five investigators' thermometers.

The five investigators then demonstrate the validity of their thermometers by measuring the temperatures of three one-liter beakers of water. The first beaker contains ice water as before. The second beaker is at "room temperature." The third beaker has been heated to a boil. The height of the column of mercury is highest for boiling water, intermediate for room temperature, and lowest for ice water thereby confirming the validity of all five thermometers: perfect validity due to the obtained correlation of 1.0.

Assume that all five investigators attend the same convention, meet each other, and tell of their highly reliable and perfectly valid thermometers. For comparison purposes they place all five instruments into a single one-liter beaker of water at room temperature and record *five different temperatures*. This difference does not disappear when the water is stirred, nor when ice is added, nor when the water is boiled. Clearly, each condition yielded a stable single temperature yet each investigator reports a different temperature!

The problem here is that no standard unit of measurement exists. Different diameters of glass tubing filled to different initial levels will rise to different absolute heights give any particular quantity of heat. Use of the same millimeter rule was only a partial solution. It is unusual for even such partial agreement to be reached within the social sciences. The essential problem is that the investigators failed to agree upon a standard unit of temperature. Calibration solves such problems. The solution to this problem is to place each thermometer in ice water and mark the glass tube at the mercury level; place each thermometer in boiling water and mark the glass tube at the mercury level; then divide the resulting interval into 100 equal parts. Placing these calibrated thermometers into a single beaker of room temperature, ice, or boiling water will now reveal very similar temperatures.

A direct *theoretical* consequence of having reinvented the centigrade thermometer is that we can conceptualize, that is define, a gram-calorie of heat energy to be the amount of energy necessary to increase the temperature of one gram (one cubic centimeter) of water one degree centigrade (from 14.5 to 15.5°C). Another conceptual advance is achieved through attention to units of measure.

Problems with Z-Score Units

The fundamental problem with Z-score units is their completely arbitrary and ever-changing nature. Z-scores are completely arbitrary because their value is determined by the standard deviation calculated on the responses of the particular subjects being measured. The unit of measure is inextricably tied to the particular sample of measurements at hand and changes as the measurement sample changes. Repeated measurement will almost certainly yield different standard deviations and therefore Z-score units of measurement. Studying additional subjects of the same general type will change the standard deviation and therefore the Z-score units. Studying different people such as men vs women or children vs adults will yield different standard deviations and therefore Z-score units. In short, the unit of measure changes constantly in unpredictable ways. Imagine the chaos that would result if one tried to study the physical world with ever-changing instruments; rulers that changed size depending upon what substance was measured for length, scales that changed depending upon what objects were placed on them. Z-score units are borne of desperation due to the absence of theoretically meaningful units of measure.

The underlying theoretical issue here is that Z-score units measure an individual against other persons rather than against a theoretical quantity or an objective criterion. It is like measuring track athletes by where they finished in comparison with the average contestant rather than timing how fast they ran their event. Each athlete's standing would reflect the behavior of other competitors as much or more than their own performance. Because selection criteria determine who participates in research studies and athletic contests, comparative units of measure are necessarily dependent upon selection criteria. Subjects who drop out and fail to complete a study or contest change the unit of measurement. In short, the unit of measurement varies over time with a multitude of factors.

Measurement Enables Theory

Science is often presented in terms of the hypothetico-deductive model, which begins the theory–measurement circle from the perspective of a hypothesis that is subjected to empirical test and possible revision. It remains unclear where original theory comes from. Science can be presented as a measurement–theory cycle where measurement sometimes provides the occasion to entertain new ideas. This is largely the case with Laennec and the stethoscope, as presented by Reiser (1979).

The prevailing theory, since the time of the Greeks, was that disease was caused by an imbalance in body fluids called humors. Correlating the sounds heard through the stethoscope with postmortem examination gave rise to the theory that disease produced anatomical changes which could be evaluated by conducting a physical examination of the patient. Modern medical theory is firmly grounded in laboratory measurements of many kinds in addition to the results of modern medical imaging techniques. Imagine what would be left of modern medical theory and practice if every concept and practice based upon instruments and their standard units of measure were eradicated.

THEORETICAL REORIENTATION

The first step toward achieving the desired theoretical orientation is to consider the topic at hand in terms of what constitutes its fundamental unit or units. Johnston and Pennypacker (1980) have reviewed this issue from the perspective of behavioral science and space prohibits reiterating their arguments here. The perspective taken here is to suggest that searching for units of measure unique to behavioral science may be misguided. Psychologists have long used clocks to measure reaction time. Activity involves motion and physics provides standard units of velocity and acceleration. A natural science orientation toward the study of behavior simply suggests expressing behavior in natural science units.

Noncomparability of Instruments

Reaction timers manufactured by different companies using different technologies (quartz crystals vs mainsprings) yield comparable results because these devices are calibrated against the standard second. Virtually all existing activity monitors have different units of measure and- or operating characteristics. There is no agreed-upon standard and no way to calibrate activity monitors to give the same readings. Ultrasound, infrared, stabilimetric chairs, tilt counters, pedometer/step counters, and accelerometer-based devices are so fundamentally different in their operation that they measure substantially different aspects of activity. Fortunately, it appears to be the case that these various aspects are positively correlated over time such that highly active persons receive higher scores than moderately active than slightly active persons. However, data from various devices are not directly comparable.

The major implication of this conclusion is that data should be reported separately by device when reviewing empirical findings. An important corollary is that results with one type of device can only weakly, not strongly, confirm or disconfirm reports based upon other devices.

Site of Attachment

It is common for psychologists, physicians, and laypersons to talk about activity as though it were some one thing. Activity is thought to be equally expressed at the wrist, ankle, and waist and therefore willingness exists to compare, without reservation, activity data taken from these sites of attachment. Modest reflection on one's own behavior, and that of others, quickly reveals counterexamples to this assertion. Persons seated at a desk are probably wrist active, may periodically be ankle active, but probably will not be waist active. Exercise on a stationary bike will produce much ankle activity, perhaps occasional wrist activity, but little waist activity which may or may not be detected depending upon the sensitivity of the device used. Walking, running, tennis, and other sports involve the entire body and hence all sites are active. The important conclusion here is that body sites are differentially active depending upon the behavior engaged in. It is unlikely that any one site is perfectly correlated with all of the others and therefore no single site can be said to reflect "general activity."

Pedometers are typically attached to the waist, actigraphs and tilt counters to the wrist and ankle, and actometers have been placed in pouches sewn to the back of a jacket. Hence, devices are differentially attached to body sites. Therefore, investigators using different devices will also probably be studying different sites of attachment.

The primary implication here is that results obtained from one site of attachment can only weakly, not strongly, confirm or disconfirm reports based upon other sites of attachment. Therefore, data should be reviewed separately by site of attachment when reviewing empirical findings.

RESEARCH DESIGN ISSUES

It is important to distinguish between repeatability of measurements under laboratory conditions and repeatability of measurements under clinical conditions when evaluating an activity monitor. The extent to which an instrument yields the same, or similar, results when measuring exactly, or nearly so, the same phenomenon we shall call *instrument reliability*. Behavioral science has traditionally evaluated instrument (psychological test) reliability by studying responses of subjects whereas natural science has traditionally evaluated measuring instruments under laboratory conditions. These matters are discussed in next section.

Treatment (intervention) research requires replicable pre- and posttreatment values (behavioral stability) in order to ascribe observed changes to the treatment rather than measurement inadequacies. A deficient understanding of behavioral variation may lead investigators to question the validity of devices when their measurement instabilities are due to small behavioral samples. These issues are discussed in the Clinical Repeatability section.

Instrument Reliability

Some investigators have erroneously evaluated the reliability of instruments (actometers in this case) on the basis of test–retest data. For example, Maccoby, Dowley, Hagen, and Dergman (1965) reported test–retest correlation coefficients 7 to 14 days apart of $r(11) = .31$ for female and $r(11) = .76$ for male wrist activity and $r(11) = .22$ for female and $r(13) = .44$ for male ankle activity. Schulman, Kaspar, and Throne (1965) reported $\rho(25) = .67$ for 1- to 3-week test–retest intervals on boys. Bell (1968) correlated activity on odd with even days for 31 females regarding ankle ($r(29) = .55$) and jacket ($r(29) = .56$) measures. Massey, Lieberman, and Batarseh (1971) reported $r(31) = .798$.

Inferences about the operating characteristics (reliability) of actometers per se, or any other instrument, cannot be sustained by such reports because they confound clinical variability with instrument variability. The reported correlations depend upon changes in behavior from one time to the next as well as upon measurement inconsistency. Laboratory evidence presented in Chapter 2 indicates that most of the test–retest variation reported by the above-mentioned investigators stems from subject variability, not instrument variability. Hence, such test–retest data estimates the extreme *lower* bound of actometer reliability. Their results are properly interpreted as indicating that actometer reliability is *greater* than the reported value. Laboratory evidence presented in Chapter 2 corroborates this position. As with any other instrument, some brands are superior to others. The literature reflects a strong tendency to overgeneralize and reject all instruments of a particular type when one brand is found to have difficulty.

It is noteworthy that the operating characteristics of psychological tests and rating scales cannot be studied independent from peoples' behavior: their reliability and validity can only be determined in conjunction with subject participation. The resulting reliability and validity coefficients are always reduced by subject instability; changes from test to retest. The operating characteristics of activity monitors are best determined under laboratory conditions where carefully controlled stimuli can be repeatedly applied to the instrument to see if it responds consistently. Clinical studies add sources of uncertainty pertaining to behavioral variations across measurement conditions due to a host of factors associated with engaging in different behaviors plus aspects of clinical disorder. This larger variability can be compared to laboratory estimates to evaluate subject variability.

Winer (1971) discusses intraclass correlation reliability coefficients and their calculation using Analysis of Variance (ANOVA) methods (cf. pp. 283–289). Winer's Table 4.5-1 (p. 284) indicates that k repeated measurements are obtained on n persons. Mean squares (MS) between and within people are calculated. The estimate of true variance (TV) is obtained by subtracting MS within people from MS between people and dividing by k. The estimate of error variance (EV) is MS within people. The intraclass reliability coefficient equals TV/(TV + EV).

Severe problems occur in this reliability analysis when people are replaced by physical instruments, such as activity monitors. High manufacturing quality produces instruments that are very similar. Calibration of these instruments further reduces their variability in that they are physically adjusted to minimize differences from one instrument to the other. Even greater homogeneity can be produced by calculating conversion constants for each device on the basis of empirical testing with standard stimuli. Data from instruments that consistently give higher-than-standard values can be multiplied by a fraction to reduce them to the standard value whereas data from instruments that consistently give lower-than-standard values can be multiplied by a number greater than 1 to increase them to the standard value. All of these commonly used methods for reducing measurement instability substantially reduce between instrument variability. When between-instrument variability equals within-instrument variability, the "true variance" estimate mentioned above equals zero resulting in *zero* reliability despite what amounts to perfect interchangeability of instruments; each instrument differs from the other by no more than any one instrument differs from itself! Should calibration and conversion reduce between-instrument variability below that of within-instrument variability, then reliability becomes *negative*. Both of these outcomes so strongly distort the true operating characteristics of physical instruments that ANOVA and correlation coefficients should *not* be used to assess reliability. Their joint deficiency is in the false assumption that a sample of instruments is as diverse as a sample of people.

Knowing that correlations can only be large given adequate variability and that high-quality instruments are so alike that differences between them cannot provide the necessary variability, it follows that the size of obtained test–retest correlation coefficients must be due to the presence of another source of variation. Such variability in the laboratory could be produced by erratic, rather than controlled, stimulation, thereby calling the entire study into question. Such variability in clinical studies is probably produced by inconsistent variation of subjects within supposedly standard test-and-retest conditions. The larger the obtained correlations the more variable subject performance probably has been, which negates the operational premise of the instrument study.

Because correlation and ANOVA reliability assessed is heavily dependent upon the diversity of the subjects studied, a psychological test or rating scale yielding inconsistent results can be made to look better by evaluating its reliability on a more heterogeneous (variable) group of subjects. Unfortunately, the high reliability result is ascribed to the psychological test or rating scale which subsequent investigators use on homogeneous as well as heterogeneous samples. This again illustrates the difficulties encountered when forced to evaluate measurement characteristics in conjunction with subject characteristics. Their confounding into one joint, inversely related system allows properties of one aspect (subject variability) to appear as the other (instrument reliability).

The coefficient of variation [$CV = (SD/Mean) \times 100$] is the preferred measure of instrument reliability because a small standard deviation of repeated measurements indicates repeatable readings assuming stability in what is being measured. The standard deviation is a root-mean-square (RMS) measure of variation commonly used by engineers. Expressing this error index as a percentage of the mean acknowledges that greater absolute uncertainty is expected when larger quantities are measured.

Because $1 - r^2$ equals error and CV equals error we can equate them and solve for $r = [1 - CV]^{1/2}$ to obtain the correlational equivalent of CV when expressed in decimal form (e.g., CV = .05; r = .9747). This practice is an improvement over the reporting used by Saunders, Goldstein, and Stein (1978), and Heiser, Epstein, and Wing (1981) mentioned below.

The above-mentioned conversion procedure allows one to compare error associated with instrumented measurements with error typically expected with psychological tests and rating scales. An instrument with CV = .19 or 19% error is equivalent to r = .90, and an instrument with CV = .36 or 36% error is equivalent to r = .80. It seems that we tolerate substantial measurement error in psychological tests and rating scales.

Clinical Repeatability

The more stable repeated measurements are in the absence of treatment, the more powerful statistical or visual analysis of intervention effects will be; and the more certain we can be that a specific individual is hyperactive or hypoactive vs normoactive.

Behavior is exceptionally dynamic from the behavioral physics perspective, where the forces associated with behavior are under consideration. Figure 1-1

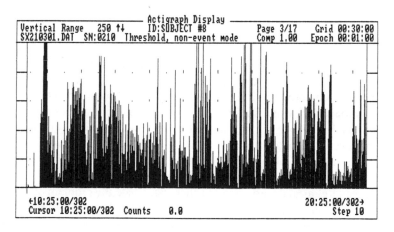

FIGURE 1.1. Normal activity is highly variable.

illustrates remarkable, and typical, variation in wrist activity between 10:25:00 and 20:25:00 of Day 302, 1989, in a normal college student using an Ambulatory Monitoring Inc. (Ardsley, NY) Motionlogger™ actigraph (cf. Chapter 2) programmed for threshold mode and a 1-minute epoch. The maximum plot is 250 counts which equals 25 seconds of activity greater than 0.1 g. The grid tics are 30 minutes apart as indicated. Further examples of Motionlogger™ output will be presented when we discuss sleep disorders in Chapter 6.

Within- and between-day variation results from lifestyle variation. Perhaps several classes are attended Monday morning and tennis is played that afternoon while Tuesday is mostly spent in the library. Variation in daily routine necessarily creates variability in daily activity. Confronted with such variability, one rapidly abandons any expectation that a single activity measurement made during a brief time period can ever be replicated.

We are now faced with determining the within- and between-day aspects of behavioral samples to insure both their repeatability (reliability) and validity.

Within-Day Samples

The amount of time per day that activity measurements should be taken partly depends upon the primary purpose for which the activity measurement is being taken. If one is concerned with activity during mathematics class then measurements should be taken only during this class. Because this time interval is already brief, measurements should be taken for the entire class period rather than the first, middle, or last few minutes. If interest resides in activity during academic periods, then all such periods should be studied. If concern exists about the child being generally overactive, then one might wish to measure all waking hours. If disturbed sleep is in question, then activity measurements should be taken at night.

Between-Day Samples

The number of days to be sampled is partly determined by the variability in daily activities. It is desirable to sample all activities at least once. Multiple samples of each behavior comprising one's lifestyle are desirable because each aspect of the lifestyle is variable. Playing tennis against a more demanding opponent may create higher activity levels than playing against a less able partner. Some recreational walks are longer than others. Sometimes one finds a closer parking spot than at others. Sometimes one takes the stairs rather than the elevator. Hence, multiple measurements of all activities should be sought.

Presence of clinical disorder may further exacerbate the problem of replicating activity measurements. Rapid cycling Bipolar Disorder, Mixed (296.6x) is a good example of where underlying pathology causes valid behavioral changes that prevent one from replicating measurements. Perhaps this is the juncture to remind ourselves that the concept of reliability requires *no intervening change*. Behavior is so dynamic that some change *always* takes place. Variability in excess of laboratory-determined measurement instability can be attributed either to the chosen independent variable or other covariate. If activity variability is impressive, then perhaps variance rather than mean level should be taken as the dependent measure. The behavior of mentally retarded persons is especially variable. Their unpredictable outbursts complicate efforts to place them in the community. Treatments that can moderate these unusually large activity changes is clinically important. Research in this area will probably not reveal stable pretreatment activity levels unless variance values turn out to be stable.

The duration of each sample will be determined by the natural frequency with which behavioral variations occur. One-week samples may be adequate if daily outbursts occur. Two-week or one-month samples may be required if outbursts are less frequent. The rule of thumb here should probably be to choose a sampling period sufficiently long to obtain a minimum of two instances of all relevant behaviors; one replication. Greater replicability can be expected with increased replications. Multiple samples of each type of activity increase both reliability and validity just like increasing the number of items on a psychological test (cf. Epstein, 1979, 1980).

Tryon (1989c) obtained 42 to 222 consecutive days of actometer data from six overweight subjects enrolled in a behaviorally oriented weight-control group plus two normal weight controls. Each subject wore a Model 108 Timex Motion Recorder (cf. Schulman and Reisman, 1959) on their dominant wrist 24 hours a day except when showering. Graphical inspection of their data indicates that treatment had little, if any, lasting influence upon their activity. It appeared as if their activity fluctuated about a set point in the same way that physiological functions such as body temperature, glucose level, and blood pressure do (Keesey, 1980). Hence, these data constitute a reasonable data set upon which to evaluate the stabilizing effects of cumulating activity measurements over 1- to 4-week intervals. Four subjects averaged 228.94 pounds ($S = 54.88$). Two normal weight subjects weighing 120 and 108 pounds also participated in this study.

The data were divided into $4 \times 7 = 28$-day months and the ability to obtain repeatable activity measurements using cumulative means beginning at the first of each month was evaluated. Monthly plots of cumulative means (Day 1, Days 1 + 2, Days 1 + 2 + 3, etc.) converged to a stable value in 6 of 8 months for Subject 1, 6 of 7 months for Subject 2, 3 of 4 months for Subject 3, 4 of 4 months for Subject 4, 2 of 3 months for Subjects 5 and 6, 2 of 2 months for Subject 7, and 1 of 1 month for Subject 8.

Cross-Situational Stability

An important aspect of clinical repeatability is the extent to which activity scores obtained in one situation predict those obtained in another situation. Activity scores will certainly vary from one situation to another but here we are concerned with a person maintaining the same relative position across activity distributions obtained from different situation. Cross-situational stability is a primary basis for drawing trait inferences.

For example, Halverson and Post-Gordon (1984) obtained free-play actometer measurements from 132 nursery school children (aged 30 to 42 months) during three daily inside and outside free play and a rest period for 1 day during each of 3 or 4 weeks. Inside Free Play correlated $r(130) = .50$, $p < .0001$ with Rest Period. Inside Free Play correlated $r(130) = .54$, $p < .0001$ with Outside Free Play. Rest Period correlated $r(130) = .69$, $p < .0001$ with Outside Free Play.

Situational Specificity

Behaviorism emphasizes environmental determinants of behavior and therefore predicts different activity levels in different situations. Every investigator who has obtained activity measurements from distinctly different situations finds different activity levels. For example, Halverson and Post-Gordon (1984) reported that 132 nursery school children (aged 30–42 months) were significantly ($p < .001$) more active during Inside and Outside Free Play than Rest Period. Further examples can be found in Chapters 3 and 4.

An extensive literature has developed around the trait vs situation debate that will not be reviewed here. Two comments are sufficient for our purposes. First, the issue of mean difference is entirely independent of maintaining the same relative position (Z-score) within two or more different distributions. Situational arguments entail mean differences whereas trait arguments entail maintaining Z-scores within distributions. Hence, one argument has nothing to do with the other despite appearances to the contrary; they are independent issues. It is therefore clearly possible to have any combination of the two positions. The data reviewed above strongly suggest that activity is both very different across situations yet predictable from situation to situation.

Situational differences are so large that they stand out immediately. Person consistency is more subtle and requires aggregation to reach substantial effect size. The Spearman–Brown prophecy formula indicates that either effect size can be made arbitrarily large depending upon the level of aggregation chosen. The implication for research and clinical practice is that one should choose the level of aggregation that provides the necessary effect size to achieve the stated purpose of the empirical inquiry at hand.

Autocorrelation

An important assumption of inferential statistics is that each observation be independent of every other observation. When repeated measurements are taken from a single individual it has traditionally been assumed that they will necessarily be autocorrelated, which means that later values can be predicted from earlier values. To calculate the Lag 1 autocorrelation coefficient, the X column is the list of repeated measurements and the Y column is a duplicate of this list placed beside the X list and slid up one position so that the first entry in list X is associated with the second entry in list Y. Every X value is correlated with the $X + $ 1st value. For Lag 2 we shift the Y list up one more value such that the first X value is paired with the second Y value. Every X value is correlated with the $X + $ 2nd value. The presence of of autocorrelation substantially changes the probabilities of making Type I (rejecting the null hypothesis when it is true) and Type II (accepting the null hypothesis when it is false) errors.

Time-series analysis typically identifies the presence of autocorrelation, models it, and then removes it leaving properly uncorrelated points for subsequent traditional statistical analysis.

Huitema (1985, 1986, 1988) has marshalled strong empirical support indicating that the distribution of autocorrelation coefficients within baseline and treatment conditions is centered about zero and ranges from strongly negative to strongly positive. This covers all possibilities. Repeated measurements can either be positively or negatively autocorrelated or they can be uncorrelated. Because the positive and negative autocorrelations are equally frequent at each degree of association, their average, median, and mode is essentially zero. We conclude, that repeated measurements are not necessarily correlated. In fact, the tendency is toward uncorrelated series.

Within-Subject Significance Testing

Significance testing is usually discussed in the context of between-groups design. Performance of subjects in an "experimental" group is compared with that of subjects in a "control" group. Several problems, both practical and theoretical, exist with this approach.

The theoretical objection emphasized here is the one traditionally proffered by advocates of the experimental analysis of behavior. Group averages do not necessarily pertain to specific individuals. This point was made especially clear by Melton (1990) when describing the irrelevance of group data to judicial decisions regarding guilt or innocence. Showing that persons of a particular type or belonging to a particular category have a significantly greater chance of committing a particular crime is insufficient evidence upon which to convict a particular individual or to deny parental visitation rights to such a person.

A second objection is that group designs minimize individual differences to the extent that they group subjects together. It is possible for half the subjects to improve and half to get worse resulting in no mean difference even though every subject changed, and perhaps changed substantially. Sometimes it is possible to divide the heterogeneous group into subgroups on the basis of sex, age, race, or score on some covariate, thereby enhancing within-group homogeneity while explaining some of the original variation. Other times, such subdivisions are not helpful and one cannot then form two groups on the basis of subjects' having improved or gotten worse. Lewis (1990) discussed another important version of the individual difference position; subject by treatment interaction. If a different 10% of the population responds substantially to each of ten different interventions, then it is possible to successfully treat everyone despite the fact that each treatment is not statistically significant when individually evaluated in moderately small samples such as are usually available to investigators.

Generalizability of results obtained through within-groups designs often exceeds that of between-groups designs when sample sizes are matched because of the much greater and more specific information available on each person.

The practical objection to between-groups designs is that they generally make demands which far exceed the resources available to most investigators. First, truly random subject samples are rarely if ever available partly because subjects have the right of informed consent and can, and sometimes do, discontinue participation before the study ends. Second, matching is often done on a group rather than individual basis. This allows a few subjects who score particularly low to balance the majority of high-scoring subjects to a value equal to a second group where a few high-scoring subjects balance the majority of low-scoring subjects. Such groups are not very well matched but will not be statistically significantly different. Third, there may not be enough subjects available who meet the inclusion criteria to meet the required sample size within the stated study or funding interval. Obtaining large sample sizes in multiple groups is a full-time job, not something that can easily be appended to daily clinical duties. As a consequence, clinical research is neglected by the vast majority of practitioners. The clients seen by clinicians is a far larger and much more representative sample than what full-time researchers study. Daily use of single-subject designs would greatly augment our knowledge base in many areas.

Within-subject designs allow each case seen to be rigorously evaluated. This commitment to assessment contributes to both the clinical accountability and research. It provides better clinical data in addition to excluding sufficient alternative interpretations as to warrant publication and acceptance by the scientific community. Such has been the core belief of the Boulder Model of training for clinical psychology (Tryon, 1990). Fitz and Tryon (1989) illustrate this approach in their analysis of nursing home restraint usage.

The above data demonstrating the lack of serial dependency in activity data, in the absence of consistent environmental constraints, authorizes the use of traditional probability theory and statistical analysis; especially after serial dependency has been shown not to exist in a particular sample. If serial dependency is found, then it can be estimated and removed using standard ARIMA methods (Nazem, 1988) and the calculations described below conducted on the residual series.

One Daily Data Point

Perhaps the first thing one is inclined to do with a time series is plot it and begin comparing aspects of the figure with clinically relevant events. A priori comparisons will be made in research contexts. Let us say that Monday through Sunday of Week 1 constitutes baseline and Monday of Week 2 begins drug treatment. The following procedures could be used to evaluate the null hypothesis that observed differences are due to chance.

The first approach assumes that one wishes to compare specific days to each other. For example, one might wish to compare baseline Monday with intervention Monday on the basis that such a comparison better controls for daily activities than comparing intervention Monday with baseline Friday or Sunday. Perhaps the subject's Friday and Sunday schedule differs from Monday. This assumption seems reasonable for most ambulatory outpatient populations that might be studied. Even institutional schedules show some variability.

In order to determine what is rare by chance, and therefore significant by definition, one must first determine what is common by chance. This context is provided by calculating all possible day-to-day differences during baseline. Given a 7-day baseline, $7(8)/1(2) = 21$ possible pair-wise comparisons, differences can be calculated. Their distribution provides an estimate of the magnitudes of daily differences that can be expected by chance. The lower 95% of these $21 = 19.95 = 20$ differences can be considered "common by chance" leaving the largest difference as "rare" by chance as it occurs but 5% of the time. This context would allow one to test for significant activity *increases*. Had the object been to test for activity *decreases*, then the largest 20 differences would be considered "common by chance" leaving the smallest difference to define "rare by chance." Such distributions can either be developed from *signed* or *absolute* differences. Signed differences are more specific in that they dictate a particular direction.

A test of intervention Monday versus baseline Monday involves comparing the obtained (signed or absolute) difference with the above-mentioned distribution to determine if it is rare or common by chance. Comparing intervention Tuesday versus baseline Tuesday means conducting a second statistical test which increments experiment-wise error beyond 5%. The general formula for calculating experiment-wise error is Equation 1 where $c =$ the number of comparisons made at the α level of statistical significance:

$$\text{Total } \alpha = 1 - (1 - \alpha)^c \tag{1}$$

To reduce total α to lower levels requires that we extend the tails of the sampling distribution to where even more rare by chance events occur. This will occur if baseline is extended as indicated below. Fifteen baseline days are needed to obtain the first 1% tail.

Having 2, 3, 4, or 5 entries in the 5% tail gives multiple examples of "significant" results thereby providing a more complete understanding of what rare chance events look like (cf. Table 1.1).

A second approach can be taken assuming that the baseline days are all essentially equivalent in the activity demand made by them. It would then be desirable to average all baseline values into a single number. Deviations of each day from this average would be limited to the number of baseline days. A total of 20 baseline days would have to be collected before having a 5% tail with 1 value. One hundred days of baseline would be required before reaching the first 1% tail with 1 value.

Having this second type of baseline distribution enables one to calculate the probability of obtaining subsequent activity readings. Let us assume that we collected 20 daily activity readings as part of a physical examination obtained while healthy. Suppose that some time later this person seeks treatment for depression. Several more days of activity could be obtained and compared to the baseline distribution in the following way. If three consecutive new data points all lay in the lower 5% tail, then one might reason that such an event could only occur $.05^3 =$ .000125 or 1.25 times in a million by chance. This compares to three other days that might each have occurred with probability of .5 such that $.5^3 = .125$, which is not at all uncommon. The accuracy of such calculations is largely dependent upon the number of baseline data points taken while healthy, which determines the accuracy of the probability values.

An interpretative caution is that it is possible to conclude that a string of common events is rare. If we ask how many ($n = ?$) events each with probability = 0.5 must occur consecutively for $p = 0.05$, we find $n = \log(0.05)/\log(0.5) = 4.3219$. The answer to how many consecutive events each with probability of 0.9

TABLE 1.1. Number of Baseline Days
Required for Significance

Baseline days	Comparisons	5%	1%
7	21	1	–
8	28	1	–
9	36	1	–
10	45	2	–
11	55	2	–
12	66	3	–
13	78	3	–
14	91	4	–
15	105	5	1
30	435	21	4
60	1770	88	17
90	4005	200	40

must occur consecutively for $p = 0.05$ we find $n = \log(0.05)/\log(0.9) = 28.4332$. Said otherwise, it is uncommon for common events to keep occurring. Nevertheless, the baseline probability distribution helps interpret the likelihood that newly collected clinical data are within chance expectation.

Daily Activity Distribution

Instruments with an inherent time base, such as the Motionlogger® and Actillume® actigraphs (cf. Chapter 2), provide additional and more powerful analytic opportunities. Using a 1-minute epoch, 60 minutes × 24 hours = 1440 data points are collected each day (24-hour period). Even restricting data analysis to 16 waking hours, assuming 8 hours of sleep, yields 960 data points. A single-day baseline activity distribution could be compared with a single-day intervention activity distribution using a 1- or 2-tailed Kolmogorov–Smirnov (K–S) test (Sigel, 1956) to evaluate the probability that the two independent distributions differ by more than chance expectation if the data are uncorrelated. A correlated-samples K–S test would be most welcome.

Distributional analysis can be extended as follows. An activity distribution from a single intervention day can be compared to the average distribution of an entire week of baseline measurements. Or, a one-week intervention distribution can be compared to a one-week baseline distribution. The power of the analysis increases as each distribution is based upon more days both because of the stability that comes with the law of large numbers and the representativeness of the behavioral sample obtained.

Temporal Measures

The following sections discuss several useful aspects of time-locked actigraphy.

Time as a Dependent Variable

Time of occurrence can be an important variable. For example, it is believed that fatigue in multiple sclerosis (MS) patients is more severe in the afternoon than in the morning. Hence, it is reasonably expected that they would be more active when less fatigued and less active when more fatigued. A test of this hypothesis requires hourly self-reported fatigue ratings in conjunction with hourly activity measures to determine if the two variables are correlated as hypothesized.

Detecting sleepwalking events with wrist or ankle actigraphy identifies the time of their occurrence. This clock time is important to the next day's interview where the person is asked if they remember being out of bed at this time. Criteria C for a DSM-III-R diagnosis of Sleepwalking Disorder (307.46) requires that the person not remember these episodes. Knowledge of their number and when each occurred both documents their occurrence and provides a behavioral focus to the interview.

Time is also an important factor when activity measures are to be taken during specific intervals such as math and reading class vs gym or recess. Knowledge of when these events occurred allows the user to inspect the actigraphic record and calculate activity scores (means, standard deviations, minimum, maximum) for just these time periods.

Time as a Measurement Parameter

In this instance time does not appear on either the X or Y axis but becomes a unit of measurement as in activity counts per minute, per 5 minutes or per hour. The activity counts recorded by the Motionlogger® actigraph constitute the numerator of the desired index while the programmed epoch of the actigraph establishes the denominator, temporal unit, of the desired index. Data are then activity counts per minute when using the zero crossing mode or seconds per minute when using the threshold mode.

The data are presented as a frequency (Y) by magnitude (X) histogram without reference to the time of day each observation was obtained. Interest is restricted to the frequency with which particular ratios occurred. An excellent example of this is provided by Urbach, Lavie, and Alster (1989) in their effort to empirically determine the activity associated with minutes of waking and sleeping. They obtained all-night polysomnograms for 7 normal subjects and had each minute scored for sleep and wake. They then sorted corresponding wrist actigraphic (Ambulatory Monitoring, Inc., Ardsley, NY) data into waking and sleep counts and plotted the frequency by value of both data sets on the same graph. The two graphs intersected at approximately 25 counts/minute. The authors specified this value as the waking threshold. Scores equal to or greater than 25 counts per minute were subsequently scored as "wake" while counts of less than 25 were subsequently scored as "sleep."

Saris, Snel, and Binkhorst (1977) took a similar approach to activity through the ambulatory assessment of heart rate. Their 63 × 94 × 22-mm device measured R–R intervals, converted them into beats/minute, and accumulated the results into one of the following 8 registers: 40–69, 70–99, 100–124, 125–149, 150–176, 177–199, 200–224, and 225–300 beats/minute. Heart-rate histograms are then calculated to summarize these results.

The central point here is that the authors were concerned with counts per minute associated with sleep at any time it occurred and with waking any time it occurred, the time these events actually occurred being irrelevant. Temporal considerations are considered as part of the unit of measurement rather than as part of the analysis.

It is quite possible that a disorder such as chronic fatigue will produce an excessive number of epochs with small activity counts but will not produce a preponderance of such epochs in the afternoon compared with the morning because of important environmental factors as needing a ride to the store which is only available in the afternoon.

Aggregation of activity distributions over time will increasingly sample the person's typical behavior patterns and thereby yield increasingly replicable results as indicated by the above discussion regarding behavioral stability and the Spearman–Brown Prophecy Formula.

Time as a Covariate

It is tempting to assume that time is unimportant and report means and standard deviations for various control and experimental conditions as if they represented stable events. However, important time-course information may exist and need to be reported if a valid understanding of the results is to be arrived at.

Consider the study by Perris and Rapp (1974) on the effects of fluspirilene on the activity (step count) of ten patients with chronic schizophrenia. Phase 1 consisted of three weeks of normal drug therapy. Phase 2 involved withholding neuroleptics but giving hypnotics. Phase 3 was a three-week trial of fluspirilene. Analysis of variance for the three conditions revealed that activity during Phase 2 was significantly greater than either Phase 1 or Phase 3 and that Phases 1 and 3 were not significantly different from each other. This result seems simple enough; neuroleptic withdrawal produced activity increase and introduction of fluspirilene reduced activity back to its original level which is indistinguishable from that associated with their initial neuroleptic.

However, inspection of their Figure 1 reveals a very different impression. Daily Phase 1 activity shows a very slight upward trend, Daily Phase 2 activity shows an approximately parallel trend but at an elevated activity level. The real surprise is the strong linear effect within the Phase 3 data. Day 1 of fluspirilene produced the lowest activity reading of the entire study; a value about 2000 steps per day less than Day 1 in either Phase 1 or 2. Day 2 was equally inactive followed by an approximately 3000-step-per-day increase by Day 7 which was greater than Day 7 in either Phase 2 or 1. It seems clear that one would want an additional week's data to determine if further activity increments are associated with fluspirilene. Their Figure 1 clearly supports the expectation that Phase 3 activity is substantially greater than that recorded during Phase 1.

Statistical Significance

A common threat to the internal validity of all empirical investigations is the possibility that the observed results came about purely by random chance events and cannot be replicated. Hence, tests of statistical significance are performed to evaluate the probability that the obtained results were due to chance. Acknowledging that any result has some probability of occurring by chance, it was decided long ago to pay special attention to rare chance events; those occurring less than 5% of the time by chance. We call these special events statistically significant and use them to support or falsify hypotheses and theories.

A special problem occurs when studying small sample sizes, a common occurrence in hospital-based medical research. The size of the statistic expected by chance when no effect is present equals or exceeds the size of the average real relationship should one be present. Only occasionally will one encounter such an enormous effect that its presence can be statistically demonstrated in a small sample. Most effects are less than gigantic and therefore capable of being mistaken for chance results in small samples.

For example, large correlation coefficients are expected by chance when calculated on small samples. Unfortunately, the size of the real underlying relationship between variables does not also increase in small samples. Hence, accurately measured important co-relationships may be dismissed as due to chance when studied in small samples. Only through further study can it be determined whether or not the correlation coefficients under study will diminish or maintain their magnitude. The problem is uncertainty. One can neither assert that a real relationship exists nor entirely dismiss the possibility of a true relationship on the basis of *large* nonsignificant correlations in small samples. More subjects will be required to reduce this uncertainty.

One must also take care to explore the full range of the independent variable before drawing conclusions about its effect upon the dependent variable(s). Restriction of range in the independent variable will predictably curtail the resulting correlation coefficient, even down to zero.

An alternative approach is to study a few subjects intensively using a within-subject experimental design (Bellack and Hersen, 1988). Replication is sought at least once for each subject. Repeatedly demonstrating an effect for each of several subjects rapidly creates convincing evidence of a functional relationship. Moreover, cause and effect relationships can be obtained in this fashion which cannot be proved by purely correlational techniques.

Equipment Used for Measuring Activity

Because measurements are taken with instruments, it is paramount that we review presently available devices for the measurement of activity. Emphasis will be given to human ambulatory activity because such measurements have the greatest clinical relevance in that they can be obtained longitudinally from the person's natural environment. Selected devices used in animal research will also be reviewed.

HUMAN AMBULATORY ACTIVITY

In addition to collecting reliable and valid information, it is important that devices used for measuring human ambulatory activity be conveniently worn and require minimal, if any, participation by the subject to facilitate longitudinal data collection. Tryon (1984a) and Pfadt and Tryon (1983) discuss these and related matters.

Actometers

Actometers are self-winding mechanical wrist watches that have been modified so that the self-winding rotor directly activates the minute hand which then drives the hour hand and calendar date in normal fashion (cf. Schulman and Reisman, 1959; Bell, 1968). Tryon (1985a; pp. 214–216) described the mechanical properties of modified Timex watches.

Unit of Measure

The average kinetic energy necessary to move the approximately 4.49-gram self-winding rotor sufficient to increment the minute hand by 1 minute marking constitutes the effective unit of measurement for actometers.

Reliability

Unstandardized Test–Retest. This method of assessing the reliability of actometers, or any other activity monitor (called instrument reliability in Chapter 1), provides a *lower* bound reliability estimate since it confounds subject instability with measurement inconsistency. The same person cannot exactly reproduce the physical properties of all their trunk and limb movements on two or more consecutive trials spaced seconds apart let alone for an entire half-hour or more on two occasions a week or more apart. Such studies actually measure behavioral stability (called clinical repeatability in Chapter 1) of the participants plus unreliability of measurement. Since person error is always present, instrument error must necessarily be less than total error. Hence, instrument reliability must always be larger than test–retest correlation coefficients imply. Because behavioral instability can be much greater than instrument inconsistency, test–retest methods can severely underestimate instrument reliability.

Consequently, investigators conducting these studies have reported widely different test–retest correlation coefficients. The use of abbreviated test periods further diminishes the "reliability" coefficients in accordance with psychometric principles discussed by Epstein (1979, 1980). Smaller samples contain proportionally more error than larger ones. Random errors tend to cancel upon aggregation leaving proportionally (not absolutely) larger "true" scores to correlate higher with themselves upon retesting of other variables. Said otherwise, abbreviated activity measurements are less reliable than are measurements based upon larger behavioral samples just as item number augments test reliability.

The following studies illustrate typical lower-bound reliability estimates obtained with the test–retest method. Maccoby, Dowley, Hagen, and Dergman (1965) reported a reliability coefficient of $r(11) = .22$, N.S. for females' ankle activity to a high of $r(11) = .76$, $p < .02$ for males' wrist activity. Schulman, Kaspar, and Throne (1965) reported $\rho(25) = .67$, $p < .001$. Massey, Lieberman, and Batarseh (1971) reported $r(31) = .798$, $p < .001$. Bell (1968) reported $r(29) = .55$, $p < .002$ for foot and $r(29) = .56$, $p < .002$ for jacket measures.

Aggregate Test–Retest. Bell, Weller, and Waldrop (1971) collected actometer data on six different days over 5 weeks. The odd- vs even-day reliability coefficient was $r(4) = .68$, N.S. Halverson and Waldrop (1973) collected actometer data on 58 children over a 6-week period. They reported odd–even correlations of $r(31) = .81$, $p < .0001$ for males and $r(23) = .92$, $p < .0001$ for females.

Buss, Block, and Block (1980) placed actometers on the wrist of the non-favored hand for 2 hours at three times when the 129 children (65 boys, 64 girls) were age 3 and again at age 4. The 1-year test–retest correlation coefficient was $r(63) = .44, p < .001$ for boys and $r(62) = .43, p < .001$ for girls indicating impressive person stability over a 1-year interval at a time when development is proceeding at a rapid rate.

Eaton (1983) studied the wrist activity, using Timex Model 108 Motion Recorders (actometers), of 27 nursery school children (13 males, 14 females) aged 42 to 62 months ($M = 50.4, S = 5.1$). Activity measurements took place for 12.2 to 39.2 minutes (median = 21 minutes) per day during free play for 1 month resulting in from 1.8 to 6.7 hours of data. A total of 14 children were studied in the morning and 13 children in the afternoon. Every day the child wore each of the 14 actometers. Reliability of single actometer readings was $r(25) = .33$, N.S. Reliability increased in a negatively accelerated fashion when calculated over 2–13 days reaching a maximum of $r(25) = .88, p < .0001$, for the 13-day aggregate. Eaton's Figure 1 indicates that further reliability increases are expected with greater aggregation. The Spearman–Brown prophecy formula (cf. Epstein, 1979, 1980) can be used to determine the number of repeated measurements to achieve any desired reliability short of unity. Hence, the question is not if actometers are reliable but how reliable they are at various levels of aggregations (behavioral sample sizes). Although the X axis of Eaton's Figure 1 is labeled "Number of actometers" it represents repeated actometer measurements.

Halverson and Post-Gorden (1984) report that Halverson attached actometers to the back of the shirt or jacket of 40 children (aged 30 to 42 months) during three daily play settings over 20 days. Reliability calculated on 1-day samples was $r(38) = .18$, N.S., whereas reliability calculated on 10-day samples was $r(38) = .96, p < .0001$.

Tryon (1984b) had 33 college students (17 males aged 21.0 years; 16 females aged 20.0 years) wear Timex Model 108 motion recorders on both wrists and ankles 24 hours a day for 14 consecutive days. Correlational analyses revealed the following: Week 1–Week 2 coefficients: left wrist ($r(31) = .49, p < .01$), right wrist ($r(31) = .73, p < .0001$), left ankle ($r(31) = .55, p < .002$), right ankle ($r(31) = .63, p < .0001$)

Further stability can be achieved when aggregating over subjects as well as time. Tryon (1984b) reported that the mean waking activity across all subjects for Week 1 of 25.86 AU/min was nearly equivalent to the mean for Week 2 of 25.76 AU/min. The difference of 0.1 AU/min is both nonsignificant ($F(1,31) = .02$, N.S.) and completely unimportant.

Simultaneous Measurement. A partial solution to the problem of subjects' not being able to replicate specific movements is to attach two sensors to the same site and correlate the pairs of measurements thus obtained over time. The rationale is that a high correlation will result if the devices respond consistently. Morrell and Keefe (1988) attached two actometers to the ankle of 7 male and 7 female chronic-pain patients aged 42 years. The behavioral sample was all waking hours for 4 consecutive days. The observed correlation of $r(12) = .997, p < .0001$ indicates a high degree of consistency.

Laboratory Assessment. A primary value of collecting data with an instrument is that its operating characteristics can be studied under laboratory conditions where the device can be repeatedly exposed to the same stimulus.

Schulman and Reisman (1959) placed their actometers (modified mens' Omega self-winding watches) on a disc from 4 in. (10.2 cm) to 7 in. (17.8 cm) from the center of rotation and spun them in the vertical plane at 2 rpm (0.2094 rad/sec) for an unspecified duration or number of revolutions. They reported one actometer reading 499 AU/hr and the second reading 500 AU/hr. The difference of 1 part error out of 499 parts of activity equals 99.8% reliability. This demonstration is problematic in that limbs do not move in continuous circular orbits and that very low levels of acceleration were used.

Johnston's (1971) replication of the above study over 24 5-minute trials resulted in reliability estimates of 98.2% and 98.4%. Spinning in the horizontal plane produced reliability estimates of 84.2% and 85.0% indicating that actometers are responsive in two planes. Placing the actometers on the carriage of an IBM electric typewriter, pressing the tab button such that the carriage moved 12.4 inches in an unknown time, and therefore with an unknown acceleration, on ten trials yielded reliability estimates of 90.1% and 92.4%. While linear motion is unrepresentative of human limb movement, the 12.4-in. length is sufficiently short that it approximates the movement of the outstretched arm or leg.

Saris and Binkhorst (1977a) rotated 10 actometers (modified Swiss Tussot watches) at 0.965 rpm for five 1-hr periods at an unstated distance, and therefore unreported acceleration, resulting in coefficients of variation equal to 0.052 to 0.155 which corresponds to error of $\frac{1}{20}$ to $\frac{1}{7}$ of 1% corresponding to 99% reliability. Apparently the self-winding rotor revolved once each time the test device rotated once. Oscillating the same actometers in an unspecified manner for five additional 1-hr periods yielded coefficients of variation of 1.24 to 2.57 indicating approximately 1 to 3% error or 97 to 99% reliability.

Tryon (1985a) constructed a mechanical oscillator and studied the reliability of four actometers under eight activity levels. The results are reprinted in Table 2.1. Coefficient of variation (CV) reliability equivalents ranged from .88 to .99.

Validity

Behavioral Observation/Rating. Halverson and Waldrop (1973) observed 58 white middle-class children (33 males and 25 females) aged 2.5 years for 5 weeks

TABLE 2.1. Means, Standard Deviations, Coefficients of Variation, Correlation Equivalents, and Analyses of Variance for Four Actometers under Eight Levels of Accelerated Movement[a,b]

G Force	Stats	1	2	3	4	F(3,36)
0.05	M	8.78	13.76	11.59	8.58	27.28**
	SD	0.29	2.55	0.96	1.21	
	CV[a]	3.30	18.53	8.28	14.10	
	r[b]	0.98	0.90	0.96	0.93	
0.25	M	25.34	31.43	35.69	23.83	9.64**
	SD	4.54	5.84	6.49	5.35	
	CV	17.92	18.58	18.18	22.45	
	r	0.91	0.90	0.90	0.88	
0.35	M	119.10	106.80	114.90	125.10	1.99
	SD	23.59	12.22	13.41	17.21	
	CV	19.81	11.44	11.67	13.76	
	r	0.90	0.94	0.94	0.93	
0.45	M	307.79	353.42	322.10	322.97	1.44
	SD	54.39	40.75	56.01	50.22	
	CV	17.67	11.53	17.39	15.55	
	r	0.91	0.94	0.91	0.92	
0.50	M	526.43	570.55	542.75	545.45	3.26*
	SD	36.23	26.04	31.30	33.27	
	CV	6.88	4.56	5.77	6.10	
	r	0.97	0.98	0.97	0.97	
0.55	M	612.30	639.08	654.37	612.91	1.56
	SD	48.21	56.60	42.63	58.46	
	CV	7.87	8.86	6.51	9.54	
	r	0.96	0.95	0.97	0.95	
0.65	M	683.3	718.88	705.83	693.78	5.67**
	SD	16.12	17.01	20.16	25.77	
	CV	2.36	2.37	2.86	3.71	
	r	0.99	0.99	0.99	0.98	
0.85	M	803.63	827.73	816.62	797.13	1.46
	SD	33.82	35.64	32.19	40.67	
	CV	4.21	4.31	3.94	5.10	
	r	0.98	0.98	0.98	0.97	

[a]Reprinted from Tryon (1985a).
[b]N = 10 trials

while they attended same-sex nursery school groups of 5 children each. Actometers were attached to the backs of each child's shorts or jacket for 90 minutes each morning during which time behavioral observations were made. Significant correlations were reported for males between actometer measurements and: observed gross motor play except for running (.67), falls (.61), runs (.80), stationary watching (−.38), shifts in play (.66), continuity of play (−.67) during outdoor play and total activity time (.47), inactivity (−.49), opposes peers (.33), withdraws from peer interaction ($-.32$), direct walking ($.48$), shifts in play ($.40$), continuity of play ($-.35$), painting ($-.34$), and mopping floor ($.47$) during indoor play. For girls the significant correlations were falls ($.65$), runs ($.82$), stationary watching ($-.62$), shifts in play ($.52$), continuity of play ($-.57$), and squeals ($.44$) during outdoor play and inactivity ($-.41$), direct walking ($.36$), and cleans self ($.42$) during indoor play.

McFarlain and Hersen (1974) reported that the senior author wore an actometer on his right leg just above the ankle with the watch face toward the opposite leg. He then counted the number of times his right foot touched the floor during 11 half-hour periods. The resulting correlation between foot counts and actometer readings was $r(9) = .97$, $p < .0001$.

Saris and Binkhorst (1977a) placed actometers on the right wrist and ankle of 9 children aged 5 to 6 years. They then walked for 10 minutes on a motorized treadmill at 0% grade at 1.0, 3.2, and 5.1 km/hr and ran for 5 minutes at 5.1 and 6.5 km/hr. The means (and standard deviations) for their right wrist over all five speeds were: 0.6 (0.5), 1.5 (1.2), 4.5 (3.6), 8.7 (1.0), and 10.9 (2.5) AU/min. The means (and standard deviations) for the right ankle over all five speeds were: 0.97 (0.5), 3.0 (0.7), 8.1 (2.9), 13.7 (3.9), and 15.7 (3.8) AU/min. Increasing wrist and ankle activity measurements are explained, and validated, by increasing average (and standard deviation) of stride frequency per minute of 107 (13.2), 142 (10.3), 163 (14.7), 203 (9.7), and 212 (14.0).

Saris and Binkhorst (1977a) also attached actometers to the right wrist and ankle of 6 males aged 21 to 31 years. They walked on a motorized treadmill for 10 minutes at 5.8, 7.2, and 8.6 km/hr and ran for 10 minutes at 7.2, 8.6, 10.1, 13.3, and 14.8 km/hr. The means (and standard deviations) for right wrist activity over all eight speeds were: 0.6 (0.4), 2.9 (1.8), 4.9 (1.6), 8.2 (0.6), 7.9 (0.6), 8.3 (0.6), 9.1 (0.7) and 7.4 (0.9) AU/min. The means (and standard deviations) for right ankle activity over all eight speeds were: 4.0 (0.6), 5.4 (0.5), 7.7 (1.9), 12.2 (1.5), 12.8 (1.3), 13.9 (1.0), 17.0 (2.4), and 20.4 (3.2) AU/min. Increasing wrist and ankle activity measurements are explained, and validated, by increasing average (and standard deviation) of stride frequency per minute of 118 (3.1), 130 (3.1), 146 (4.4), 152 (10.7), 157 (4.4), 158 (5.0), 168 (6.8), and 176 (2.6).

Running clearly and consistently produced greater activity measurements in both children and adults than did walking. Saris and Binkhorst (1977b) reported a correlation of $r = .89$, $p < .01$ between ankle actometer and waist pedometer measurements and $r = .78$, $p < .05$ between wrist actometer and waist pedometer measurements.

Ullman, Barkley, and Brown (1978) placed actometers on the wrist and ankle of hyperkinetic boys, aged 5 to 12 years, who were on drug holiday and 18 normal control children while they played in a grid-marked playroom. For the hyperkinetic boys, wrist and ankle activity correlated $r(16) = .72$, $p < .001$ and $r(16) = .88$, $p < .0001$, respectively, with the number of quadrant changes. For control boys, wrist and ankle activity correlated $r(16) = .83, p < .0001$ and $r(16) = .44, p < .05$, respectively, with the number of quadrant changes.

Fitzpatrick and Donovan (1979) placed actometers on all four extremities of 44 residents between the ages of 70 and 90 residing in a home for the aged. Behavioral ratings from two trained raters were obtained using the Motor Activity Rating Scale (MARS). The following significant correlations were reported between total actometer scores (the sum of all four actometers) and MARS body movement (.28), intensity (.33), arm and leg movements (.45), arms (.43), and legs (.32).

Buss, Block, and Block (1980) placed actometers on the wrist of the non-preferred hand of 129 children (65 boys, 64 girls) for 2 hours on each of three occasions when they were 3 and again when they were 4 years of age. Three nursery school teachers with a minimum of 5 months' experience with these children rated their activity. At age 7, one teacher and two examiners rated the children's activity. The actometer measurements taken at from girls at age 3 correlated $r(64) = .50, p < .0001$ with average ratings at age 3, $r(62) = .34, p < .01$ with average judge ratings at age 4, and $r(62) = .35, p < .05$ at age 7. The actometer readings taken from girls at age 4 correlated $r(62) = .36, p < .01$ with ratings at age 3, $r(62) = .48, p < .0001$ with ratings at age 4, and $r(62) = .28, p < .05$ with ratings taken at age 7.

The actometer measurements taken at from boys at age 3 correlated $r(63) = .61, p < .0001$ with average ratings at age 3, $r(63) = .56, p < .0001$ with average judge ratings at age 4, and $r(63) = .19$, NS at age 7. The actometer measurements taken at from boys at age 4 correlated $r(63) = .66, p < .0001$ with average ratings at age 3, $r(63) = .53, p < .0001$ with average judge ratings at age 4, and $r(63) = .38, p < .01$ at age 7.

Halverson and Post-Gorden (1984) report that Halverson found a 1-day correlation between number of runs and actometer score of .15 to .44 depending upon which day was used. Aggregating across 10 days yielded a correlation of $r(130) = .77, p < .0001$ between actometer scores and number of runs.

Morrell and Keefe (1988) asked 7 male and 7 female adult (aged 42 years) chronic pain patients to walk 5 laps each measuring 32 yards and recorded ankle actometer readings from the dominant leg after each lap. Eight of the within-subject correlations between distance walked and actometer scores were $r(3) = .999, p < .0001$. The lowest correlation was $r(3) = .973, p < .01$.

Laboratory Assessment. Table 2.1 also clearly demonstrates the validity of actometers. Without exception, higher G-force values resulted in higher actometer scores across eight activity levels in all four actometers. However, a disordinal relationship emerged. Actometer 2 gave the highest reading under $G = 0.05$, the second highest reading under $G = 0.25$, and the lowest reading under $G = 0.35$, etc. Individual conversion constants were calculated for a sample of 59 actometers at six G-force levels and empirical equations presented for converting arbitrary actometer units to acceleration values (cf. Tryon, 1985a; Table 7.3, pp. 229–230). These constants further testify to the validity of actometers in that a perfect rank order correlation coefficient was obtained across between six G-force levels and actometer units for all 59 actometers.

Because longer limbs produce greater acceleration when moved the same angular distance in the same time, higher actometer, accelerometer or other directly proportional sensor, readings are expected. Eaton (1983) reported a nonsignificant correlation of $r(25) = .28$, $p < .19$ between forearm length and actometer score. Tryon (1984b) reported a point biserial correlation of equivalent of wrist-ankle actometer differences of $r(31) = .8406$, $p < .0001$ thereby demonstrating the importance of limb length.

Johnson (1971) placed two actometers, "in tandem," on a subject's arm and took readings after each set of 10 4-inch arc strokes. Apparently they were placed side by side rather than on top of each other as they reported that "The more distally placed watch recorded nearly twice as many units as the proximally placed watch." (p. 2109) Although intended as a reliability study, these data indicate that greater distance from the axis of rotation produces larger actometer readings.

Other Modified Watches

Bloom and Eidex (1967) began with the observation that the knee is bent 90 degrees when sitting but is straight when standing. They inserted a weighted arm into a mechanical wristwatch such that it stopped the gears from moving when the person was sitting but allowed the gears to move while standing. The watch was attached to an aluminum holder that was attached to the leg, just above the knee, with a standard perforated rubber strap. The watch holder allowed the watch to be turned such that it did not run when sitting. Since the devices were worn from getting out of bed in the morning until retiring to bed in the evening, a record of bedtime at night was also available. The major dependent variables were the amount of time spent in the upright position and the percent of time out of bed spent standing, the posture which consumes the largest number of calories.

Unit of Measure

The unit of measure is the minute as this timer operates as a normal clock while the individual is standing.

Reliability

No data were provided regarding the reliability of this instrument. However, attachment to the leg involves rotating the watch so that it operates when the individual stands up. It is likely that repeated standings and sittings will cause the device to start and stop.

Validity

No data were provided regarding the validity of this device except that attachment to the leg involves rotating it so that it begins running when the person stands up and stops running when the person sits down. Hence, validity is a function of proper attachment.

Pedometers

Vertical movements at the waist activate a mechanism that advances an analog or digital mileage indicator according to a stride setting. More vertical movements are required to register 1 mile with a 3-foot stride setting than with a 5-foot stride setting. Unfortunately, it is generally difficult to accurately read fractions of a mile. This problem is overcome by the step counters reported below.

Unit of Measure

The unit of measurement with pedometers is the mile or kilometer. These units are enabled either through calibration of the device or conversion from arbitrary to standard units.

Calibration is achieved by walking the person a measured distance, such as one-half mile or one mile, comparing the pedometer reading, adjusting the stride index up or down, and rewalking the measured distance until the pedometer reading corresponds to the measured distance. This procedure is problematic in that subjects sometimes refuse to make the necessary walks.

Conversion is achieved by setting the stride index to its largest setting to maximize the pedometer's sensitivity and walking a measured distance once. If the pedometer indicates one-half miles after having walked one mile then subsequent "mileage" readings are divided by 1.5 to obtain real miles walked. Data can then be converted into kilometers by multiplying by 1.6093.

Instrument Reliability

The only way to determine the consistency with which a device measures an event is to repeatedly measure *the same* event. Evaluation of instrument operating characteristics can only be done in the laboratory, where stimulus control can be exerted.

Saunders, Goldstein, and Stein (1978) reported that 36 pedometers (Digi Manpo, Mitchell Mogul Co., NY) could be adjusted to read within 0.5 mile of each other after having been vibrated on an Eberbach single-speed reciprocating power unit for 30 minutes to an average mileage reading of 37.5, yielding a measurement error of but $0.5/37.5 = 0.013$ or 1.3%.

Heiser, Epstein, and Wing (1981) performed two reliability studies. In study 1, 55 pedometers (Taylor Company, Arden, NC), with stride adjustment set to 1 foot, were vibrated for 60 minutes on an Eberbach Lateral Shaker on each of two trials. The results were that 85% of the pedometers gave values of within 5% of 3 miles (range $= 2.85 - 3.14$ miles). In study 2, the same pedometers, with stride adjustment set to 2 feet, were vibrated for 30 minutes, readings taken, and vibrated for another 30 minutes where upon final readings were taken. Two such trials were run. The results were that 91% of the pedometers were within 5% of 6 miles (range $= 5.7 - 6.3$ miles).

Tryon, Pinto, and Morrison (1990) used the mechanical oscillator described by Tryon (1985a) to study the reliability of 19 Digitron™ Jog-Walk digital pedometers (Gutmann Co., Inc., 120 South Columbus Avenue, Mount Vernon, NY, 10553; 1-914-699-4044) over 7 trials of 7000 oscillations (stride index = 5 ft). The average CV was found to be 4.75% ($S = 2.16$). The correlational equivalent of the average CV is .98. The least reliable pedometer had a CV of 9.39 which equals a test–retest correlation coefficient of .95.

Clinical Repeatability

Simultaneous Measurement. This approach seeks to examine the consistency with which two or more instruments yield the same reading when attached to the same site of an individual. Constant differences between devices can be corrected by calculating conversion constants. Hence, it is important that devices correlated with each other at the same site of attachment.

Gottfries, Gottfries, and Olsson (1966) placed two pedometers (Feinmechanische Apparatenbaugesellschaft Kasper u. Richter, Uttemruth, Germany) on the same leg of 20 female student nurses aged 20 to 33 years (median = 23 years). The correlation between these readings was very high as well as significant ($r(18) = .95$, $p < .0001$).

Washburn, Chin, and Montoye's (1980) Experiment I involved 20 subjects aged 13 to 57 years (mean = 27.2 years) walking six 1-mile walks on a motor-driven treadmill at 0% grade; 2 walks at 2, 3, and 4 mph while wearing four Edgemark Digimeter pedometers (vendor unspecified). Two pedometers were attached to the subject's shorts or belt and two more were attached to a second belt worn slightly higher. The stride adjustment of all pedometers was set to the middle setting and taped into place.

The results were expressed in ratio to activity recorded during the 3-mph walk. During the 2-mph walk, the four pedometers ranged from 0.57 to 1.06 that of the 3 mph walk. During the 4-mph walk, the four pedometers ranged from 0.75 to 0.92 that of the 3 mph walk. These results were obtained from their Figure 1 using a millimeter rule. The authors rightfully called attention to the wide variability in results as evidence of poor quality control in the construction of Edgemark Digimeter pedometers.

Test–retest reliability coefficients were calculated for pedometers 1–4 under all three walking conditions. For the 2-mph condition they were: .61, .53, .26, and .56 for a mean of .49. For the 3-mph condition they were: .85, .42, .78, and .75 for a mean of .70. For the 4-mph condition they were .86, .60, .51, and .66 for a mean of .66. Evidence on validity reported below shows that these pedometers were capable of revealing significant activity, subject, and subject-by-activity effects despite their limited reliability.

That correlation coefficients are inappropriate for the determination of instrument reliability stems from the well-known fact that the correlation between two variables is zero when the variability in either X or Y approaches zero (cf. Chapter 1 regarding instrument reliability). If all pedometers yielded the same value, in either the test or retest conditions or both as is ideally desired, then the test–retest correlation coefficient would be *zero*! Hence, the above correlations mainly reflect between-subject differences; they reveal the extent to which subjects behaved differently within and between the test and retest conditions. Such large between-subject variability helps explain why their Figure 1 results are so variable.

Standard Walk. Stunkard (1960) reported that pedometer (New Haven Clock Company, New Haven, CT) measurements were within 15% of measured distance walked. The correlation needed to cause $1 - r^2$ to be .15 is .922.

Gayle, Montoye, and Philpot (1977) investigated the reliability of three analog and three digital pedometers (brand and vendor unspecified) via a series of controlled walks. Eight males walked 1 mile at 0% grade at 3 mph on 6 occasions while wearing two pedometers on the left hip and two others on the right hip. The stride adjustment was set to 66 cm on all pedometers. Conversion constants based upon a standard walk were used to minimize absolute errors as follows: if the pedometer read 1.1 miles after walking a standard mile, then all subsequent readings were multiplied by $1/1.1 = .909$; if the pedometer read 0.9 miles then all subsequent readings were multiplied by $1/0.9 = 1.11$. The results showed a reproducibility error of 13.2% for pedometers with analog displays (Brand I) and 5.9% for pedometers with digital displays (Brand II). Significant left- vs right-hip differences were reported for pedometers with analog ($F(1,14) = 619.58, p < .0001$) but not digital ($F(1,14) = 3.65$, N.S.) displays further emphasizes the importance of the site of attachment.

Washburn, Chin, and Montoye's (1980) Experiment II involved 20 subjects aged 18 to 28 years (mean = 21.5 years) who performed two measured 1-mile walks: a) around a 400-meter track, and b) along a jogging trail. They then twice ran the 1-mile jogging trail at their own comfortable pace. Resting was permitted if they remained stationary during the rest period. Subjects wore an Edgemark Digimeter on their right waist, an Eschenbach pedometer at their left and right waist, and a Schritte Watch type pedometer at their left and right ankles (vendors unspecified).

The results were expressed in ratio to activity recorded during the standard 400-meter track walk. Results from the trail walk ranged from 0.92 to 1.2 that of the standard walk. Data from the trail run ranged from 0.79 to 1.5 that of the standard walk.

Test–retest reliability coefficients were calculated for pedometers 1–4 under all three walking conditions. For the standard 400-meter track walk condition the reliabilities of pedometers 1–5 were: .61, .14, .42, .39, and .81 for a mean of .47. For the trail walk condition the reliabilities of pedometers 1–5 were: .31, .04, .50, .90, and .65 for a mean of .48. For the trail-run condition the reliabilities of pedometers 1–5 were: .59, .38, .51, .66, and .60 for a mean of .55. As mentioned above, these test–retest correlations mainly reflect within- and between-test and retest subject variability rather than pedometer unreliability.

Tryon, Pinto, and Morrison (1990) examined the clinical repeatability of pedometer readings in adults (39 college men and women) while twice walking a measured quarter-mile around an indoor track while wearing a Digitron Jog-Walk digital pedometer with its stride index set to the maximum of 5 feet. They found an average CV of 3.39% with a correlation equivalent of .97. Individual CVs ranged from 0% to 14.29% with corresponding correlational equivalents of 1.0 to .93.

While the average CV of 3.39% for college students is numerically less than the mean CV of 4.65% reported above under laboratory conditions, the standard deviation of 6.27% is larger than the 2.16% value reported above. Hence, students on a standard walk yield somewhat less reproducible values than do laboratory conditions.

The present data correspond favorably with 5.9% (Brand 1) and 13.2% (Brand 2) errors reported by Gayle, Montoye, and Philpot (1977) for subjects repeatedly walking at 3 mph on a 0% grade and Stunkard's (1958) report of 15% error in obese people.

Tryon, Pinto, and Morrison (1990) also examined the repeatability of pedometer readings in 11 normal and 11 mildly hyperactive boys. Groups were established via Factor IV of the Conners Teacher Rating Scale (Conners, 1969, 1973) and the Motor Excess Subscale of the Revised Behavior Problem Checklist (RBPC) (Quay and Peterson, 1987). All subjects wore a Digitron Jog-Walk digital pedometer with the stride index set to 5 feet while walking a measured half-mile away from and back to their school. The average CV for normal boys was 12.54% ($S = 18.78\%$) with a correlational equivalent of .94. Mildly hyperactive children displayed an average CV of 28.76 ($S = 40.06\%$) with a correlational equivalent of .84. It therefore appears that normal children are less behaviorally consistent than normal adults and mildly hyperactive children are less behaviorally consistent than mildly hyperactive children.

Unstandardized Test–Retest. Plomin and Foch (1980) reported the test–retest reliability coefficient for 1-week pedometer (brand and vendor unspecified) measurements on 30 boys and girls averaging 7.6 years of age to be $r(28) = .67, p < .0001$. The pedometer measurements were age corrected by predicting them from age and calculating the residual. The just mentioned correlation coefficient is between test and retest residual values.

Validity

Saris and Binkhorst (1977a) placed Russian-built pedometers on the left and right hip plus left ankle of 9 children aged 5–6 years while they walked for 10 minutes at 0% grade on a motorized treadmill at 1.0, 3.2, and 5.1 km/hr and ran for 5 minutes at 5.1 and 6.5 km/hr. The right waist means (and standard deviations), in unknown units, for the three walking speeds were: 34 (21.5), 173 (19.8), and 205 (15.1). Corresponding values for the two running speeds were 219 (18.1), and 225 (10.3). The means (and standard deviations) for the left ankle regarding the three walking speeds were: 56 (7.1), 167 (27.7), and 217 (48.9). Corresponding values for the two running speeds were 259 (4.2) and 250 (3.9). Faster speeds yield higher values because mean (and standard deviation) stride frequency per minute increased from 107 (13.2) to 142 (10.3), to 163 (14.7) during walking as the treadmill speeds increased. Running produced further increases in stride frequency of 203 (9.7) and 212 (14.0) respectively.

Saris and Binkhorst (1977a) also placed pedometers on the left and right waist and left ankle of 6 males aged 21 to 31 years and had them walk at 5.8, 7.2, and 8.6 km/hr for 10 minutes and run at 7.2, 8.6, 10.1, 13.3, and 14.8 km/hr for 10 minutes. The right waist means (and standard deviations), in unknown units, for the three walking speeds were: 121 (12.2), 144 (16.8), and 183 (39.1). Corresponding values for the five running speeds were 155 (8.8), 155 (4.2), 163 (5.2), 170 (6.5), and 192 (12.4). The means (and standard deviations) for the left ankle regarding the three walking speeds were: 125 (19.2), 137 (12.4), and 206 (18.8). Corresponding values for the five running speeds were: 213 (13.5), 202 (24.0), 169 (45.1), 212 (85.0), and 76 (27.5). Faster speeds yield higher values because mean (and standard deviation) stride frequency increased from 118 (3.1) to 130 (3.1) to 146 (4.4) during walking as the treadmill speeds increased. Running produced further increases in stride frequency of 152 (10.7), 157 (4.4), 158 (5.0), 168 (6.8), and 176 (2.6) respectively. Notice that while waist pedometer readings continued to accurately track increased stride frequency, ankle readings did not. The authors indicated that the impact forces at the ankle overloaded the pedometer at higher stride frequencies.

Epstein, Wing, and Thompson (1978) had 16 nonobese college females wear a pedometer for an entire week while simultaneously keeping an activity log. They reported a significant correlation ($r(14) = .59, p < .05$) between these two activity measures.

Wong, Webster, Montoye, and Washburn (1981) attached a pedometer to the trunk of 15 subjects while walking on a motor-driven treadmill with 0% grade for 3 minutes at 2, 3, and 4 mph; running for 3 minutes at 6 and 8 mph; and stepping up onto an 8-in. bench and down again for 3 minutes at the rate of 80, 120, and 140 repetitions per minute. Evaluation of the relationship between pedometer readings and normalized oxygen consumption (ml of O_2/kg/min) was restricted to graphical presentation but clearly indicated a strong linear relationship.

Washburn, Chin, and Montoye's (1980) Experiment I involved 20 subjects aged 13 to 57 years (mean = 27.2 years) walking six 1-mile walks on a motor driven treadmill at 0% grade; two walks at 2, 3, and 4 mph while wearing four Edgemark Digimeter pedometers. Two pedometers were attached to the subject's shorts or belt and two more were attached to a second belt worn slightly higher. The stride adjustment of all pedometers was set to the middle setting and taped into place.

Separate analyses of variance were conducted for each pedometer and the following F ratios were reported for speed condition: 94.36, 4.28, 3.19, and 7.62; all $p < .05$. The correlation equivalents of these F ratios (cf. Hunter, Schmidt, and Jackson, 1982; p. 98) are .92, .76, .60, and .93 respectively. The F ratios for subjects were: 13.99, 4.28, 3.19, and 7.62; all $p < .05$. The correlation equivalents of these F ratios are .66, .44, .39, and .55. The F ratios for subjects by conditions were: 4.18, 2.37, 1.74, and 2.23; all $p < .05$. The correlation equivalents of these F ratios are: .43, .34, .30, and .33. Hence, Edgemark Digimeter pedometers were able to distinguish among walking speeds and individuals, and to detect individuals by walking speed differences despite their questionable reliability (see above). The correlation effect size estimates of .92 and .93 regarding walking speed are admirable by psychometric standards. The .76 and .60 effect sizes are also high by psychometric standards.

Washburn, Chin, and Montoye's (1980) Experiment II involved 20 subjects aged 18 to 28 years (mean = 21.5 years) who performed two measured 1-mile walks: a) around a 400-meter track, and b) along a jogging trail. They then twice ran the 1-mile jogging trail at their own comfortable pace. Resting was permitted if they remained stationary during the rest period. Subjects wore an Edgemark Digimeter on their right waist (pedometer 1), an Eschenbach pedometer at their left (pedometer 5) and right waist (pedometer 4), and a Schritte Watch type pedometer at their left (pedometer 3) and right (pedometer 2) ankles.

Separate analyses of variance were conducted for each pedometer and the following F ratios were reported for the speed condition for pedometers 1–5: 11.50, 2.33, 96.94, 3.98 and 11.37; all $p < .05$. The correlation equivalent of these F ratios (cf. Hunter, Schmidt, and Jackson, 1982; p. 98) are .62, .34, .92, .43, and .62. The F ratios for subjects regarding pedometers 1–5 were: 5.73, 1.18, 3.39, 6.35, and 7.72; all $p < .05$. The correlation equivalents of these F ratios are .49, .25, .40, .51, and .55. The F ratios for subjects by conditions for pedometers 1–5 were: 1.56, 1.56, 2.16, 3.89, and 3.23; all $p < .05$. The correlation equivalents of these F ratios are: .28, .28, .33, .42, and .39. Hence, these various pedometers were able to distinguish among walking speeds and individuals, and could detect individuals by walking speed differences despite their limited reliability (see above). The correlation effect size estimates of .92 and .62 regarding walking speed are admirable by psychometric standards. The .43 and .34 effect sizes for walking speed are acceptable by psychometric standards.

A laboratory study of pedometer validity could easily be accomplished by oscillating or vibrating a set of pedometers 1000, 2000, 3000, 4000, 5000 times. Very likely, all instruments would show increasingly large readings and therefore perfect validity given the traditional correlational approach to this topic.

A more important question is how small an activity increment the pedometers could capture say 95% or 99% of the time. This question remains unanswered for pedometers as well as for all other currently available activity monitors. Perhaps this issue should be termed *sensitivity* rather than validity. Pedometers (and all other activity monitors) are perfectly valid against suitably large activity differences, but how sensitive are they? In short, the physical properties (construction validity) of activity monitors insure their validity against suitable activity differences. The issue of sensitivity remains open.

Step Counters

Step counters are very similar to pedometers in that they key on the vertical movements associated with ambulation. Whereas pedometers use energy in the vertical plane to mechanically increment either an analog or digital display, modern step counters use the same energy to increment a liquid crystal display (LCD) of steps taken.

Marsden and Montgomery (1972), Barber, Evans, Fentem, and Wilson (1973), and Fentem, Fitton, and Hampton (1976) described an early version of the step counter as a load transducer that can be placed in the heel of a shoe to sense pressure changes associated with footfalls.

Sanders (1980) modified a Casio Pocket Watch-PW 80 stopwatch/calculator to interface with a mercury tilt switch. The tilt switch is taped to the subject's outer thigh, where the palms touch when arms hang easily at the sides, with 5.3-mm-wide rubber elastic bandage with Velcro sewn onto both ends. Leg movements which tilt the switch more than 5 degrees from the horizontal plane will be counted.

Modern step counters clip to waist band or belt and measure steps taken by sensing vertical acceleration at the waist as do pedometers. L.L. Bean sells a "Digital Electronic Pedometer" (Catalog number 6052PP; $16.50) measuring 2 in. wide by 1.5 in. high by .7 in. deep that weighs 3 oz. It consists of two parts: a waist-worn base unit with sensor, and an 8-digit LCD calculator that slides into the top of the base unit and counts the steps recorded by the sensor. This device rarely needs to be reset because it can count up to 99,999,999 steps. This instrument can be operated in either a step-count mode or a pedometer mode where steps are converted either to miles or kilometers depending upon the stride constant entered. It requires one G10 battery or equivalent.

Radio Shack sells two interesting waist-worn devices. The less expensive model (Catalog number 63–671; $14.95 as of 8/88) is called a Micronta Walk-Mate® and features only a step-count mode. It measures 1.75 × 1.75 × 0.5 inches and has a 5-digit liquid crystal display that counts up to 99,999 steps before it must be reset by pressing a button. The folding case both conceals and protects the step-counter display. It runs on one RS386A battery.

The second and somewhat more expensive Radio Shack device is an electronic pedometer (Catalog number 63-681; $24.95) that has a programmable stride length for converting steps into miles walked. By adjusting the stride index for walking when walking and for jogging when jogging, a more accurate estimate of distance traversed can be obtained. It can record up to 999.9 miles and it runs on one RS386A battery.

A full-feature electronic pedometer is available through Innovative Time ($39.90 + $3 P&H: DSK Industries Inc. Summer 1988 catalog). It is reported to calculate distance walked and calories burned (estimated by a table look-up procedure), and beeps when a particular distance has been traversed (specified number of steps taken).

Unit of Measurement

The basic unit of measurement for the step counter/pedometer's is the step. Some models (Radio Shack #63–681 Jog-Mate, $24.95; Free Style, FS790 Digital Quartz Pedometer sold by L.L. Bean, Inc., Freeport, Maine, 04033, as a Digital Electronic Pedometer, #6052KE, $16.50) feature a programmable stride-length memory which the device multiplies by steps taken to determine distance walked. These devices can be calibrated like pedometers. Less expensive step counters (e.g., Radio Shack Micronta #63-671 LCD Pedometer, $14.95) do not have stride-length adjustments, but steps can be converted into miles or kilometers as described above.

It can be argued that the step is the preferred unit of measure because it is a natural unit of ambulation. Recall the fairly common scene of a parent crossing the street with his or her young child. The parent walks at a comfortable pace taking relatively few steps to cross the street while the child hurriedly takes many steps to keep up with the parent. I submit that the child was relatively more active than the adult when crossing the same street and so should rightfully receive a higher score. The calibration and conversion processes explained above would cause them to receive the same score.

Reliability

The essential similarity of the activity sensor contained in electronic step counters/pedometers and in traditional mechanical pedometers strongly argues that reliability data for one device generalizes to the other device. Since no reliability data are currently available for step counters/pedometers, we infer their reliability from the above pedometer data.

The fourth experiment reported by Tryon, Pinto, and Morrison (1990) evaluated the repeatability of step-counter data in normal, mildly hyperactive, and clinically hyperactive children. Sixty boys attending six parochial schools aged 6 to 12 ($M = 9.67$, $S = 1.62$) were divided into three groups: 31 normal, 7 mildly hyperactive, and 22 clinically hyperactive, on the basis of norms (Goyette, Conners, and Ulrich, 1978) established for the hyperactivity Factor (IV) of the Conners Teacher Rating Scale (CTRS) (Conners, 1969). Each subject wore a Free Style USA electronic step counter (from L.L. Bean, Inc.) on his waist while he walked a measured half-mile away from school and back again. Step-count readings were taken at the half-way point (Walk I) and upon returning to school (Walk II).

The average and standard deviation of the CV's for normal ($M = 8.75\%$, $S = 8.64\%$), mildly hyperactive ($M = 8.89\%$, $S = 14.59\%$), and clinically hyperactive ($M = 11.78\%$, $S = 11.19\%$) children correspond to correlation equivalents of .96, .95, and .94 respectively. While all of these reliability coefficients are acceptable by psychometric standards, the clinically hyperactive children, as expected, are less behaviorally consistent than either mildly hyperactive or normally active children.

It is recommended that the measured walk be conducted twice or that one long walk be divided in half for the purpose of obtaining two measures in order to assess behavioral consistency. Such information is useful when interpreting subsequent variability. Persons with larger walk–rewalk differences will probably show greater behavioral variability under natural conditions than persons with lesser walk–rewalk differences.

Validity

The essential similarity of the activity sensor contained in electronic step counters/pedometers and in traditional mechanical pedometers strongly argues that validity data for one device generalizes to the other device. Since no data are currently available for electronic step counters/pedometers, we infer their validity from the above-mentioned pedometer data.

The more accurate the stride length estimate, the more accurate the distance traversed value will be. The longer the measured walk is the more accurate the stride length (steps per mile) conversion constant will be. Hence, it is desirable to use as large a measured walk as possible. Also at issue is the accuracy with which the walk route is measured. Having subjects walk around the inner perimeter of either an outdoor track or indoor track is a good reference. A wheeled tape measure used by lawn-maintenance and real estate people is a good device for measuring distances along a sidewalk.

Gayle, Montoye, and Philpot (1977) indicated that pedometers are sensitive to movement style; the way the foot makes contact with the ground. Either of the calibration or conversion procedures described above will compensate for these individual differences.

Tilt Counters

Foster, Kupfer, Weiss, Lipponen, McPartland, and Delgado (1972), McPartland, Foster, Kupfer, and Weiss (1976), Foster, McPartland, and Kupfer (1977) describe a tilt sensor capable of detecting departures of ± 5 degrees or more from the horizontal plane. The sensor consists of a small tube wrapped with fine copper wire containing a small ferromagnetic ball. Movement of the ball inside the tube changes the tube's inductance which occasions FM transmission of a pulse signal to a nearby receiver that movement has begun. Movement beyond the first 5 degrees will not be registered. Only when the device is tilted in the opposite direction and the ball rolls to the other end of the tube will another pulse be transmitted. The forcefulness of the movement plays no role. Mild and vigorous tilts are counted alike.

The device described by Stevens (1971) uses a mercury switch that closes when tilted 5 degrees of more from the horizontal plane. It contains a small ball of mercury that opens or closes an electric circuit depending upon position. Its functional characteristics are like the ball in tube sensor described above.

Schulman, Stevens, and Kupst (1977) describe a three-dimensional version of Stevens (1971) using three mercury switches mounted 120 degrees relative to each other. In this way, movement in all three planes will close at least one switch. A further variation on this theme is provided by Taylor, Kraemer, Bragg, Laughton, Miles, Rule, Savin, and DeBusk (1982), who placed one liquid mercury switch on each of six sides of a cube.

McPartland, Kupfer, and Foster (1976) have developed a third-generation motor-activity recording monitor (MARM) measuring $4.0 \times 2.0 \times 2.0$ cm. It is built around a single mercury switch sensor that closes whenever it is tilted more than 5 mm. Activity counts, number of tilts, are accumulated over a 1.875-, 3.75-, 7.5-, 15-, or 30-minute selectable epoch. The resulting sum is written to one of 512 memory locations thereby allowing data collection to continue from 16 hours to 10.7 days depending upon the selected epoch. Data are subsequently downloaded from the MARM to a computer. This device is commercially available from GMM Electronics, Inc., 1200 Riverview Drive, Verona, PA 15147, (412) 624-2354.

Unit of Measure

The unit of measure is the frequency of a 5-degree tilt from the horizontal plane or from any plane in the case of the triaxial device. It is unclear how the 5-mm displacement regarding the MARM was determined.

Reliability

McGowan, Bulik, Epstein, Kupfer, and Robertson (1984) placed two tilt counters, called large scale integrated (LSI) units, on a carriage shaker set at 160 horizontal movements per minute for two 30-minute trials. Hence 30 × 160 = 4800 movements were executed. The LSI display increments by one for every 16 activity counts sensed due to a scaling circuit. The readings for the first device were 306 and 304. Readings for the second device were 298 and 298. Multiplying by 16 yields 4896 and 4864 activity counts for the first device and 4768 counts for both trials for the second device. These values have a built in uncertainty of 15 counts due to the scaling circuit. The difference of 32 counts divided by the average of 4880 for the first device equals error of 0.00656 which can be expressed as 99.34% consistency. The second device displayed 100% consistency.

The first device overcounted by 96 on the first trial and 64 on the second trial assuming an exact 30-minute test interval. Their average of 80 divided by 4800 is but 0.01667 error or 98.33% accuracy. The second device undercounted by 32 on both trials which when divided by 4800 equals 0.00667 error or 99.33% accuracy.

Foster, McPartland, and Kupfer (1978) describe human and mechanical studies of the reliability of their mercury-switch-based system. The human studies were conducted under both laboratory and field conditions. Motion sensors were attached to the nondominant wrist and ankle of 3 female (24 to 26 years) and 4 male (19 to 24 years) subjects so that they recorded horizontal movement. Two additional sensors were attached to the trunk to measure horizontal and vertical movement. Subjects then performed the following behaviors. They walked on a motor-driven treadmill at 2 mph at 0% grade for 2 minutes, stopped for 2 minutes to record data, and began again at 3 mph for another 2 minutes. This progression increased through the transition of walking to running at 5 mph and continued to 8 mph. The retest began with running at 8 mph and decreased to walking at 2 mph.

Significant test–retest correlations were obtained across the 7 subjects ($df = 5$) at the ankle, wrist, and trunk under every condition. Ankle test–retest correlations ranged from a low of .78 to a high of .94. Wrist test–retest correlations ranged from .76 to .95. Horizontal trunk correlations ranged from .78 to .99 and vertical trunk correlations ranged from .85 to .99.

Williamson, Calpin, Diorenzo, Garris, and Petti (1981) reported perfect reliability after oscillating such sensors an unspecified number of times.

Validity

Subjects 1 and 2 from the Foster, McPartland, and Kupfer (1978) study walked 12 consecutive 0.25-mile laps at 0% grade and recorded their activity at the end of each lap. Activity counts correlated $r(10) = .998$, $p < .001$ with distance walked. Subject 1 repeated the 3-mile course but running instead of walking. Activity counts correlated $r(10) = .998$, $p < .001$ with distance ran. Variability in activity counts was within 11%. Absolute values varied within 5% between subjects.

LaPorte, Kuller, Kupfer, McPartland, Matthews, and Caspersen (1979) placed an activity sensor at the waist and wrist of 10 Physical Education majors and 10 control students (9 Psychology and 1 English majors). Data were recorded four times each day (0930, 1300, 1630, and 2000 hours) for two days. The mean trunk activity count per hour for Physical Education majors ($M = 199.41$) was significantly greater ($F(1,18) = 13.23$, $p < .01$) than for the control subjects ($M = 99.02$). The mean ankle activity count per hour for the Physical Education majors ($M = 192.43$) was also significantly greater ($F(1,18) = 23.37, p < .01$) than for the control subjects ($M = 101.11$).

All 20 subjects self-rated energy expenditure. The correlation between average waist activity counts per hour and average energy expenditure was $r(18) = .69, p < .001$. A lesser correlation was observed between ankle activity counts per hour and energy expenditure ($r(18) = .43, p < .07$). The trunk is more highly correlated with energy expenditure because it approximates the center of gravity.

A laboratory test was performed involving the shaking of three sensors at rates ranging from 50 to 440 movements per minute. The results yielded a correlation of $r(20) = .99, p < .0001$ between activity counts and horizontal movements. A minimum motion of 5 degrees is necessary to stimulate the sensor. All activity counts were within 2% of the actual number of movements made.

Webster, Messin, Mullaney, and Kripke (1982) compared the Vitalog Corporation (1058 California Avenue, Palo Alto, CA 94396) tilt-switch, Grass Instruments (Quincy, MA) single-axis accelerometer and a custom made multiaxial accelerometer (Kripke, Mullaney, Messin, and Wyborney, 1978). The Vitalog tilt-switch contained an array of six mercury switches arranged such that one complete rotation around either the X, Y, or Z axes would cause four switches to close. All three devices were mounted in a single box and three experiments were performed. Experiment I indicated that the accelerometer detected movement not discerned by the tilt-switch. This includes all movements too small to rotate the mercury switches through an adequate arc to close at least one of them. Experiment II indicated that the custom multiaxial accelerometer detected all motion sensed by the Grass single-axis device plus additional movements not detected by the Grass instrument.

Experiment III pertained to the site of attachment issue. Nine subjects completed 22 nights of activity recording with a custom made piezo-ceramic accelerometer taped to the left and right wrists, one ankle, and forehead. Two raters agreed that the left wrist indicated the greatest amount of activity and therefore was the preferred site for detecting movement and wakefulness.

Klesges, Klesges, Swenson, and Pheley (1985) obtained 1-hour activity measurements with the CALTRAC and LSI wrist activity monitor (McPartland, Foster, Kupfer, and Weiss, 1976) from 50 adults (25 male; 25 female) aged 18 to 41 years ($M = 21.5$, $S = 4.68$). The correlation between these two devices was $r(48) = .83$, $p < .0001$.

The validity of these activity counters is also supported by clinically meaningful covariation with presenting condition described primarily in Chapter 3 with mood-disordered adults. For example, depressed inpatients are found to be less active than matched controls as expected.

Motionlogger™ Actigraph

Colburn, Smith, Guarini, and Simons (1976) described the first solid state wrist-worn actigraph. Its sensor was a piezoelectric bilaminar bender element whose free end generates a voltage proportional to its deflection. This voltage is input to a circuit which, when it exceeds a set threshold, emits a fixed duration pulse at a fixed rate. The resulting activity counts, up to 192, are accumulated over a 15-minute memory cycle and written to one of 256 8-bit memory locations. Four Mallory WH-1 mercury cells provide 1500–2000 hours of recording.

Redmond and Hegge (1985) described the second generation actigraph and various preliminary studies that went into technical decisions regarding its construction. A bandpass of 0.25 to 2.0 Hz was chosen. Eliminating frequencies above 2 Hz removes vibrational artifact such as is associated with holding onto a power lawn mower. Eliminating frequencies below 0.25 Hz prevents electronic baseline shifts from being mistakenly counted as activity. The activity-sensing threshold ranges from 0.05 to 0.10 g (where $g = 9.80616$ m/s/s at sea level at 45 degrees latitude; the rate with which freely falling bodies accelerate toward earth). A single-axis sensor was chosen because the root-mean-square (RMS) power intercorrelations among the three axes correlate increasingly from approximately .60 with a 1-sec epoch to approximately .98 with a 256-sec epoch. Power consumption of then available analog-to-digital converters excluded serious consideration of this option for converting sensor output into activity counts. A more practical solution was to count zero crossings in between peaks reached as the sensor beam oscillates in response to movement (zero crossing mode). Alternatively, time above threshold can be determined by onsetting a 10-Hz counter when suprathreshold activity is detected. Calibration is achieved by attaching the actigraph to a pendulum with adjustable periods ranging from 2.0 to 0.5 sec (0.5 to 2.0 Hz) and "trimming" the analog circuitry to achieve predetermined values. User-defined counter settings of up to 16 bits = 65,535 thereby greatly expanding the capabilities of the Colburn *et al.* (1976) device. Battery life was estimated at 1000 hours.

Some design modifications were implemented by Precision Control Design, Inc. (Ft. Walton Beach, FL) during construction of the commercial version of this device retailed by Ambulatory Monitoring, Inc. (Ardsley, New York 10502, (914) 693-9240) under the trade name Motionlogger™. This device has been extensively tested by U.S. Army basic research with field infantry. This solid state accelerometer-based wrist-worn device measures 2.5 × 3.5 × 0.75 in. and weighs 3 oz. It attaches to the wrist or ankle with a Velcro wristlet but can also be worn at the waist. It can be programmed to run in either a zero-crossing or threshold mode as indicated above. In the zero-crossing mode the number of times acceleration related voltages cross zero, when movement changes from being accelerated (+), faster, to being decelerated (−), slower, or vice versa, are counted. In threshold mode, a 10-Hz counter is turned on whenever acceleration exceeds 0.01 g and the number of counts is recorded. Hence, counts divided by 10 equal time above threshold in tenths of a second. Both modes employ programmable epochs ranging from 1 second to 99 minutes and 99 seconds. Selecting a 1-minute epoch allows data to be continuously collected 24 hours a day for 8 days. The subject can record the occurrence of an event by pressing a button on the Motionlogger™ which records the incident in 1 bit of memory. The Motionlogger™ is programmed, and data are downloaded, through an interface attached to the serial port of an IBM or compatible computer running MS-DOS.

The next-generation actigraph, known as the AMA-32, has become available too late for a full description to be included in this book, but a few of its properties are known. Its size has been reduced through hybrid chip technology to that of a diver's watch. The sensor is a lollipop-shaped piezoelectric element. It is a fully programmable device with a 32K memory of which approximately 28K is available for data storage after programming is loaded. High and low dynamic sensitivity ranges are available. Of particular interest is the autogain feature which automatically increases amplifier sensitivity under low activity conditions, such as sleep, and records the new amplifier setting. Maximum sensitivity is reported to be able to detect heart rate and respiration if placed on the sternum. The user can specify one of 20 filter bands ranging from 0.1 to 10 Hz to customize the actigraph's response characteristics. Red and green flat-panel switches on the face of the device can be used as event buttons. It runs on less costly, easier to obtain "coin" batteries.

Unit of Measure

The Motionlogger™ has two units of measure depending upon the mode of operation selected when the device is initialized. The more sensitive zero crossing mode counts the number of times that the voltage changes sign from positive to negative and vice versa associated with the up-down vibrations of the accelerometer beam sensor. The frequency with which these voltage changes occur is partly dependent upon the behavior performed, though hardware filters considerably restrict such variability (cf. Redmond and Hegge, 1985). Because these zero crossing values are independent of intensity of movement, the Motionlogger™ is essentially a movement detector. Given the fixed duration of data epochs, say 1 minute each, the zero crossings observed can be expressed as a proportion of the maximum possible counts per epoch to determine the proportion of the epoch during which suprathreshold activity was present.

The somewhat less sensitive threshold mode has more straightforward units of measurement. It enables a 10-Hz counter whenever suprathreshold activity is sensed. The total possible counts in a 1 minute epoch is 60 seconds $\times$ 10 Hz = 600. Dividing observed counts by 10, moving the decimal point to the left one space, gives the number of seconds per epoch for which suprathreshold activity was sensed. When using a 1-minute epoch, the units of measure become seconds of activity per minute. More generally we have seconds of activity per epoch length of time; e.g., seconds of activity per 2 minutes given a 2-minute epoch. These unusual units can be scaled back to seconds per minute.

Reliability

The reliability of the Motionlogger™ is best studied using a Precision Control Design, Inc., precision pendulum. The actigraph is attached to the pendulum, which is displaced from the vertical plane by 10 degrees, where it is held by a catch. The actigraph is then initialized with an IBM or compatible computer for immediate data collection. The trigger button on the pendulum is pressed and the arm plus actigraph swing freely about a low friction point for approximately 10 minutes.

The two square top portions of Figure 2.1 presents the output from a single actigraph in zero crossing mode over two consecutive pendulum tests. The impressive similarity of response to the two virtually identical pendulum tests is strong evidence of the Motionlogger's™ reliability. The preceding portion of the figure represents handling the actigraph between programming and attachment to the pendulum. The final spike is associated with removing the actigraph from the pendulum prior to downloading data. The horizontal bar indicates no data.

Figure 2.2 presents the output from the same actigraph in threshold mode over two consecutive pendulum tests. Again, the impressive similarity of response to two virtually identical stimulations is strong evidence of Motionlogger™ reliability. The reasons for the particular and different shapes of the figures is discussed in the next section on validity.

Validity

Figure 2.1 also provides validity data. The gradual decay of simple sinusoidal motion of a low friction pendulum is well known and can be rigorously described mathematically. The periodicity of the pendulum remains constant as the amplitude

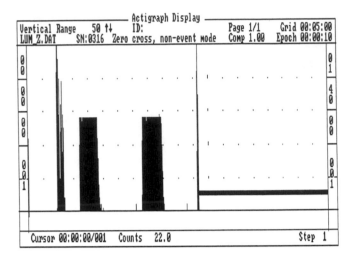

FIGURE 2.1. Pendulum test with Motionlogger™ actigraph programmed for zero crossing mode.

of swing decreases. Hence, pendulums provide a constant rate of zero crossing over time; swinging back and forth producing positive, zero, and negative acceleration in one direction and vice versa in the opposite direction. Figure 2.1 shows that the Motionlogger™ actigraph accurately tracks this constant rate of zero crossing when set in zero crossing detection mode.

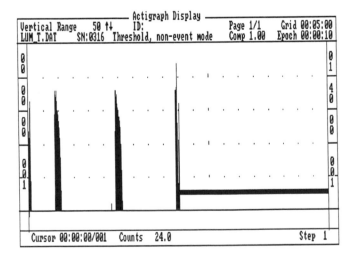

FIGURE 2.2. Pendulum test with Motionlogger™ actigraph programmed for threshold mode.

The amplitude of the pendulum swing gradually decays over time thereby reducing the portion of the pendulum trajectory during which acceleration exceeds the threshold of the Motionlogger™ actigraph set in threshold mode. Figure 2.2 shows that the Motionlogger™ actigraph responds to this reduced amplitude by recording less time above threshold, fewer activity counts.

That the zero crossing mode is more sensitive than threshold mode is seen by comparing the horizontal distance (time) for the tracings in Figures 2.1 and 2.2. The Motionlogger™ actigraph responded to small swings near the end of the test, when set to zero crossing mode, that were not sensed in threshold mode.

Chapter 3 contains evidence that the behavior of mood-disordered adults differs significantly in the predicted direction from normal control subjects. Chapter 4 provides validity evidence for actigraphs. For example, Porrino, Rapoport, Behar, Ismond, and Bunney (1983) reported significantly greater activity in children diagnosed as hyperactive than in matched-control boys. In Chapter 6, on sleep activity, records spanning one or more 24-hour intervals provide contrasting sleep and wake periods. Without exception, activity during the wake periods vastly exceeds that recorded during the sleep periods as expected.

Accelerometers

Unit of Measure

The standard unit of measure of acceleration is the rate with which bodies freely fall due to gravity. The accepted value is $g = 9.80616$ meters/second/second at sea level at 45 degrees latitude. A practical demonstration of this value is easily arranged by dropping any object while observing it.

Reliability

The reliability of accelerometers is best evaluated under laboratory conditions, where they yield highly repeatable values.

Validity

The validity of accelerometers is also best evaluated under laboratory conditions, where they are typically shown to be linear to within a few percentage points.

Accelerometers have been used to measure animal (Mundel and Malmo, 1979) and human (Morris, 1973) activity. Cotes and Meade (1960) measured vertical acceleration about the waist while subjects walked on a treadmill. They reported that the acceleration produced during the lift portion of the walking cycle times body weight times step frequency correlated $r = .98$ with oxygen consumption. It is therefore possible to estimate relative oxygen consumption by counting steps assuming constant step characteristics and body weight.

Wong, Webster, Montoye, and Washburn (1981) described the use of a portable accelerometer device for measuring energy expenditure in humans. They begin by indicating that such devices should exclude the contribution of gravity (0 Hz = DC); they used a 0.21-Hz high pass filter. They did not expect significant human activity above 10 Hz and therefore recommended a 11.8-Hz low pass filter. They began by attaching a 255-mg ball bearing to the tip of a Calectro S2-294 (GC Electronics, Rockford, IL) piezoelectric monaural phonocartridge. This accelerometer was attached to the trunk of 15 subjects while walking on a motor-driven treadmill with 0% grade for 3 minutes at 2, 3, and 4 mph; running for 3 minutes at 6 and 8 mph; and stepping up onto an 8-in. bench and down again for 3 minutes at the rate of 80, 120, and 140 repetitions per minute. Evaluation of the relationship between vertical acceleration and normalized oxygen consumption (ml VO_2/kg/min) was restricted to graphical presentation but clearly indicated a strong linear relationship. Simultaneous pedometer readings also indicated a strong linear relationship With oxygen consumption.

Montoye, Washburn, Servais, Ertl, Webster, and Nagle (1983) attached the 400-g 14 × 8 × 4-cm accelerometer developed by Wong et al. (1981) to the waist, at the back, of 21 healthy subjects aged 20 to 60 years. Subjects performed each of the following 14 exercises, 4 minutes each, on two separate days while oxygen uptake (ml VO_2/kg/min) was monitored: walking on a motor-driven treadmill at 2 mph at 0%, 6%, and 12% grades; walking on the same treadmill at 4 mph at the same grades; running on the treadmill at 6 mph at 0% and 6% grades; stepping up on and down from an 8-in. bench 20 and 35 times per minute; half knee-bends at 28 and 48 repetitions per minute; and floor touches while bending knees at the rate of 24 and 36 touches per minute.

The results indicated that first and second trial accelerometer readings taken from 4 subjects during each of the 14 activities ($N = 56$) correlated $r(54) = .94$, $p < .0001$. Correlation of all $N = 14 \times 21 = 294$ acceleration and oxygen readings was $r(292) = .74$, $p < .0001$. The average within-subject correlation over 14 data points was $r(12) = .79$, $p < .001$.

Wong, Webster, Montoye and Washburn (1981) cite a Yugoslavian symposium presentation by Reswick, Perry, Antoneilli, Su, and Freeborn (1978) showing that both vertical acceleration, and its integration over time, correlate well with oxygen consumption. Although their results were limited to graphical presentation, Wong et al. estimated that their figure represented at least $r = .90$.

Brouha (1960) reported a correlation of $r = .83$ between the temporal integral of vertical platform acceleration and oxygen consumption by office and industrial workers.

Kripke, Mullaney, Messin, and Wyborney (1978) compared wrist acceleration and polysomnography during sleep. They reported a correlation of $r(3) = .954$, $p <$

.05, between sleep period measurements, $r(3) = .982, p < .01$, between sleep time measurements, and $r(3) = .851, p < .05$, between wake time within sleep measurements in 5 normal sleepers.

CALTRAC™

Servais, Webster, and Montoye (1984) provide a detailed rationale for estimating energy expenditure due to movement with an accelerometer based device that they constructed and tested in various ways. CALTRAC™ is a commercially available device (Hemokinetics, Inc., 2923 Osmundsen Road, Madison, Wisconsin 53711; 608-274-0877) for measuring caloric expenditure due to activity. This device also estimates calories expended as a result of resting metabolic rate (RMR) on the basis of weight, height, and age as explained in Chapter 5.

Klesges, Klesges, Swenson, and Pheley (1985) obtained 1-hour activity measurements with the CALTRAC™ and wrist activity (McPartland, Foster, Kupfer, and Weiss, 1976; GMM Electronics, Inc., Verona, PA) devices from 50 adults (25 male; 25 female) aged 18 to 41 years ($M = 21.5, S = 4.68$). The correlation between these two devices was $r(48) = .83, p < .0001$.

Klesges and Klesges (1987) validated CALTRAC™ against the Fargo Activity Timesampling Survey (FATS) (cf. Klesges, Coates, Moldenhauer, Holzer, Gustavson, and Barnes, 1984) which was partially validated against wrist (tilt) activity counts. The activity of 28 children aged 24 to 48 months ($M = 33.87, S = 8.01$) was observed from breakfast until 1 hour after the evening meal using the FATS with new observers every 2 hours. Caltract activity counts were obtained every hour. Hourly correlation coefficients between FATS and CALTRAC™ ranged from .55 to .95.

Actillume™

The Actillume™ is an improved version of the Motionlogger™ actigraph described above (cf. Cole, Kripke, Gruen, and Nava, 1990). It is built around a Motorola CMOS 6800 series microprocessor with a 256-byte RAM (random access memory), 2K-byte EEPROM (electrically erasable programmable read only memory), ROM bootstrap loader, 32K-byte RAM disk, clock, and an RS232 interface.

Activity is sensed by a precision linear accelerometer ($0.1-5$ g; drop resistant) and digitized by a 4-channel 8-bit A/D (analog-to-digital) converter twenty times per second (20 Hz). The 8-bit A/D capability enables the device to distinguish among $2^8 = 256$ intensities of movement on a ratio (equal interval + absolute zero) scale. Two aspects of activity are recorded. The first, called Sum, is the total of all activity measurements made during an epoch; whose length is user selectable from 2 seconds to 1 hour. This mode largely corresponds to the Motionlogger™ actigraph except that the results are now directly proportional to activity intensity. The second mode, called Max, is the largest single activity measurement recorded during each epoch.

Light exposure is sensed with a precision photodiode photometer traceable to the National Bureau of Standards (0.01–100,000 lux with green filter). The microprocessor samples light once each second (1 Hz). Light intensities are measured in log lux and the geometric mean is computed for each epoch.

The Actillume℗ runs on a $1/2$ AA lithium battery for approximately 3 weeks that can be changed in the field without data loss. The system automatically switches to a low-power wait state when a low battery condition is detected to prolong data preservation. It measures $2^3/4 \times 1^1/2 \times 7/8$ in. ($7 \times 3.8 \times 2.2$ cm) and weighs 3.1 oz (100 gm). Its nickel-plated aluminum case is water resistant (not submersible). It contains a real-time event marker which can be used to signal the beginning and/or end of a predefined event.

The Actillume's℗ microprocessor is fully programmable. The user downloads his or her program into the Actillume's℗ RAM through the RS232 port of an IBM or compatible computer connected to a Data Retrieval Unit (DRU) which also displays percent of full battery voltage. A small bootstrap program then further downloads the program from RAM into the EEPROM and finally passes control to this code. The user can select recording epoch length as with the Motionlogger℗ plus additional flexibility. Activity and light data are uploaded through the same DRU.

The primary benefit of the Actillume℗ is that the data are directly proportional to the forcefulness of the behavior being monitored.

Reliability. Figures 2.3 and 2.4 present the results of four pendulum tests with the same actigraph. Figure 2.3 displays the Sum results while Figure 2.4 displays the Max results. Notice the high degree of similarity across all plots indicating a high degree of repeatability under standard stimulus conditions.

Validity. The decaying amplitude of the pendulum provides a well-defined smoothly changing series of accelerations across a considerable range. Notice that the Actillume℗ responds as expected by reporting a decreasing series of activity intensity.

SIBIS

Linscheid, Iwata, Ricketts, Williams, and Griffin (1990) describe the Self-Injurious Behavior Inhibiting System (SIBIS). They programmed the device to respond to a 1.5-g impact, which is sufficient to detect a forceful slap. The attached 9-V battery then produced 16 pulses, each lasting 5 ms over a 0.2-s interval at an intensity of 0.007 W/s. Their Table 1 indicates that these parameters are comparable

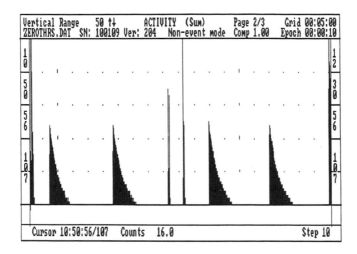

FIGURE 2.3. Pendulum test with Actillume™ actigraph reporting in Sum mode.

to those used by other investigators. A more limited device for detecting SIBIS was described by Ball, Sibbach, Jones, Steele, and Frazier (1975).

Unit of Measure. The unit of measure is the frequency with which 1.5 *g* or greater impacts occur.

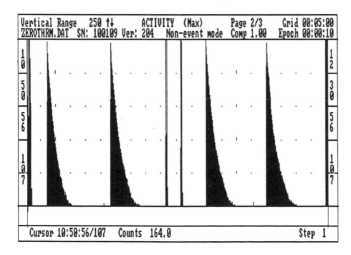

FIGURE 2.4. Pendulum test with Actillume™ actigraph reporting in Max mode.

Reliability. Apparently all impacts above 1.5 *g* are responded to.

Validity. Here we engage the question of whether all impacts above 1.5 *g* are due to self-injurious behaviors. The answer to this question largely depends upon the activities in which the person engages. Wearing this device during contact sports such as football and rugby would present a problem. Wearing it under normal residential settings leaves mainly the problem of one resident striking another.

Heart Rate

Bradfield (1971) and Warnold and Arvidsson-Lenner (1977) recommended using heart rate as a measure of activity. Stott (1977) describes methods for recording and analyzing ambulatory electrocardiograms and blood pressure. The resulting data are primarily summarized in terms of histograms of frequency by interbeat interval. Ambulatory monitoring of blood pressure is also discussed.

Saris, Snel, and Binkhorst (1977) described a portable heart-rate distribution recorder capable of recording 8 levels of heart rate over a 24-hour period. Two chest electrodes are connected to a 63 × 94 × 22-mm stainless steel box weighing 220 gm carried in a pocket attached to a belt around the waist. The associated electronic circuit detected, timed, and expressed R-R waves in terms of beats per minute (four hearing aid batteries last 3 weeks). The results of each R-R wave measurement incremented one of 8 counters each capable of recording two million events. One counter was dedicated to each of the following heart rate bands: 40–69, 70–99, 100–124, 125–149, 150–176, 177–199, 200–224, and 225–300. Data are visually displayed using a readout console and recorded by hand.

Taylor, Kraemer, Bragg, Miles, Rule, Savin, and Debusk (1982) describe a system for the ambulatory recording and processing of heart rate and physical activity in outpatients. Richardson (1971) describes the use of heart rate to measure activity in middle-aged men. Goldsmith, Miller, Mumford, and Stock (1976) discussed the use of heart rate to measure energy expenditure.

Relatively inexpensive pulse monitors are increasingly available. L. L. Bean (Freeport, ME, 04033) retail a Casio PulseCheck Watch (Catalog # 5764RL) for $56. Similar devices are the Pulse Tach Watch (Microcomputer Technology, Inc., 3304 West MacArthur, Santa Ana, CA, 92704) and Insta-Pulse (from Biosig, Inc; available through The Sharper Image, 260 California Street, San Francisco, CA, 94111).

Unit of Measure

One normally thinks of measuring heart rate in beats per minute. However, Khachaturian, Kerr, Kruger, and Schachter (1972) persuasively argue for measuring heart rate in terms of milliseconds for each interbeat interval. They report a nonlinear relationship between interbeat interval and beats per minute. The authors hold that phasic relationships between a stimulus and cardiac response are more clearly discernible when measured as milliseconds of interbeat interval than beats per minute. The authors also report that interbeat interval data contain from 1.9 to 4.6 times less skewness than beat per minute data. These differences are especially noticeable at high heart rates typical of performance under stress, children, and small animals.

Reliability

No studies expressly testing the reliability of heart-rate monitors were found. Because data can be no more valid than they are reliable, we can infer from the next section that heart-rate monitors are highly reliable. Their common usage in hospitals for monitoring vital signs also testifies to their reliability.

Validity

Webster, Messin, Mullaney, and Kripke (1982) validated a heart-rate recorder by scoring electrocardiogram tapes using the recorder and a standard acoustic monitor for 8 subjects. The recorder reported an average of 5874 beats vs the 5870 beats recorded by the acoustic monitor for Tape 1. For Tape 2, the recorder registered an average of 3459 counts vs the acoustic monitor's 3419 counts. The two scoring methods were highly correlated ($r(23) = .99, p < .0001$). Pedometer data indicated that 20 fifth-grade children (9 boys, 11 girls) were equally active on the one day that they wore the heart rate monitor as they were on three previous days thereby indicating that the monitor does not alter natural activity.

Reviews of heart-rate monitoring are provided by Horton (1984) and Brun (1984). Horton (1984) and Torun (1984) insist that each subject must be calibrated under laboratory conditions to determine the particular relationship between heart rate and activity that currently exists for them. This functional relationship is different across people and changes within an individual as a result of conditioning and other factors. Horton (1984) further asserts that this method is much more accurate for high than low heart-rate levels as change in posture and anxiety will create larger percentage changes in low than high heart rates.

Oxygen Consumption

Katch and McArdle (1988) indicate that metabolism requires oxygen and that approximately 1 liter of oxygen is required to produce 4.82 kcal of heat energy. Hence, caloric expenditure can be calculated once oxygen consumption is known. The authors illustrate the use of a portable spirometer for ambulatory oxygen measurements (pp. 98–100).

Consolazio, Johnson, and Pecora (1963), and Consolazio (1971), describe the portable collection of expired gases to measure activity level. Horton (1984) discusses a method of indirect calorimetry using a portable respirometer to capture expired breath for later analysis. Oxygen (O_2) consumption is determined by comparing the oxygen in expired air vs fresh air. Carbon dioxide (CO_2) consumption is calculated the same way. The relative proportions of carbohydrates, lipids, and proteins being oxidized is estimated using the aforementioned measurements in conjunction with N_2 excretion.

Ambulatory Monitoring Inc. (731 Saw Mill River Road, Ardsley, NY 10502; 914 693-9240) sells a lightweight battery-operated device called Oxylog™ which measures and records oxygen consumption in tenths of a liter of oxygen consumed. A sensing head determines the amount of oxygen consumed by subtracting the oxygen content of expired from inspired air. A recorder jack permits recording by a built-in Solicorder sampling once per minute or to a 4-channel Medilog recorder.

Decker, Hoekje, Kingman, and Strohl (1989) describe a portable system for the ambulatory monitoring of arterial oxygen saturation. This device is a modified battery powered pulse oximeter connected to an analog recorder that runs for 30 hours between battery changes. The accuracy of this device is such that the mean difference between its readings and those obtained by an IL282 CO-oximeter was -1.12% with a 95% confidence interval of $\pm 2.75\%$. Continuous records from 6 healthy subjects over an average of 19 hours ($S = 5$ hr) yielded a mean of 89% ($S = 7\%$) usable data.

Schulman, Kaspar, and Throne (1965) measured oxygen consumption in behavior-disordered boys. Waxman and Stunkard (1980) measured oxygen consumption in obese boys while they performed various activities to estimate the caloric requirements of these activities.

Unit of Measure

Gases are measured in liters and flow rate in liters per minute.

Reliability

Reliability studies were not found. Consistency of mechanical operation supports the reliability of such equipment.

Validity

Validity is best determined under laboratory conditions. Calibration procedures establish the validity of such equipment. Data on the linearity of the above-mentioned equipment was unavailable at press time.

Body Temperature

Exercise raises body temperature. CorTemp™ (Human Technologies, Inc., 300 Third Avenue North, St. Petersburg, FL 33701; 1-800-274-4600) is a miniature disposable temperature sensor, developed by The Applied Physics Laboratory of The Johns Hopkins University under a NASA grant, that telemeters temperature data (Fahrenheit or centigrade) to a nearby solid state memory receiver along with the time the temperature reading was taken and display the same information on the screen of the CorTemp™ Ambulatory Monitor worn by the patient. The "Pill" (as it is known) is expected to remain in the digestive system for 24 to 72 hours. It can be rectally or vaginally implanted, where it will remain active for 10 days. The Monitor is capable of recording data for up to 250 days depending upon how often temperature samples are taken and stored.

Romanczyk, Crimmins, Gordon, and Kashinsky (1977) describe an inexpensive alternative for measuring body temperature. They recommend attaching a small thermistor to the armpit area using an adhesive pad with a lead connected to a small digital voltmeter. This allows either the wearer or an independent observer to record voltage readings at prescribed times and subsequently convert them to temperature readings on the basis of calibration data provided by the thermistor manufacturer.

Unit of Measure

Temperature is measured either in degrees centigrade or Fahrenheit.

Reliability

Reliability studies were not found. It is very likely that modern thermistors yield highly repeatable measurements.

Validity

Validity of thermistors is established in the laboratory through calibration procedures. No data were available on the linearity of the above-mentioned devices.

Integrated EMG

Activity requires muscle contraction. Electromyography measures the electrical correlates of muscle contraction.

Unit of Measure

Needle-electrode EMG is typically measured in microvolts whereas surface-electrode EMG is measured in microvolts per square centimeter.

Reliability

No reliability studies were found. It is important to ask about reliability under what conditions. Reliability of detecting activity in a frog-leg preparation is expected to be much higher than reliability of activity estimates in ambulatory subjects for many reasons; partly due to inconsistency in subject movements.

Validity

Harding and Sen (1970) recommended measuring activity via integrated electroymography (EMG). Globus, Phoebus, Humphries, Boyd, and Sharp (1973) used integrated EMG to measure activity in college students as part of a circadian rhythm study. However, Horton (1984) concludes: "It [integrated EMG] is entirely unsatisfactory for studies of energy expenditure during physical exercise and should not be used for this purpose." (p. 123)

HUMAN LABORATORY ACTIVITY

Stabilimeters

In this section we review devices that a person can sit (chair) or lie (bed) on and have subsequent body movements automatically recorded.

Chair

Foshee (1958) described a device consisting of a deskchair mounted on a platform supported by rubber supports at each of the four corners. A lever attached to the back of this platform mechanically amplified all longitudinal movements. Chair movement caused the bar magnet, mounted on this lever, to move inside a steel core wound with 4000 turns of copper wire thereby creating voltage changes which were integrated and recorded as condenser discharges per unit time.

The Cromwell, Palk, and Foshee (1961) ballistographic chair was constructed somewhat differently. The chair is attached to a platform which is suspended by cables. A lever attached to the back of this platform works as described above.

Sprague and Toppe (1966) describe a desk chair mounted on a platform supported by a central bolt projecting from the floor allowing for a $1/4$-in. tilt in the forward–backward or left–right planes. Microswitches count tilts in both directions.

Farrall Instruments (P.O. Box 1037, Grand Island, NE 68801) sells "The Wiggle Chair." A similar instrument can be purchased from the Lafayette Instrument Company (P.O. Box 1279, Lafayette, IN 47902).

Christensen (1975), Edelson and Sprague (1974), Juliano (1974), and Montagu and Swarbrick (1975) employ a stabilimetric cushion containing microswitches. The subject sits on the cushion. Position changes open some switches and close others.

Bed

The crib is the natural habitat for infants. Lipsitt and DeLucia (1960), Campbell (1968), and Lewis and Wilson (1970) describe the construction of devices suitable for human infants. A related device is described by Griffiths, Chapman, and Campbell (1967). Word and Stern (1958) describe a related device for use with the rat.

Behavioral sleep studies (cf. Cox and Marley, 1959; Kleitman, 1963, pp. 85–86; Stonehill and Crisp, 1971) connect the bed springs to a strip chart recorder to indicate the presence of body motility. These devices can be made extremely sensitive; sufficient to record respiration. Figure 1 from Stonehill and Crisp (1971) indicates a strong positive relationship between body weight and motility counts. They recommend correcting observed motility scores to a single weight using the following regression score: Motility $= 8.20$ W $+ 0.42$.

Cairns, Thomas, Mooney, and Pace (1976) connected a large electric clock to a switch activated by bed spring movement such that the clock would run when no one sat on or lay down in the bed. It served as a measure of "up time" on a chronic pain ward.

Unit of Measure

The unit of measure for chair stabilimeters is the change in moment (weight times distance from center of platform) necessary to tilt the platform sufficient to cause either a microswitch closure or enough voltage to produce one activity count.

The unit of measure for bed stabilimeters is the distance (in millimeters) the spring must move in order to activate the recording instrument. In the case of Cairns's up-time indicator, the fundamental unit of measure is the second; degrees of movement and/or when they occur are not of interest.

Reliability

The reliability of stabilimeters reduces to the consistency with which weight transfers and bed spring movements close microswitches or otherwise activate recording instruments. As with all other mechanical instruments, choosing to repeatedly stimulate the device with forces well above threshold produce highly reliable results. No such study of stabilimeter reliability has been located to date.

Validity

Stabilimeters measure what they were designed to measure. As with other instruments, it is important to restrict one's concept of activity to that which the stabilimeter measures when employing such a device.

Photoelectric Cells

Well-focused light beams are placed along two adjacent walls and corresponding photocells are placed opposite them on the other two walls thereby dividing the floor space into square blocks (cf. Ellis and Pryer, 1959). Movement from one block to another interrupts one or more light beams and increments the counter associated with that light source–photocell pair.

The video camera approach, described below, provides a much more flexible and comprehensive method of dividing an area into square units and tracking movement.

Unit of Measure

The unit of measurement pertains to the distance necessary to trigger a photoelectric beam. If square areas are used then the unit of measurement can be as small as one side or as large as the diagonal which equals the square root of twice the square of the length of one side. Perhaps one could settle for the average of these two values. Using rectangular areas increases the difference between the two unit estimates and therefore is undesirable.

Reliability

The question of reliability reduces to the consistency with which particular movements completely intersect specific light beams. A device that totally blocks light will be found to produce 100% reliable results.

Johnson (1972) examined the reliability of a photoelectric device in the following way. First, an adult subject walked a predefined course at a slow speed for 3 minutes. Activity counts per 15 seconds were recorded and yielded $N = 12$ values with a mean of 59.42 and a standard deviation of 3.78 yielding a coefficient of variation of 6.36. Second, the subject sat quietly for another 3 minutes yielding 11 counts of zero and one count of 1 yielding near perfect reliability. The basic limit to this approach is the extent to which the person could walk consistently and sit quietly. The results are more informative regarding the person than the apparatus.

Validity

The validity of a photoelectric cell device is directly dependent upon the accuracy with which the beam–detector pairs are installed and aligned.

Ultrasound

Peacock and Williams (1962) describe an apparatus that floods the room with an audio standing wave of 41 kHz, over twice the human threshold of hearing. Movement within the standing wave field alters the standing wave pattern (cf. Crawford and Nicora, 1964; Montagu and Swarbrick, 1975; Ray, Shotick, and Peacock, 1977). Transducers sense such changes and generate activity counts in direct proportion to them. Unfortunately, this device is known to be directionally sensitive. Dabbs and Clower (1973) indicated that the highest " . . . rates occurred when the movement was fast, close to, or directly toward or away from the motion detector." (p. 475) Activity counts are directly proportional to being head on and near the transducer and inversely proportional to the distance from the transducer. Movement parallel to the transducer produces fewer activity counts than movement towards or away from the transducer.

Unit of Measure

The unit of measure for ultrasonic instruments can be expressed either as the degree of displacement necessary to be detected or as the rate of movement necessary to be detected.

Reliability

Reliability is relative to the amount of displacement or rate of displacement. If substantially suprathreshold values are used then very high levels of reliability can be expected. As the stimulus magnitude approaches threshold, reductions in the consistency of response are expected.

Johnson (1972) constructed a mechanical walker with two 50.8-cm-long legs that oscillated in opposite directions at 7 rpm. He reported that an ultrasonic detector gave five different counts when placed in five different locations consistent with Dabbs and Clower's (1973) description. The coefficients of variation (error) ranged from 14.86% to 35.9%.

Validity

The reliability data suggest that ultrasonic activity monitors are nonlinear measuring devices. Moreover, they will respond to all movements including curtains blowing from a fan or pets moving about in addition to the human motion in question. Activity from two or more people will be fused into one set of activity counts.

ANIMAL LABORATORY ACTIVITY

Video Camera

The Columbus Instruments International Corporation [P.O. Box 44049, Columbus, OH 43204; 1-800-669-5011] "Videomex-V"™ system takes data from a TV camera or videocassette recorder (VCR), scans it with a 256 × 192 binary frame grabber at 15 to 30 frames per second. Both a low light and true infrared viewing option are available. Horizontal and/or vertical movements from one or more cages can be separately recorded on VCR for subsequent analysis by a single Videomex-V™ system.

Subjects can be rodents, other animals, or insects behaving in land or water mazes, open field areas, or cages; even fish in an aquarium where infrared beam systems cannot penetrate water and where visible light beam systems might alter behavior.

Once data are recorded, the investigator can run any of the following programs and print results to an Epson-compatible printer. The Multiple Zone Distance Traveled program allows the user to define 95 different zones and select one zone as the goal. Total time to goal plus route taken and how far it traveled in each zone can be determined.

The Multiple Zone Motion Monitor divides the digitized image into 768 blocks comprising a 32 × 24 matrix. Each block contains 64 picture elements (pixels) arranged in an 8 × 8 matrix and can be assigned one of 95 labels. Nesting areas can be labeled "N," food areas "F," and water areas "W." All other areas are assigned another symbol such as a "+." The program calculates the number of pixels turned on by activity as time spend in the zone and calculates the number of pixels changing in an area as the activity associated with the zone. It therefore allows observations of much time spent but little activity in one zone.

The Multiple Motion Monitor is a special case of the above program. It measures general activity in the entire field by counting the number of pixels that change from one image to the next. One can determine the number of moving animals in each image by dividing the total number of pixels on by the average number of pixels stimulated by a single animal.

By placing an angled mirror to the side of the cage, it is possible to measure vertical movements as well as horizontal ones. Clockwise and counterclockwise rotations can be calculated.

The Social Contact monitor detects proximity by calculating the smallest rectangle that will completely enclose two animals. The diagonal of this rectangle is the distance measure. Distances below a defined level constitute contact. The time the contact began and its duration are computed. Any of 5 relays can be activated upon contact to excite a VCR so that only the times when contact occur are recorded.

The Distance Traveled and Pattern of Movement program tracks the route taken by an animal and its total distance. By tagging subjects with colored tags, the Videomex-X™ Color Video Image Analyzer can track up to 6 individuals at 60 frames per second each with 240 × 240 pixels resolution. The distance between colored markers can also be tracked.

Unit of Measure

The unit of measure common to all of the above measurements is the pixel. Its physical width as projected into the cage or experimental area constitutes the basic unit of measure upon which all subsequent calculations are based.

Reliability

No specific reliability data were available.

Validity

No validity studies were found.

Capacitive Plates

Stoff, Stauderman, and Wyatt (1983) describe an alternative approach to monitoring the behavior of a single animal in a cage. Four independent electric fields are established along the inside walls of the animal's cage ($+X$ East, $-X$ West, $+Y$ North, $-Y$ South). The rat makes contact with ground through the floor grid and distorts each field proportional to its distance from each wall, which is noted as a capacitance change. This arrangement will respond to fine 5-mm movements as well as large 150-mm movements. Position data are available up to 6 times per second. A PDP 11-03 computer was used to monitor the results of 16 such cages.

Unit of Measure

The unit of measure can be expressed either as the degree of displacement necessary to be detected or as the rate of movement necessary to be detected.

Reliability

No specific reliability data were available.

Validity

No validity studies were found.

Infrared Emitter/Detector

Silverman, Chang, and Russell (1988) describe the construction of an apparatus for measuring activity in small animals using relatively inexpensive solid state infrared emitter-detector arrays coupled to a TRS-80 Model III or IBM PC compatible microcomputer.

Unit of Measure

The unit of measure is the size of square or rectangle determined by the position of the infrared emitters/detectors.

Reliability

No specific reliability data were available.

Validity

No validity studies were found.

Activity Wheel

An extensive literature exists regarding animal activity and variables that influence it. Virtually every article provides a description of their apparatus and accordingly such information will not be repeated here. Richter (1965) extensively describes the apparatus he used for many years. Other descriptions are given by Rusak and Zucker (1975), Terman and Terman (1970, 1975), Richter (1976), Elsmore and Hursh (1982), and Terman (1983).

An important feature of an activity wheel is that it is the animal's complete habitat meaning that activity is recorded whenever it occurs.

Unit of Measure

The unit of measure can be expressed either as the degree of displacement necessary to be detected or as the rate of movement necessary to be detected depending upon how wheel turns are sensed.

Reliability

No specific reliability data were available.

Validity

No validity studies were found.

Activity, Mood Disorders, and Schizophrenia

Affective disorders and schizophrenia were among the first behavioral abnormalities to be expressed in terms of activity measurements. The first edition of the Diagnostic and Statistical Manual (DSM-I) (APA, 1952, p. 25) included increased motor activity among the formal inclusion criteria for Manic Depressive Reaction, Manic Type (000-x11). Manic Depressive Reaction, Depressed Type (000-x12) was said to be characterized by "motor retardation and inhibition." The term "stupor" was also used in contrast with agitation (p. 25).

The less severe neurotic emotional disorder, Depressive Reaction (000-x06), was differentially diagnosed from its psychotic counterpart by the absence of "severe psychomotor retardation" and by "stupor." (p. 34)

Activity measures pertained to Schizophrenic Reaction, Schizo-affective Type (000-x27) because of the previously defined affective disorders. Schizophrenic Reaction, Catatonic Type (000-x23) was partly diagnosed by "marked generalized inhibition (stupor, mutism, negativism, and waxy flexibility) or excessive motor activity and excitement." (p. 26) We were told that Schizophrenic Reaction, Acute Undifferentiated Type (000-x25) was often "accompanied by a pronounced affective coloring of either excitement or depression." (p. 27)

MOTOR ACTIVITY

Various references to abnormal motor behavior are made within DSM-III-R. The purpose of this section is to review and clarify these references to motor activity.

Psychomotor Agitation

DSM-III-R (APA, 1987) defines psychomotor agitation as "excessive motor activity" (p. 404) that is observable. DSM-III-R emphasizes the need for objective measurement by indicating that psychomotor agitation must be "observable by others, not merely subjective feelings of restlessness . . ." (p. 222) Examples include "Inability to sit still, pacing, wringing of hands, (and) pulling at clothes." (p. 404) The term "restless" is sometimes used to describe such purposeless activity. Akathesia is a drug-induced form of this type of psychomotor agitation.

Psychomotor Retardation

DSM-III-R (APA, 1987) defines psychomotor retardation as "Visible generalized slowing down of physical reactions, movements, and speech." (p. 404) DSM-III-R emphasizes the need for objective measurement by indicating that psychomotor retardation must be "observable by others, not merely subjective feelings of . . . being slowed down." (p. 222) Depressed mood is an indirect way of referring to decreased activity. When activity is particularly diminished in the presence of schizophrenic symptoms, the term catatonic stupor is used. Further reduction in motor activity is referred to as semicoma, coma, or torpor.

Mood Shifts

Mood shifts refer to changes from psychomotor retardation to agitation and vice versa. They are documented by the same criteria as discussed above plus a pattern of alternation. The terms "excitement" and " expansive mood" are also used. Hypervigilance is a less common but still-used term. If schizophrenic symptoms are present, the term "catatonic excitement" is used. Sometimes increased activity can refer to enhanced purposeful activity such as increased work or recreational activities all of which involve higher levels of motor activity.

DSM-III-R MOOD DISORDERS

The purpose of this section is to describe the ways in which actigraphy can assist in the diagnosis and assessment of mood disorders as conceptualized by DSM-III-R (APA, 1987). Mood disorders involve a prolonged depression or elation; they were called Affective Disorders by DSM-III. It is important to notice that activity and mood are substantively equated at many points. Hence, objective mood assessment has become activity measurement. Mood Disorders are divided into Bipolar Disorders and Depressive Disorders.

The "x" associated with diagnoses such as 296.2x (Major Depression, Single

Episode) refer to the "fifth digit" which is used to quality the diagnosis. Fifth-digit codes for Manic Episode (p. 218) and Major Depressive Episode (p. 223) include: 1 = mild, 2 = moderate, 3 = severe, 4 = with psychotic features, 5 = in partial remission, 6 = in full remission, and 0 = unspecified.

The diagnostically relevant period for disorders such as Cyclothymia and Seasonal Pattern of Major Depressive Episode encompasses 1 to 3 years. It is not expected that treatment will be delayed for such an interval while activity data are collected to first verify the correctness of the diagnosis. It is presumed that once the importance of behavioral measurements to accurate diagnosis is more widely appreciated, that activity measurements will become part of the basic medical record established through periodic visits for various reasons including prophylactic physical examinations to provide background information against which subsequent DSM-III-R related concerns can be better evaluated.

Bipolar Disorders

"The essential feature of Bipolar Disorders is the presence of one or more Manic or Hypomanic Episodes (usually with a history of Major Depressive Episodes)." (p. 214) Activity-related inclusion criteria for mania (pp. 217–218) specify "decreased need for sleep, e.g., feels rested after only three hours of sleep" and "increase in goal-directed activity . . . or psychomotor agitation." The two types of Bipolar Disorder are: 1) Bipolar Disorder and 2) Cyclothymia.

Bipolar Disorder

The essential feature of Bipolar Disorder is a history of one or more Manic Episodes (as defined above) plus one or more Depressive Episodes. A Hypomanic Episode is like a Manic Episode except that it is less severe, such that hospitalization is not required and delusions are never present.

Data presented in Chapter 6 indicate that actigraphy can easily document the presence of three hours of sleep. Increased activity can also be measured, though actigraphy cannot discern whether this increased activation is purposive or not.

Bipolar Disorders can be Manic (296.4x), Depressed (296.5x), or Mixed (296.6x). The inclusion criteria for Bipolar Disorder, Mixed (p. 226) specify that the "Current (or most recent) episode involves the full symptomatic picture of both Manic and Major Depressive Episodes (except for the duration requirement of two weeks for depressive symptoms) (pp. 217, 222), intermixed or rapidly alternating every few days" (p. 226), plus "Prominent depressive symptoms lasting at least a full day." (p. 226)

Actigraphy can document the presence of consistent activity excesses (mania) or deficits (depression) as well as estimate sleep efficiency in depressed persons (Reich, Kupfer, Weiss, McPartland, Foster, Detre, and Delgado, 1974). Actigraphy can also track the course of a Mixed disorder showing depression for a full day and cycles every few days.

McFarlain and Hersen's (1974) Patient 1 is a 54-year-old white male manic-depressive, circular type treated with a combination of lithium carbonate and thioridazine. Activity was measured at the right ankle with an actometer (modified 17-jewel calendar wrist watch) 24 hours each day. The device was read and reset each morning at 0815. Unfortunately, the activity units were reported in "arbitrary units." Nonetheless, their data show a substantial and systematic reduction in activity across 5 lithium carbonate–thioridazine combinations spread over 14 days.

Urinary MHPG. Urinary 3-methoxy-4-hydroxyphenyl-ethylene glycol (MHPG) is a major metabolite of brain norepinephrine (noradrenaline). Ebert, Post, and Goodwin (1972) examined the relationship between activity and MPHG depression to follow-up on previous reports that this metabolite is lower than control values for depressed persons, higher than in depressed or other patients in manic persons, and essentially normal during remission. Six patients on a NIMH metabolic ward served as subjects. Twelve-hour urinary excretion of MHPG was measured for three control and one exercise day. Eight to 12 hours of activity was obtained between 0700 and 1900. Baseline excretion was 0.96 mg/12 hours vs 1.96 mg/12 hours for the exercise day ($p < .01$ using a one-tail correlated t-test).

Wehr, Mucettola, and Goodwin (1980) based their research on two observations: 1) most physiological, biochemical, and behavioral processes follow circadian rhythms, and 2) the sleep of depressed subjects resembles that of normals when shifted several hours earlier (phase advanced) relative to their normal sleep period. Ten depressed bipolar subjects and 14 normal controls on different NIMH research wards served as subjects. Nondominant wrist activity was measured with a Colburn, Smith, Guarini and Simons (1976) actigraph (Ambulatory Monitoring Inc., Ardsley, NY prototype) using 15-minute epochs. Urine samples were collected every three hours over a 24-hour period on the two days such specimens were obtained.

A repeated measured ANOVA indicated a significant ($p < .001$) temporal variation of MHPG with time that accounted for 16% of total variance compared with a nonsignificant ($p < .10$) 8% effect between patients and controls. A cosine function [$f(t) = u + a \cos (\omega t + \phi)$, where u = mean, a = amplitude, ω = frequency = 1 cycle per day, and ϕ = phase-angle] was fitted, using a least squares criterion, to each subject's MHPG data and used to determine the time at which maximum (acrophase) excretion occurred. (The time of day that acrophase [peak activity] occurs estimates phase-angle.) These times were averaged (± SE mean) across subjects. MHPG excretion was maximal, on average, at 1838 ± 46 minutes for controls and at 1608 ± 31 minutes for depressed subjects ($p < .05$ vs controls) and at 1512 ± 64 minutes for manic subjects ($p < .02$ vs controls). This is a 2-hour

20-minute phase advance for depressed subjects and a 3-hour 26-minute phase advance for manic subjects. None of the manic vs depressed comparisons were significant. These data are consistent with the phase-advance hypothesis.

Fitted cosine functions to activity data revealed that peak activity occurred at 1547 ± 19 minutes for controls, 1510 ± 40 minutes for depressed subjects ($p < .05$ vs controls), and 1337 ± 29 minutes for manic subjects ($p < .001$ vs controls). This is a 37-minute phase advance for depressed subjects and a 2-hour 10-minute phase advance for manic subjects. None of the manic vs depressed comparisons were significant. Again, phase advance was observed. Activity was higher for manic patients than controls at all times of day. For the 8 patients observed during both manic and depressed phases, activity was always greater during the manic than during the depressive phase.

The authors mentioned two particularly interesting implications of their phase advance finding. First, lithium is known to be effective for manic-depressive disorder and it is one of a very few agents known to slow biological clocks. Hence, the therapeutic effects of lithium may be mediated through the biological clock (suprachiasmatic nucleus of the hypothalamus; cf. Moore, 1978). Second, failure of dexamethasone to completely suppress urinary free cortisol output may partly be due to a phase advance relative to midnight, when suppression is usually at a maximum. The Kripke, Mullaney, Atkinson, and Wolf (1978) study described below suggests that lithium prevents the dysynchronization of activity and temperature cycles through clock slowing. Perhaps influences that speed up the central clock introduce instability (dysynchronization).

An unstated implication of the above results is based upon the observation that both activity and MHPG were phase advanced. It is easier to obtain 24-hour activity data in the natural environment through actigraphy than to obtain quality MHPG data, which requires collecting urine every 3 hours for 12 hours and freezing the samples at $-20°C$. Activity phase advance is more conservative and therefore probably more clinically significant when it occurs. The availability of a large data set over as many days as desired increases statistical power and compensates for the smaller phase-advance effect size.

Matussek, Romisch, and Ackenheil (1977) measured MHPG excretion and ankle activity via pedometer in 14 endogenously depressed female patients 30 to 57 years of age ($M = 43.6$, $S = 8.4$ years) when 14 days free of neuroleptic medication, 5 days free of tricyclic antidepressants, and 4 weeks free of MAO inhibitors and lithium. Control subjects were 5 female laboratory assistants aged 34 to 54 years ($M = 43.2$, $S = 8.4$ years). The correlation between ankle activity and MHPG excretion was $r(12) = 0.1371$, N.S. The failure to find a significant relationship could be explained either by the low power due to a small sample size or to restricted range regarding either pedometer or MPHG values. The presence of $r(12) = -.7949$, $p < .005$ between MPHG excretion and self-ratings of depression suggests that any range-restriction problems are associated with pedometer data.

The absence of a mean and standard deviation for the pedometer precludes further analysis of this situation.

Circadian Rhythms. Wehr and Goodwin (1980) noted strong similarities between the rest–activity cycles of nine of ten rapidly cycling manic-depressive patients and normal subjects living in isolation from external temporal cues. When normal subjects are deprived of daily time cues (zeitgebers), their usual 24-hour sleep–wake and temperature cycles extend to approximately 25 hours. After several days or weeks, the activity cycle breaks away from the temperature cycle (they become desynchronized; also called uncoupling and internal desynchronization) and slows to a period of 40 or 50 hours per cycle during which the subject continuously stays awake without feeling drowsy. The temperature and activity cycles oscillate in and out of phase while the activity cycle attempts to catch up to the temperature cycle. This results in the superimposition of 25-hour temperature variation upon 40-50 hour rest–activity variation, which "beat" against each other.

This research reports that rapidly cycling manic-depressive patients show break-away desynchronization in the absence of environmental isolation; they seem to be naturally insulated from environmental cues. The onset of a manic period, in nine out of ten studied patients, corresponded to the break-away point where the patient remained awake more than 48 consecutive hours (1–4 nights) with no subjective sense of drowsiness.

Wehr, Wirz-Justice, Goodwin, Duncan, and Gillin (1979) tested the hypothesis that phase advance of the circadian sleep–wake cycle would function as an anti-depressant in four depressed manic-depressive patients. Continuous 24-hour wrist activity was monitored throughout the study. Treatment consisted of changing the usual sleep period from 2300–0700 to 1700–0100; moving the sleep period 6 hours earlier in time. One subject, a 57-year-old women experienced a complete remission of depression replaced by a normal to hypomanic condition lasting approximately 2 weeks prior to the return of her depressive symptoms. Durable treatment is not expected from a circadian phase change any more than jet lag produces permanent changes. The return of depressive symptoms strengthens the hypothesis that thera-peutic effects are mediated by changes in circadian phase relationships. A second phase advance produced another temporary clinical remission of depressive symp-toms. A third phase advance was performed just prior to predicted relapse but did not prevent the return of depressive symptoms. A fourth phase advance was unsuc-cessful in relieving depression. The authors explained this by a failure of her temperature cycle to advance this time as it had previously done during both the first and second sleep changes.

A 65-year-old unipolar man partially improved after a sleep phase advance. A 28-year-old bipolar I woman completely remitted after a phase advance. A 49-year-old bipolar II woman switched to hypomania after a sleep advance.

Kripke, Mullaney, Atkinson, and Wolf (1978) represent Halberg's (1968) two-oscillator-beat model of rapidly cycling manic depression. Oscillator A runs with 24-hour periodicity. Oscillator B runs somewhat faster. The B/A ratio becomes especially large and near zero every few days as the two oscillators go in and out of phase with each other. Kripke *et al.* (1978) obtained longitudinal hourly wrist activity (cf. Kripke, Mullaney, Messin, and Wyborney, 1978) and 3 to 6 times daily oral 5-minute body temperature from five male and two female patients with manic depression, circular type. The case-by-case results are too extensive to be presented here. The main finding was that evidence was found for a free-running oscillator in support of Halberg's (1968) beat-oscillation hypothesis.

Depression, Euthymia, and Mania. Weiss, Foster, Reynolds, and Kupfer (1974) obtained wrist activity from 3 manic patients (1 man aged 22 years; 2 women aged 50 and 60 years) who were continuously monitored 24 hours per day. All patients were maintained on a drug-free baseline for 2 weeks. During this time their daytime (0800 to 2300 hours) activity hovered about the 75 counts/min mark. Thereafter, activity steadily declined to a low of approximately 5 counts/min around 0400–0500 and then rose back to the 75 counts/min level by 0800.

The effects of lithium carbonate were investigated on the above 3 patients plus 3 bipolar depressives (1 man aged 50 years; 22 women aged 24 and 39 years). Despite 1500 mg of lithium carbonate daily resulting in serum levels of 0.9 to 1.2 mEq/liter during the second week of active treatment, no significant wrist activity changes resulted. Significant differences might have been obtained had waist activity been monitored, which is sensitive to ambulation. Wrist activity could have remained at the same level but have been more productive after vs before treatment.

Henninger and Kirstein (1977) studied the wrist activity of 15 Bipolar I and II and unipolar depressive male and female inpatients aged 25 to 67 years. Treatment with lithium carbonate ranged from 12 to 40 days with doses between 900 and 2100 mg/day resulting in serum lithium concentrations of from 0.71 to 1.69 mEq/liter. However, no significant activity changes were reported. This result replicates that reported by Weiss, Foster, Reynolds, and Kupfer (1974) reviewed above.

Weiss, Foster, Reynolds, and Kupfer's (1974) report results from a 5-month-long case study of a 22-year-old manic depressive patient who passed through all phases of her disorder. Most impressive was the sixfold activity increase during the night (0000–0700 hours) between her hypomanic and florid periods ($p < .001$). Lithium carbonate produced a 20% decrease in daytime (0700–2400 hours) activity.

McFarlain and Hersen's (1974) Patient 2 is a 44-year-old white male manic-depressive, depressed type. Family and financial matters appeared to precipitate his depression. During the first 3 baseline days, all hospital privileges were available to him. Then he was transferred to a token-economy program for 6 days where he earned points as a member of an Escort Service with which to purchase privileges. Three more days of baseline ensued followed by 4 more days of token economy.

Activity was measured at the right ankle with an actometer (modified 17-jewel calendar wrist watch) 24-hours each day. The device was read and reset each morning at 0815. Unfortunately, the activity units were reported in "arbitrary units." Nonetheless, the results indicated substantially greater activity during the token economy compared with baseline. This activity increase was due to his work-related responsibilities.

Kupfer, Weiss, Foster, Detre, Delgado, and McPartland (1974) examined wrist activity in seven unipolar depressives and four bipolar but currently depressed patients. Three weeks of pharmacotherapy (150 mg for unipolars and serum lithium level of 0.9 to 1.2 mEq/liter for bipolars) did not produce any significant activity increases. However, daytime activity (0700 to 2100 hrs) increased from a mean of 34.48 counts/min ($S = 4.31$) to a mean of 42.87 counts/min ($S = 7.54$) but this 24.3% activity increase was not significant with such a small sample size.

Prior to pharmacotherapy, the 7 unipolar patients were found to be significantly more active from 0700 to 1200 hours and from 2100 to 0700 hours than bipolar patients. While all patients increased activity during treatment, the bipolar patients increased enough more than the unipolar patients to make all differences between the two groups nonsignificant.

Foster, McPartland, and Kupfer (1978) obtained wrist activity counts on 7 severely depressed inpatients aged 19 to 33 years who had been maintained drug-free for 14 days and 7 age-matched controls. Significantly ($p < .05$) lower wrist activity counts were obtained from the depressed ($M = 357.8$ counts/day) than controls ($M = 562.8$ counts/day). Significantly less ($p < .001$) nighttime activity was reported for the depressed ($M = 7.4$) than control ($M = 26.5$) subjects. The percentage of activity occurring at night was significantly ($p < .01$) less for the depressed ($M = 2.2\%$) than control ($M = 5.1\%$) subjects. Significantly ($p < .05$) less 24-hour activity was recorded for the depressed ($M = 365.2$ counts/day) than control ($M = 589.8$ counts/day) subjects.

Post, Stoddard, Gillin, Buchsbaum, Runkle, Black and Bunney (1977) obtained wrist activity data on a rapidly cycling manic depressive woman over approximately 110 days of hospitalization. They reported that 24-hour activity increases significantly ($p < .001$) predicted the patient's switch into stage I mania (hypomania) and subsequent 24-hour activity decreases significantly ($p < .001$) predicted the patient's switch back to depression. More pronounced activity changes could well occur if a more severe manic condition existed.

Wehr and Goodwin (1979) studied tricyclic antidepressant-induced rapid cycling between mania and depression in five female bipolar patients under two no tricyclic and two tricyclic medication conditions. The mean manic-depressive cycle off tricyclic medication was 127 days ($S = 50$ days). Tricyclic medication significantly ($p < .001$) reduced this period to an average of 33 days ($S = 14$ days). Case-by-case presentations of 24-hour activity records clearly indicates substantial differences in activity among manic, euthymic, and depressed clinical states in all 5 patients.

Wolff, Putnam, and Post (1985) studied activity in 5 unipolar subjects aged 20 to 35 years (mean = 27.6, S = 5.7 years), 25 bipolar subjects aged 22 to 69 years (mean = 42.1, S = 12.9 years), and 18 normal volunteer control subjects aged 19 to 57 years (mean = 23.6, S = 9.0 years) in an inpatient setting. He obtained 24-hour nondominant wrist activity data with a Colburn, Smith, Guarini and Simons (1976) actigraph (Ambulatory Monitoring Inc., Ardsley, NY prototype) using 15-minute epochs. Each persons activity profile was based on a minimum of three days. The average number of days per profile was 24, S = 16 days. Profiles were collected representing depressed, euthymic, and manic states, each patient being used as his or her own control.

The 24-hour activity counts by time distribution displayed the same shape in the depressed, euthymic, and manic conditions but differed in activity level with depressed being lowest, euthymic in the middle, and manic being the most active. Activity ranged from approximately 175 to 260 counts per 15 minutes at 0700 to a high of approximately 325 to 385 at 1300 then gradually tapering off to a low of 25 to 50 counts per 15 minutes during the night back to the 175 to 260 range by 0700 the next morning.

In 23 patients the average 24-hour total activity during depression was found to be significantly less (mean difference = 665 counts/15 min) than during euthymia (p < .0003). This effect was entirely due to daytime differences (mean = 602 counts/15 min) between 0700 and 2200 hours (p < .0001) as no significant differences (mean = 63 counts/15 min) were found regarding nighttime activity (2200 to 0700 hours). In 9 patients, 24-hour total activity was found to be significantly (p < .02) greater (mean difference = 1599 counts/15 min) during mania than depression (p < .02). This difference holds both during the day (mean difference = 1226 counts/15 min; p < .05) and during the night (mean difference = 373 counts/15 min; p < .003). However, no significant differences were found between mania and euthymia in the 11 subjects where such comparisons could be made. Differences of 643 counts/15 minutes for 24-hour activity, 417 counts/15 minutes for daytime activity (0700–2200), and 226 counts/15 minutes for nighttime activity (2200–0700) activity were all in the predicted direction but not significant.

The average 24-hour activity profiles of 30 euthymic affective disorder subjects was significantly less than the activity of 18 normal control subjects during 12 of the 24 hourly periods. Most of the differences were located between 1400 and 2400 hours. In all 48 subjects, age was negatively correlated with 24-hour activity ($r(46)$ = −.33, p < .02), and nighttime activity ($r(46)$ = −.39, p < .007) but not daytime activity ($r(46)$ = −.27, N.S.). This latter correlation would have been significant (p < .05) given N = 54; just 6 more subjects. Apparently this relationship is significant only for women ($r(19)$ = −.59, p < .006).

Cyclothymia (Bipolar II)

The essential feature of Cyclothymia (301.13) is one of repeated mood swings that qualify for Hypomanic, but not Manic, Episodes and fail to qualify as Major Depressive Episodes over a period of at least two years for adults; one year for children and adolescents. There cannot be a symptom-free period of longer than two months.

The demanding criteria of demonstrating systematic activity swings over a two-year period without more than two months in between "up" and "down" phases can best be done through instrumentation. The emphasis placed on intermediate level of severity also is best evaluated though instrumented measurement (actigraphy).

Foster, McPartland, and Kupfer (1976) reported a case study of a 29-year-old woman with severe cyclothymia. Her 63-day premedication baseline yielded an average of 1245 wrist activity counts per day ($S = 324$). Treatment with lithium and tranylcypromine reduced her activity to an average of 429 counts per day ($S = 149$) over the next 56 days.

Depressive Disorders

Depressive Disorders are divided into Major Depression and Dysthymia.

Major Depression

Inclusion criteria for Major Depressive Episode (pp. 222–224) specify "insomnia or hypersomnia nearly every day," "psychomotor agitation or retardation nearly every day (observable by others, not merely subjective feelings of restlessness or being slowed down)." (p. 222) These symptoms must occur "for most of the day, nearly every day, during at least a two-week period" (pp. 218–219). A further distinction is made between Major Depression, Single Episode (296.2x) or Major Depression, Recurrent (296.3x).

Chapter 6 reviews research indicating that actigraphy can consistently identify sleep–wake periods. Therefore, actigraphy can be used to evaluate complaints of insomnia for the indicated two-week period. Such data could be collected at the person's home prior to admission.

Psychomotor agitation and retardation are perhaps best considered against the person's prior behavior when healthy. For this reason it is desirable to obtain activity baselines as part of regular physical examinations. In cases where activity is extremely and consistently elevated or depressed, data from age- and sex-matched general medical and surgical patients plus hospital or clinic staff may be sufficient to demonstrate abnormality. The ability to review actigraphic data according to the time of its occurrence makes it possible to determine if the necessary daily consistency is present.

Inclusion criteria for the Melancholic type specify "depression regularly worse in the morning" and "early morning awakening (at least two hours before usual time of awakening)," and "psychomotor retardation or agitation (not merely subjective complaints)." (p. 224) Actigraphy can assist with the diagnosis of Melancholic type because it can document the presence of early morning awakening (cf. Chapter 6) as well as whether less activity occurs in the morning hours; i.e., psychomotor retardation is worse.

Seasonal Pattern is another subtype of Mood Disorders that is also referred to as Seasonal Affective Disorder (SAD). Inclusion criteria (p. 224) specify depression onset between the beginning of October and the end of November and offset between mid-February to mid-April. This seasonal pattern must exist for three years, two of which must be consecutive. Actigraphy is useful in documenting the preseasonal activity level and how it is disrupted near the beginning of October through the end of November and normalized between mid-February and mid-April.

Inpatient Studies. Kupfer and Foster (1973) obtained longitudinal EEG and 24-hour nondominant wrist activity (using the Kupfer *et al.*, 1972, device) on a 54-year-old black female suffering from psychotic depression. Her recovery after treatment with amitryptyline was associated with spending more than 37.5 hours sleeping. Periods of insomnia were associated with activity increases whereas periods of hypersomnia were associated with activity decreases.

Foster and Kupfer (1975) report longitudinal nocturnal EEG and 24-hour nondominant wrist activity (using the Kupfer *et al.*, 1972, device) on 33 hospitalized patients (11 women, 6 men) of mean age = 47.5, $S = 2$ years. Subsamples included 12 unipolar, 5 bipolar, and 16 Acute Cognitive Disorganization (ACD). Results indicated that depressed subjects ($n = 17$) were significantly ($p < .01$) more active at night (0000–0700) than were the ACD ($n = 16$) subjects. Depressed subjects displayed a significantly ($p < .001$) larger percentage (8.3%) of their 24-hr activity at night (0000–0700) than did the ACD subjects (4.5%). This difference was explained as the result of "a fundamental change in the phasing of psychomotor rhythms" (p. 930) rather than as a primary sleep disorder.

A curious aside is the significant ($r = .54$, $p < .05$) correlation between clinician ratings of anxiety and 24-hr wrist activity measurements in the ACD patients.

Benoit, Royant-Parola, Borbely, Tobler, and Widlocher (1985) obtained longitudinal (hospitalization ranged from 15 to 71 days; mean = 34 days) nondominant wrist activity measurements in 10 female patients diagnosed as major unipolar depressives by DSM-III. Their ages ranged from 40–68 years (mean = 53.2 years). The activity instrument was a small (30 × 51 × 17 mm) lightweight (87 g) accelerometer-based device sensitive to 0.1 g. Data were collected using 15-minute epochs. Results indicated significant ($t(8) = 5.4$, $p < .001$) reductions in Hamilton (1967) ratings of from $M = 20.7$, $S = 6.5$ upon admission to $M = 6.5$, $S = 5.2$

upon discharge. Significant ($t(8) = 3.54$, $p < .01$) 24-hour activity increases from $M = 40.3$, $S = 12.4$ counts upon admission to $M = 63.0$, $S = 12.3$ upon discharge. Periods of immobility (no activity for 15 minutes) significantly ($t(8) = 3.0$, $p < .02$) decreased during the day from $M = 21.7$, $S = 10.8$ upon admission to $M = 12.0$, $S = 6.8$ upon discharge. Immobility also significantly ($t(8) = 6.1$, $p < .001$) decreased during the night (0000–0600) from $M = 10.9$, $S = 4.4$ on admission to $M = 6.3$, $S = 2.9$ upon discharge. Patients considered to be endogenously depressed showed more immobility than did patients thought not to be endogenously depressed. The authors concluded that "Immobility appeared as a sensitive indicator of the intensity of this depressive state. With partial improvement, immobility first decreased at night, then when improvement was completed, diurnal occurrences of immobility also disappeared." (p. 590)

Godfrey and Knight (1984) placed actometers (modified Swiss Olympic model 10768 wrist watches) on the dominant wrist of 5 major depressive and 4 hypomanic patients between 0800 and 0900 every morning and took them off 12 hours later and recorded the day's activity. This routine was followed every day of hospitalization, which ranged from 7 to 27 days (average = 15.2 days) for the depressed patients and 8 to 15 days (average = 10.5 days) for the hypomanic patients. College-student control subjects were used but will not be reported here because though matched for age and sex, they did not live on the ward and therefore their activity scores are not at all comparable to those of the other two groups of subjects. The dependent variable appears to be Activity Units (AU = minutes of apparent elapsed time) per 12 hours.

Analysis of variance revealed a significant increase in activity for the 5 depressed patients from a pretreatment average of 273.60 AU to a posttreatment average of 540.9 AU ($F(1,8) = 11.84$, $p < .01$). However, the decrease from a pretreatment average of 387.50 AU to a posttreatment average of 237.62 AU for the hypomanic 4 patients was not significant ($F(1,6) = 2.16$, N.S.). Several qualifying comments are relevant. First, the very small sample of hypomanic patients causes this analysis to have extremely low power and therefore very likely to overlook positive results. It took an enormous improvement by the depressed subjects to reach significance. Second, the posttreatment hypomanic mean is substantially below the depressive pretreatment mean. Could it be that the "cure" for hypomania was to induce depression greater than what depressed subjects were initially treated for? It seems unlikely that one could expect the hypomanic posttreatment mean to decrease further. Hence, further effect size increases must come from more elevated hypomanic pretreatment means, which seems quite likely given these data. Notice that the hypomanic pretreatment mean is *below* the posttreatment depressive mean. Hence, these "hypomanic" patients do not seem to evidence much by way of activity excess. A covariance analysis controlling for State Trait Anxiety Inventory scores did not change the above-mentioned result pattern.

Teicher, Lawrence, Barber, Finklestein, Lieberman, and Baldessarini (1988) used time-based actigraphy (early version of current Motionlogger™; Ambulatory Monitoring Inc., Ardsley, NY) to monitor activity of 2 men and 6 women aged 69 to 80 years (M = 75.0 years, S = 4.2 years) during their third and seventh days of hospitalization for unipolar depression. Activity was monitored from the nondominant wrist using 15-minute epochs for 48 to 64 continuous hours. Eight healthy volunteers (4 men, 4 women) living on a similar ward served as control subjects. The results indicated that the depressed subjects (M = 370, S = 77 counts) were significantly ($F(1,90)$ = 18.18, $p < .001$) *more* active than the control subjects (M = 286, S = 27 counts). This result was found during both the day and night. Diurnal activity in depressed subjects (M = 129, S = 26 counts) was significantly ($t(14)$ = 3.06, $p < .02$) greater than that of controls (M = 97, S = 13 counts). Nocturnal activity for depressed subjects (M = 21, S = 10 counts) was also significantly ($t(14)$ = 3.28, $p < .02$) larger than for controls (M = 9, S = 2 counts). Circadian acrophase, point of greatest activity, occurred significantly ($t(14)$ = 4.67, $p < .001$) later at an average of 1554 hours (S = 67 min) for depressed subjects versus at 1351 hours (S = 28 minutes) for control subjects.

These data indicate that depressed geriatric patients are agitated. Clinical observation indicates the presence of much pacing and purposeless handwringing. The approximately 29% activity excess observed here is close to the 28% activity excess found for hyperactive boys [cf. Porrino *et al.* (1983a,b)]. Bipolar depressed patients have lower than normal activity. These geriatric patients were phase delayed rather than phase advanced as would have otherwise been expected.

Woggon, Angst, Curtius, Niederwieser, Levine, Borbely and Tobler (1985) reported positive treatment effects associated with tetrahydrobiopterin (BH₄) in three therapy-resistant endogenous depressed patients was easily discernible using a solid-state wrist-worn activity monitor. No activity data were presented.

Outpatient Studies. The above studies were all conducted within the confines of a hospital setting using inpatients. The Futterman and Tryon (1985) study was designed to determine if behavioral evidence of depression could be found in an outpatient sample at a Community Mental Health Center. They studied 11 depressed, Major Depressive Episode, outpatient women aged 20 to 40 years plus 10 age-matched normal control subjects. All subjects took the Beck Depression Inventory (BDI) to both confirm that the patients were depressed and to document that the control subjects were not depressed. All subjects wore actometers on their dominant wrist, in order not to underestimate their activity level, upon getting out of bed in the morning until going to bed in the evening for two consecutive weeks because DSM-III-R specifies this length of time. They recorded the time of day that the actometers were put on and taken off. Data were expressed in terms of activity units per minute (AU/min). The results indicated that the depressed group was significantly less active during the day than was the control group ($F(1,19)$ = 9.53, $p < .01$). However, nighttime activity was not found to be significantly greater in depressed than control subjects ($F(1,19)$ = 1.74, N.S) despite the fact that the means were in the expected direction. A larger sample size may well produce significant nighttime results. Analyzing 24-hour activity again found depressed subjects to be significantly less active than control subjects ($F(1,19)$ = 9.25, $p <$ .01).

Creatine Phosphokinase. Meltzer (1969a,b) and Meltzer, Elkun, and Moline (1969) have demonstrated that elevated serum levels of the skeletal muscle isozyme creatine phosphokinase (CPK) are an index of acute psychotic disturbance. Approximately 50 times normal CPK is found in 70% of the patients. Meltzer and Moline (1970) reported that 25% of the first-degree relatives of patients show exaggerated increases in CPK in response to exercise. The purpose of the present study was to investigate the extent to which ambulatory activity could account for CPK elevations. Twice-weekly CPK and 24-hour nondominant wrist activity measures (using the Kupfer *et al.* 1972 device) on 23 (15 women, 8 men) consecutive admissions to a research ward (average age = 40.4 years) were obtained. At least 7 CPK values were available for all subjects. Degrees of freedom associated with reported correlation coefficients indicates that repeated measurements for all 23 patients were pooled. The correlation of preceding 24-hour activity (mean counts per minute) correlated $r(282)$ = .14, $p < .05$ with CPK (IU/ml). Dividing the day into three periods, we find a nonsignificant relationship between the preceding day-time (0700–2100) activity and CPK ($r(304)$ = .04, N.S.), but significant relationships between the preceding evening (2100–2400) activity and CPK ($r(302)$ = .25, $p <$ .001) and between preceding nocturnal (0000–0700) activity and CPK ($r(302)$ = .27, $p < .001$). The authors conclude that "in addition to sex, race, age, and muscle mass, motor activity during the preceding evening and night is probably a major determinant of base line serum CPK activity levels." (p. 756) The strong implication is that future investigators should obtain activity measures when conducting research on serum CPK and statistically control for activity variation in their CPK analyses.

Foster and Kupfer (1973) examined the relationship between serum creatine phosphokinase and motor activity in 23 consecutive inpatients (15 women, 8 men) aged 40.4 years, on average, and having a wide variety of diagnoses. Most patients had some form of affective disorder. Wrist activity counts were obtained continuously from admission to discharge. Activity counts were summed over daytime (0700–2100), evening (2100–2400), and night (0000–0700) as well as over all 24 hours. CPK measurements were obtained within 48 hours of admission, again during the first 7 days, and then 2–3 times per week thereafter. A significant positive correlation of $r(282)$ = .14, $p < .05$ was reported between the preceding 24-hour activity and CPK measurement. Another significant positive correlation of $r(302)$ = .27, $p < .001$ was obtained between preceding nocturnal activity and CPK.

Goode, Meltzer, Moretti, Kupfer and McPartland (1979) reviewed literature establishing a rise in serum creatine phosphokinase (CPK) in psychotic patients, especially during the early acute phase. Because CPK is elevated in normals by strenuous activity and because activity appears elevated during acute psychotic episodes, these authors obtained daily blood samples and 24-hour nondominant wrist activity (using the Kupfer et al. 1972 device) data for 4 to 12 days from 10 patients selected from a larger group of 30 hospitalized psychiatric patients (15 with schizophrenia, 8 with affective psychosis, 3 with schizo-affective psychoses, 2 with unspecified psychosis, and 2 with psychosis secondary to drug abuse). Only 4 of 10 daytime activity CPK correlations were significant. They ranged from $r(4) = -.56$, N.S. to $r(7) = .750, p < .05$. The same number of nighttime activity CPK correlations were significant and they ranged from $r(2) = -.61$, N.S., to $r(2) = .642$, N.S. For only 1 subject were the day- ($r(2) = .975, p < .05$) and nighttime ($r(2) = .998, p < .05$) correlations both significant. The extremely low statistical power, due to small sample size, associated with these results precludes firm negative conclusions.

Meltzer and Holy (1974) reported significant sex and race correlations with serum CPK with black males highest and white females lowest. Analysis of the same black/white and male/female 4-group design revealed significant ($F(3,29) = 3.558, p < .05$) differences but a different group order (Black males: $M = 340.6, S = 140.1, n = 9$; White females: $M = 393.8, S = 88.3, n = 5$; Black females: $M = 271.1, S = 138.1, n = 6$; White males: $M = 270.8, S = 146.3, n = 10$). Categorizing the present subjects into high vs low activity did not yield significant CPK differences ($F(1,28) = 1.164$, N.S.). The authors indicated that they did not place activity sensors on the most agitated patients for fear of damaging the device yet acknowledged that these are the very patients who would be expected to show the predicted relationship. They essentially argue that their correlations have been truncated due to activity range restriction.

Biogenic Amines. Detre and Jarecki (1971) recommended that motor activity be monitored for depressed persons. Van Praag and Korf (1971) suggested that levels of homovanillic acid (HVA) in cerebrospinal fluid (CSF) may differentiate retarded from nonretarded depressions. Both Post, Kotin, Goodwin, and Gordon (1973) and Ebert, Post, and Goodwin (1972) reported an increase in this biogenic amine in urine and CSF after increased activity or simulated manic behavior in depressed subjects. Weiss, Kupfer, Foster, and Delgado (1974) sought to further investigate the relationship of biogenic amines and activity in 11 patients (7 females, 4 males) aged 25 to 60 years (mean = 48.4 years) who were hospitalized for various depressive disorders. The authors reported correlations of $-.48, .39, -.43$, and $-.44$ between HVA and activity between the hours of 0700–0900, 0900–1200, 1200–1900, and 24 hours respectively. These data raise the *possibility* of a HVA decrease, followed by an increase, followed by a further decrease as qualified below. The correlations for 5-HIAA (5-hydroxyindoleacetic acid) over these same four time periods was 0.20, 0.34, $-.28$, and .13 respectively. HVA/HIAA ratios produced the following correlations with activity over the same time intervals: 0.38, 0.20, $-.13$, and 0.29 respectively.

The rationale for cautiously interpreting large correlations found in small samples was presented in Chapter 1. In short, while correlations are inflated by chance in small samples, true relationships are not. Hence, chance results equal or exceed large real relationships in small samples. Increasing sample size causes chance correlations to decrease but legitimate relationship measures to remain constant. One must always consider the possibility that large correlations obtained from small samples will be preserved in larger samples. The problem is uncertainty. One can neither assert that a real relationship exists or entirely dismiss the possibility of a true relationship on the basis of *large* correlations in small samples.

Post, Kotin, Goodwin, and Gordon (1973) reasoned that differences in activity level could help explain why some investigators have found significantly lower CSF 5-HIAA levels in depressed patients than in neurological controls whereas other researchers have not. A baseline lumbar puncture was taken in 7 moderately depressed patients at 0500. Then subjects simulated the complete manic mood, including motoric and verbal manic behavior, for four hours, and another puncture was taken at 0900. All subjects had previously observed manic behavior and therefore knew how to behave. Two other patients mimicked only manic physical activity.

The results indicated that all patients showed substantial increases in CSF values. Activity produced a 45% ($p < .01$) increase in 5-HIAA from 29.2 to 42.2 ng/ml and a 150% ($p < .01$) increase in HVA from 16.9 to 42.1 ng/ml. The 90% increase in MHPG was nearly significant only because of marked reversal in 1 patient. Patients simulating only activity increased as much as patients who simulated the entire manic mood thereby demonstrating the importance of activity measurements to this line of research.

Dysthymia

The activity related inclusion criteria for Dysthymia (300.40) specify "insomnia or hypersomnia" and "low energy or fatigue." Symptoms must persist for at least two years for adults and one year for children and adolescents (p. 230). No symptom-free period must last for more than two months (p. 230).

Diagnosing Cyclothymia presents a formidable challenge to behavioral assessment in that it requires from one to two years of data. Longitudinal behavioral measurement is highly relevant to such an undertaking, for it will provide the necessary documentation that cycles exist and that symptom-free periods do not last longer than two months.

Subtypes of Endogenous Depression

Science is usually portrayed in terms of the hypothetico-deductive approach where a carefully constructed theoretical prediction is put to empirical test. Theory is presumably revised on the basis of observation and modified predictions are once again submitted to empirical test. This view subordinates measurement to theory and ignores the issue of where theoretical conjecture originates from experience. A more balanced account of the creative process, called science, gives method at least an equal footing with theory. The history of science reveals that sometimes important fundamental theoretical advances result primarily because of measurement issues.

Prior to Laennec, disease was thought to result from imbalances in bodily fluids called humors, and the diagnostic role of the physician was limited to interviewing the patient about his or her symptoms. Sounds heard through the first stethoscope (Reiser, 1979) correlated with postmortem examination set the occasion for Laennec to propose an anatomical theory of disease based upon physical examination of the patient. Subsequently, a broad array of physical/chemical analyses of physical specimens collected from diseased and normal patients allowed for *Clinical Diagnosis by Laboratory Methods*; the name of a medical text by Davidsohn and Henry (1974). The advent of various imaging technologies (e.g., CAT, NMR, PET scans, computerized EEG) has provided a rich basis for theoretical development. Actigraphy may well provide the necessary measurements about behavior to also facilitate new theoretical developments. Lawrence, Teicher, and Finklestein (1989) indicate that the computer may be to activity measurements what the microscope is to specimens where methods of time series analysis, like biological stains, highlight particular structures; dynamic configurations in the case of activity.

Evidence of the theoretical value of activity measurements is exemplified by Teicher, Barber, Lawrence, and Baldessarini's (1989) proposal to diagnose subtypes of endogenous depression into two categories: Agitated and Retarded, as illustrated in Table 3.1.

The first defining characteristic is that activity is increased over normal in agitated depression and decreased below normal in retarded depression. Sleep decreases in agitated depression and increases in retarded depression. Appetite and weight are similarly affected except that they can decrease in retarded depression if severe enough or if associated with high stress. Agitated depression includes what is now called unipolar depression. Retarded depression includes what is now called Bipolar I or II, Seasonal Affective Disorder, and Pseudounipolar Depression. Agitated depression usually onsets after age 40 whereas retarded depression usually begins before age 30. A family history of Involutional Melancholia is sometimes present in agitated depression and usually present in retarded depression. The preferred pharmacologic treatment of agitated treatment includes sedating antidepres-

TABLE 3.1. Agitated and Retarded Subtypes of Endogenous Depression[a]

Features	Clinical clusters	
	Agitated	Retarded
Locomotor activity	Increased	Decreased
Sleep	Decreased	Increased
Appetite–weight	Decreased	Increased (can be decreased if depression is very severe or associated with high stress)
Clinical polarity disorder	Unipolar (can be confused with dysphoric mania)	Bipolar (Bipolar I or II, Seasonal Affective Pseudounipolar depression)
Onset age	Older (> 40) (Involutional melancholia)	Younger (< 30)
Family affective history	Sometimes	Usual
Preferred treatments	Sedating antidepressants amitriptyline imipramine doxepin trazodone amoxapine	Stimulating antidepressants nortriptyline desipramine protriptyline tranylcypromine
Additional treatments	Neuroleptics added	Lithium salts, anticonvulsants; stimulants sometimes used

[a]Reprinted from Teicher, Barber, Lawrence, and Baldessarini (1989).

sants such as amitriptyline, imipramine, doxepin, trazodone, and amoxapine. Neuroleptics may also be added. The preferred pharmacologic treatment of retarded depression includes stimulating antidepressants such as nortriptyline, desipramine, protriptyline, tranylcypromine. Lithium salts, anticonvulsants, and other stimulants may occasionally be used.

Circadian distribution of activity is a property common to animals and man. This point of equivalence allows one to explore animal models of depression in terms of disturbed rest–activity cycles and normalizing treatments (cf. Barber, Teicher, and Baldessarini, 1989; Teicher, Barber, Baldessarini, and Shaywitz, 1988). Of special interest is the similar behavioral effect of amphetamine withdrawal and cocaine withdrawal in animals and humans and likeness to bipolar patients with retarded depression discussed by Teicher, Barber, Lawrence and Baldessarini (1989).

DSM-III-R Schizophrenic Disorders

The diagnostic criteria for Schizophrenia are presented on pages 194–195 of DSM-III-R, including the following "fifth-digit" extensions: 1 = Subchronic, 2 = Chronic, 3 = Subchronic with Acute Exacerbation, 4 = Chronic with Acute Exacerbation, 5 = In Remission, 0 = Unspecified. The principle activity-related symptom of schizophrenia is "catatonic behavior." (p. 194)

Catatonic Type

The inclusion criterion of catatonic stupor is defined as "marked decrease in reactivity to the environment and/or reduction in spontaneous movements and activity." (p. 196) The inclusion criterion of catatonic excitement is defined as "excited motor activity, apparently purposeless and not influenced by external stimuli." (p. 196)

Actigraphy can document the reduction of spontaneous movements and activity and even reactivity to the environment in Catatonic Type (295.2x) if one also knew the time at which activating stimuli were present. Time-based actigraphy could be used to compare the person's activity during times activating stimuli were present with when they were absent.

Differential diagnosis concerns exclusion criteria for the following disorders which require that catatonia *not* be present: Disorganized Type (295.1x), Paranoid Type (295.3x), and Undifferentiated Type (295.9x).

Schizophrenia

Perris and Rapp (1974) used 100,000 capacity step counters (they called them pedometers) to examine the effects of fluspirilene in 10 randomly chosen chronic schizophrenic inpatients. Mean steps taken during 7 baseline days of normal drug treatment was 9,079.985. This value increased significantly ($p < .01$) to 9,746.185 during the next week when normal chemotherapy was withdrawn thereby indicating either that schizophrenia is associated with increased activity or that medication withdrawal produces an activity increase. Administration of Fluspirilene produced a weekly average of 9,089.8 steps which was not significantly different from baseline. However, their Figure 1 indicates substantial activity reduction on Day 1 compared to the other two conditions followed by a strong linear increase. By Day 7 fluspirilene resulted in slightly more activity than was seen on Day 7 of drug removal.

ACTIVITY THERAPY

Depression often accompanies post-myocardial infarction. Naughton, Bruhn, and Lategola (1968), Kavanaugh, Shephard, Tuck, and Qureshi (1977), Stern and Cleary (1982), and Stern, Gorman, and Kaslow (1983) have reported that exercise may help to alleviate such reactive depression.

Treatments that work when depression is secondary to another medical problem may not work when depression is the primary disorder. Simons, McGowan, Epstein, Kupfer, and Robertson (1985) reviewed seven studies treating depressed patients with multiple exercise sessions using at least a quasi-experimental design. The results of their review indicate that all studies significantly reduced depression through exercise.

Johnsgard (1989) discusses what he calls "the exercise prescription for depression and anxiety." In Chapter 6 (pp. 119–150), Johnsgard reviews research on the antidepressive effects of activity. Brown (1987) divided 600 undergraduates into depressed and nondepressed groups. Some students in each group elected to remain sedentary, others elected to exercise three times per week, and the rest elected to exercise five times per week. The results showed no change in depression for subjects electing to remain sedentary but significant reductions in depression for subjects exercising five times per week. The lack of random assignment to groups obviously limits causal conclusions. However, either exercise or willingness to participate in exercise seems implicated in depression reduction.

Berger and Owen (1983) reported significant mood changes following 40 minutes of swimming versus no significant changes following 50 minutes of lecture.

Sime (1987) conducted a within-subject study on 15 moderately depressed men and women aged 26 to 53 years. Depression was assessed before and after a two-week baseline period during which time they met for the purpose of nonaerobic calisthenics and stretching exercises. They then participated in a gradually more demanding walk-run program for the next 10 weeks during which three subjects dropped out. However, depression scores for the remaining 12 subjects were significantly reduced and remained so at a 6- and 21-month follow-up.

Greist, Klein, Eischens, and Faris (1978) randomly assigned University Counseling Center clients to one of three groups: 1) running therapy, 2) time-limited (12 weeks) psychotherapy, or 3) time-unlimited psychotherapy. The results indicated that 10 weeks of 30 to 40 minutes of running three times per week had approximately the same effect as 12 weeks of either type of psychotherapy. Greist, Klein, Eischens, and Faris (1979) reported successfully treating 24 of 30 psychiatric referrals for depression with running. Of the 6 nonresponders, 4 never became runners.

Klein, Greist, Gurman, Neimeyer, Lesser, Bushnell, and Smith (1985) randomly assigned 60 carefully selected depressed persons to one of three groups:

1) twice weekly 45-minute walk-jog sessions preceded and followed by stretching plus warming up/down, 2) cognitive-interpersonal psychotherapy, and 3) meditation-relaxation therapy. Completing rates over 12-weeks were 56%, 67%, and 48% for groups 1–3 respectively. All three groups showed significant reductions in depression by the end of treatment. These data show that exercise therapy is as effective as more traditional psychological treatment.

McCann and Homes (1984) selected 43 mildly depressed women from 250 university students and randomly assigned them to one of three 10-week treatments: 1) aerobic dance, jogging, and running for 1 hour twice a week, 2) 5 minutes of walking followed by relaxation exercises, and 3) wait list. All subjects were given the cover story that this was a study of stress management rather than depression reduction. Subjects were initially matched regarding depression and expectation of benefit. All subjects showed significant depression decreases between selection and beginning of treatment indicating the uniform presence of placebo effect. By the fifth week, significantly greater depression reduction occurred in the aerobic than walk-relax group and even larger differences occurred by the tenth week.

Martinsen (1987) treated 49 patients aged 17 to 60 years currently experiencing a major depressive episode. Thirty-three patients were symptomatic for at least the previous 6 months. The average number of prior depressive episodes was 8. All subjects received individual psychotherapy and occupational therapy, and some of them were on antidepressant medication. Half of the subjects were randomly chosen to also undergo a 9-week exercise program including walking, jogging, bicycling, skiing, and swimming at 50 to 70% of their aerobic capacity for 1 hour three times per week. As a result of random assignment, 38% of the subjects in the exercise group and 73% of the control subjects were on antidepressant medication. This bias favored the control group. However, the results indicated significantly lower depression scores for the patients who exercised than for those who did not.

Kupfer, Sewitch, Epstein, Bulik, McGowen, and Robertson (1985) investigated the extent to which no exercise, regular exercise, and double exercise influenced the mood of 10 young males aged 22 to 27 years ($M = 24.8$, $S = 2.0$) scoring in the good to excellent to superior range of aerobic fitness due to jogging 2.5 to 4 miles per day, 5 days per week for the past 3–6 months. Large-scale integrated sensor (LSI) activity measurements taken from the nondominant hip confirmed the no exercise, regular exercise, and double exercise conditions. No changes were seen on the KDS-1 or KDS-2 (cf. Kupfer and Detre, 1971) self-rating scales concerning depression, mania, anxiety, cognitive disorganization, and organicity. Perhaps these very active subjects were already maximally benefitting from exercise, and a brief period of under- and over-activity was insufficient to influence their mental health.

Actigraphy can be used to monitor exercise participation and thereby document the extent to which exercise recommendations are carried out. Time-based systems can further document when exercise began and ended, and some (cf. Actillume™

Ambulatory Monitoring Inc. Ardsley, NY) can even evaluate the intensity of exercise. Hence, information regarding the frequency, intensity, and duration of exercise can now be unobtrusively monitored while the subject behaves in his or her natural environment.

If exercise can reduce depression, it follows that more active persons should be less depressed than less active persons. It would therefore be informative to correlate depression scores and one- or two-week activity measurements.

DEPRESSION IN CHILDREN AND ADOLESCENTS

Teicher, Glod, Harper, Magnus, Brasher, Pahlavan, and Wren (1989) obtained 72 hours of nondominant wrist activity data from 41 inpatient children/adolescents aged 5 to 15 years ($M = 11.4$, $SEM = 0.48$ years) and 9 normal controls (5 male; 4 female) aged an average of 11.8 years ($SEM = 1.3$). Twenty-nine of the 41 children (15 male; 14 female) were diagnosed as having definite depression, possible depression, or nonaffective illness such as ADHD, conduct disorder, or oppositional disorder without evidence of a concurrent affective disorder.

The results were that patients with definite depression were approximately 14% less active than normal controls whereas nonaffective disordered children were 24% more active than controls ($F(3,34) = 3.68$, $p < .05$). The amplitude of the circadian rhythm, corrected for differences in average activity, were approximately 15% below controls in patients with definite or possible depression whereas the affectively ill patients were normal in this regard ($F(3,34) = 9.76$, $p < .001$). The amplitude of the hemicircadian rhythm (half day) was 50% greater than controls in patients with definite and possible depression but equal to controls in non-affective disordered children ($F(3,34) = 8.63$, $p < .001$). Dividing the amplitude of the hemicircadian rhythm by the amplitude of the circadian rhythm allowed nearly complete discrimination between normal controls plus nonaffective disorders versus definite and possible depression.

Activity and Hyperactivity–Attention Deficit Disorder

Activity level is consistently featured as a primary component of infant and child temperament (Buss and Plomin, 1975, 1984; Hubert, Wachs, Peters-Martin, and Gandour, 1982; Thomas and Chess, 1977). Consequently, disorders of childhood often impact activity level. Hyperactivity is among the most common behavior disorders in childhood and has become widely studied (Barkley, 1981; Winchell, 1981; Conners, 1986).

Controversy exists over whether hyperactivity exists as a separate factor from conduct disorder. Lahey, Green, and Forehand (1980) argued that hyperactivity does not exist as a distinct disorder. Achenbach and Edelbrock (1978) reported that hyperactivity has been reported as a distinct narrow band spectrum in 12 studies and that it pertains equally well to girls and boys. Achenbach (1980) further supports this view. Loney, Langhorne, and Paternite (1978) reported oblique factors for Aggression and Hyperactivity ($r = .27$) indicating that it is both feasible and desirable to distinguish between these two factors. Milich and Loney (1979) indicate that drug responsivity is related to Hyperactivity whereas Aggression is associated with adolescent outcome.

Milich, Loney, and Landau's (1982) validated the hyperactivity/aggression distinction against systematic behavioral observations, including wrist and ankle actometers plus playroom floor grid crossings, in 90 boys aged 6 to 12 years 11 months referred to the Child Psychiatry Service at the University of Iowa. They report that "the Hyperactivity factor made a unique contribution in accounting for the variance of numerous dependent variables, beyond the variance it shared with the Aggression factor." (p. 183)

Next we will consider definitions of hyperactivity–attention deficit disorder.

Then we shall review what little developmental information is available. A discussion of what we know about children on the basis of various instruments will then be reviewed. Because the results of each device are not directly comparable, a separate section is provided for each type device. Not all instruments have been used to address the same questions. Organizing by instrument results in unavoidable topic changes when moving from instrument to instrument. Having carefully considered the more traditional approach of using topics as headings and subordinating measurement concerns, I have decided that the measurement priorities require that I endure the resulting topical discontinuity and ask for the reader's indulgence as well. I hope that this presentation will serve to highlight areas in which future research needs to be concentrated. It is hoped that de facto standards will emerge in a future where most investigators will use comparable equipment, thereby facilitating comparison and obviating the necessity to divide material by instrument used.

A final section, on the validity of rating scales, is included for three reasons. First, rating scales are the single most common approach to assessment of this disorder. Second, it is refreshing to find that instrument measurements validate the use of these tests. Third, the discrepancies between ratings and instrumented measurements indicate that substantial clinical "mistakes" are probably being made daily. It is recommended that an economical "second opinion" be obtained using behavioral measurement.

DIAGNOSTIC CRITERIA

DSM-II

Concern with excessive activity in children was formally incorporated into the catalog of mental disorder for the first time by the second edition of the Diagnostic and Statistical Manual (DSM-II) (APA, 1968). The official entry was Hyperkinetic Reaction of Childhood (or Adolescence) (308.0). "This disorder is characterized by overactivity, restlessness, distractibility and short attention span, especially in young children; the behavior usually diminishes in adolescence. If this behavior is caused by organic brain damage, it should be diagnosed under the appropriate nonpsychotic organic brain syndrome." (p. 50)

DSM-III

DSM-III (APA, 1980) revised the above conception into Attention Deficit Disorder with Hyperactivity (314.01) and Without Hyperactivity (314.00). This distinction elevated measurement of motor activity to a point of singular differential diagnostic importance. Because the diagnostic decision pertained to the child's extraclinic behavior, ambulatory monitoring became of critical importance. Clinic tests of activity while taking psychological tests or waiting to be seen are small behavioral samples thought to reflect natural activity, but ambulatory measures remained the theoretical criterion.

DSM-III required that two of the following five operational definitions of hyperactivity be satisfied over a 6-month period prior to the seventh birthday and not meet the inclusion criteria for Schizophrenia, Affective Disorder, or Severe or Profound Mental Retardation in order to reach a positive diagnosis for ADHD (314.01):

1. "Runs about or climbs on things excessively."
2. "Has difficulty sitting still or fidgets excessively."
3. "Has difficulty staying seated."
4. "Moves about excessively during *sleep*."
5. "Is always 'on the go' or acts as if 'driven by a motor'."

Ambulation is clearly referred to by criteria 1 and 5 and is reflected in wrist, waist, and ankle activity thereby allowing one to choose any available device and place it at any of these sites of attachment. fidgeting excessively very likely is reflected in excessive wrist movement though currently no method exists for separating constructive wrist activities, such as coloring, from fidgeting. Having difficulty sitting still may be reflected at the waist depending upon how much vertical movement occurs. Movements of an inch or two during partial attempts to leave the seat are probably detectable by a Motionlogger™ actigraph or a step counter. If item 3 indicates that the child actually gets out of his or her seat then this behavior can also be measured at the wrist, waist, or ankle.

Activity during sleep (item 4) is best monitored at the wrist as discussed in Chapter 6. A time-based device such as the Motionlogger™ actigraph or the Actillume™ is desirable because one can more certainly separate activities occurring immediately before bedtime and immediately upon awakening from those occurring during sleep. It is overly optimistic to assume that parents will always be present when the child awakes to take readings from a general accumulator-type device and will consistently reset the device after that last glass of water or trip to the bathroom before going to bed. The time-based device allows one to exclude those portions of the record from analysis by visual inspection.

It is not strictly necessary to obtain sleep activity measures because one needs but 2 of 5, or 4 if sleep is excluded, to diagnose ADHD (314.01). However, 4 of 5 categories refer to waking hours and only 1 to sleeping hours. Sleep constitutes a major portion of everybody's day and should therefore be sampled to reach truly representative conclusions. Sleep is also well defined and therefore quite easily interpreted. Unlike daytime, when activities are dependent upon other people (someone to play tennis with), the weather (not going for a walk because it is raining), and circumstances (can't find a close parking spot), sleep activity is not confounded by such variables. The normal condition is easy to define; small periodic bursts of activity due to changes in body position. All these features makes diagnosing hyperactivity during sleep fairly straightforward, especially in children, where restless leg syndrome is not found. These issues are discussed further in Chapter 6.

It is important to note that one cannot accurately diagnose Attention Deficit Disorder *without* Hyperactivity (314.00) until the above-mentioned activity measurements have been made and found not to be problematic.

Achenbach (1980) challenges DSM-III on the basis that empirical investigations regarding the nature of childhood disorders " . . . revealed little reliable evidence of attention deficit disorders without hyperactivity . . . " (p. 407)

DSM-III-R

DSM-III-R (APA, 1987) reasserts Attention Deficit Hyperactivity Disorder (314.01) as a singular disorder with somewhat different characteristics than DSM-III. The DSM-III Attention Deficit Disorder without Hyperactivity has been placed within Undifferentiated Attention Deficit Disorder (314.00), about which the following is said: "Research is necessary to determine if this is a valid diagnostic category and, if so, how it should be defined." (p. 95)

Regarding Attention Deficit Hyperactivity Disorder, DSM-III-R stipulates: "The essential features of this disorder are developmentally inappropriate degrees of inattention, impulsiveness, and hyperactivity. People with the disorder generally display some disturbance in each of these areas, but to varying degrees." (p. 50) Achenbach (1980) concluded that a review of empirical studies of childhood disorders indicates that " . . . a separate syndrome of attention deficit without hyperactivity has not been reliably detected . . . " (p. 411) DSM-III-R de-emphasized these empirical studies when developing the following guidelines, though residual references to activity remain.

At least 8 of the following 14 criteria must be met for at least 6 months before the child reaches his or her seventh birthday and does not meet the criteria for a Pervasive Developmental Disorder before a positive diagnosis for 314.01 can be made (cf. DSM-III-R pp. 52–53):

1. "Often fidgets with hands or feet or squirms in seat." (In adolescents, may be limited to subjective feelings of restlessness.)
2. "Often has difficulty remaining seated when required to do so."
3. "Is easily distracted by extraneous stimuli."
4. "Has difficulty awaiting turn in games or group situations."
5. "Often blurts out answers to questions before they have been completed."
6. "Has difficulty following through on instructions from others (not due to oppositional behavior or failure of comprehension), e.g., fails to finish chores."
7. "Has difficulty sustaining attention in tasks or play activities."

8. "Often shifts from one uncompleted activity to another."
9. "Has difficulty playing quietly."
10. "Often talks excessively."
11. "Often interrupts or intrudes on others, e.g., butts into other children's games."
12. "Often does not seem to listen to what is being said to him or her."
13. "Often loses things necessary for tasks or activities at school or at home (e.g., toys, pencils, books, assignments)."
14. "Often engages in physically dangerous activities without considering possible consequences (not for the purpose of thrill-seeking), e.g., runs into street without looking."

These items are listed in the order of importance found for diagnosing Disruptive Behavior Disorder. Item 1 directly refers to measurable activity at the wrist (hands) and ankles (feet). Waist activity may also be present and perhaps may better distinguish persons with this disorder because normal waist measures may be near zero whereas normal wrist measures may be fairly high. Remember, physical sensors cannot make social discriminations between productive activity and fidgeting. Ankle measurements may also provide high discriminability in that fidgeting probably extends to the ankles whereas productive activity does not. These empirical questions remain to be answered.

It is important to note that disordered adolescents may not be measurably more active than normal control subjects as indicated by the caveat that only subjective feelings of restlessness may exist.

Item 2 about difficulty remaining seated may involve actually leaving one's seat repeatedly or frequently making partial efforts at leaving one's seat. In either case waist activity would likely be the preferred site of attachment because low waist activity should be associated with normal control children. Foot activity should also increase during efforts to leave one's seat. Wrist activity again is confounded with purposive activity while seated. It is unlikely that periodic efforts to leave one's seat would substantially increase wrist activity above normal control levels.

All other 12 items refer to attentional deficits. No longer are the following DSM-III blanket references to generally elevated activity made: "Runs about or climbs on things excessively," "Moves about excessively during *sleep*," "Is always 'on the go' or acts as if 'driven by a motor.'" However, we are told that "Hyperactivity may be evidenced by difficulty remaining seated, excessive *jumping about*, *running* in the classroom, fidgeting, manipulating objects, and twisting and wiggling in one's seat." (emphasis added) (p. 50) Activities such as jumping about and running should yield elevated waist and ankle activity in addition to increased wrist activity.

DSM-III-R refines reference to activity in the "Age-specific features" sections on pages 50–51. "In preschool children, the most prominent features are generally signs of gross motor overactivity, such as excessive running or climbing. The child is often described as being on the go and "always having his motor running." (p 50) Because the age of onset in approximately half of the cases is before 4, ambulatory activity measures can play a large diagnostic role in younger children. "In older children and adolescents, the most prominent features tend to be excessive fidgeting and restlessness rather than gross motor overactivity." (p. 50)

Under "Associated features," DSM-III-R (p. 51) indicates "temper outbursts." Excessive wrist, waist, and ankle activity are very likely associated with such incidents. Isolating these events in time is greatly facilitated by time-based instruments such as the Motionlogger™ and Actillume™ actigraphs where 1- or 2-minute epochs can readily be selected. Temper outbursts would likely be revealed as unusually intense activity having a rapid onset. Because intensity is an important defining characteristic, an instrument like the Actillume™ capable of measuring 256 activity intensities is the preferred instrument.

A positive diagnosis for Attention-Deficit Hyperactivity Disorder cannot be made until differential diagnosis has excluded: (1) age-appropriate overactivity, (2) Mental Retardation, (3) Pervasive Developmental Disorders, (4) Mood Disorders, and (5) Undifferentiated Attention Deficit Disorder.

The most difficult differential diagnosis is with "age-appropriate overactivity" which, we are told, "does not have the haphazard and poorly organized quality characteristic of the behavior of children with Attention Deficit Hyperactivity Disorder." (p 52) Physical sensors cannot presently distinguish one "quality" of activity from another. They either measure the presence of activity or its intensity. Two possible solutions exist. First, persons with "organized" and "disorganized" activity should have their activity measured with fully proportional triaxial accelerometric devices placed at the wrist, waist, and ankle in order to sample various behaviors, settings, and sites of attachment. Perhaps a physical "signature" exists characteristic of "organized" and "disorganized" activity. One might expect "disorganized" activity to show greater discontinuities than "organized" activity. Included here would be frequent shifts from quiet to highly accelerated behavior such as were suggested to be characteristic of tantrum behavior, which we presume would be classified as "disorganized." Such rapid behavioral changes would emerge as peaks in a power spectrum analysis. The equipment for such a study currently exists. Silicon [IC Sensors, 1701 McCarthy Blvd., Milpitas, CA; (408) 432-1800] accelerometers can be used in conjunction with Medilog recorders [Ambulatory Monitoring, Inc., 731 Saw Mill River Road, Ardsley, NY 10502; (914) 693-9240] to obtain the necessary raw data.

A second approach would be to have trained clinicians, teachers, and/or parents make qualitative judgments about how well organized the child's behavior is and obtain simultaneous behavioral measurements to determine the intensity and distribution of activity over time. In this way one capitalizes upon the strengths of human observers and physical instruments.

NORMAL ACTIVITY DEVELOPMENT

Developmental changes in activity are of interest in their own right as part of a comprehensive understanding of child development. Information on normal development provides a perspective from which to discuss hyperkinesis. Hence, we now consider what is currently known regarding normal activity development of boys and girls.

Documenting developmental changes requires that the same type of instrument be used with boys and girls of varying ages or prospectively with the same children over time. The necessity of using the same instrument is the reason why the following material is organized by the instrument used. Very few studies meet these criteria.

A general limitation shared by all of the studies we will review is that they have been conducted under very specific situations for brief time periods. For comparability, only data relating to free play settings is reviewed below. The use of short measurement intervals is directly analogous to using few test items; both tend to decrease reliability which attenuates correlations with other variables. The use of specific "test" situations restricts generalizability to similar natural settings. Generalizations from test taking to free play and vice versa are probably unwarranted. A desirable aspect of using test situations is that they have a greater chance of being replicated by other investigators.

The following discussion places primary emphasis upon comparing 95% confidence intervals to stress the issue of measurement precision. Psychology has too long labored against the null hypothesis handicap (cf. Bakan, 1966; Meehl, 1967; Rozeboom; 1960; Morrison and Henkel, 1970). Investigators have limited their aspirations to showing that their data are not entirely random noise rather than obtaining accurate quantitative information and carefully comparing results across studies and with theoretical predictions. Current emphasis upon statistical power (Cohen, 1977; Kraemer and Thiemann, 1987; Lipsey, 1990) is desirable in that it stimulates concern for quality measurement among other issues. Lipsey (1990) is especially strong in his call for routinely reporting confidence intervals in treatment effectiveness research (pp. 172–174). The uninformative width of some confidence intervals begs for larger sample sizes and/or longer measurement periods to better estimate the individual's typical activity level.

Actometers

Days 1 to 4

Campbell, Kuyek, Lang, and Partington (1971) attached actometers to the right leg of 30 boys and 29 girls randomly selected from the nurseries of the Kingston General Hospital during the first four days after birth. Unfortunately, they used the following units of measure: "The watch scores were turned into decimal numbers. 'Days' shown on the calendar became integers, and 'time' shown by the hands became the decimal. These quantities were then divided by the time during which observations had been made and the results expressed as activity/h." (p. 110) It appears that numbers to the left of the decimal point equals days of apparent time. Numbers to the right of the decimal point could either mean hours and minutes or fractional hours. For example, a reading of 5.21 could mean 5 days, 2 hours 1 minute or 5 days and .21 days. Such unit uncertainty should be avoided by future investigators.

Their Figure 2 results indicated significant activity increases over the first four days of life ($F(3,117) = 6.3, p < .01$). The means (and standard deviations) for the first four days are 0.45 (0.20), 0.59 (0.32), 0.73 (0.35), 0.91 (0.50). Unfortunately, data were not presented separately for boys and girls thereby obviating any conclusions regarding sex effects.

Weeks 1 to 10

Campbell, Kuyek, Lang, and Partington's (1971) Figure 4 indicated that activity dropped markedly during the first three weeks at home such that the average second plus third week was approximately 0.55 units. A steady activity increase to approximately 0.65 units occurred during weeks 4 and 5 reaching the predischarge level of about 0.9 units during weeks 6 and 7. Activity then reached about 1.15 units during weeks 9 and 10 which marked the end of this study.

Mack and Kleinhenz (1974) investigated activity during the first 8 weeks of life in 5 black female infants by placing actometers (modified Tissot self-winding wrist watches) on both wrists (dorsal surface) and ankles (lateral aspects) for 24 hours when the infants were 8, 16, 28, and 56 days old. Unfortunately, activity was summed over all four attachment sites. Inspection of their Figure 1 reveals that activity was flat across all four measurement points for Infants 1 and 2. On Day 56, Infant 1 obtained a total of 283 AU across all four actometers over 24 hours equal to $283/4/1440 = 0.049$ AU/min per actometer. The corresponding value for Infant 2 was 0.030 AU/min. Infants 3 and 5 showed modest activity increases over time to where they achieved totals of 834 AU and 783 AU respectively on Day 56 equalling 0.145 and 0.136 AU/min per actometer respectively. Infant 4 displayed a dramatic activity increase achieving a total of 2,849 AU on Day 56 equalling 0.495 AU/min per actometer.

No sex differences were possible since all subjects studied were female.

Months 4 to 6

Rose and Mayer (1968) placed one actometer on the left wrist and ankle of 31 infants (16 females, and 12 males) aged 4 to 6 months. Twenty-four hours later, the same actometers were attached to the right wrist and ankle. Twenty-four hours later, the same actometers were moved back again to the left side. Measurements continued for 2 consecutive days and nights. They summed data for two consecutive nights across four actometers and divided by four. They defined each day registered on the actometer as one unit of activity. This makes their AU $60 \times 24 = 1440$ times larger than the usual AU unit. But they also expressed their data in AU per day which contains 1440 minutes thereby equating to the present AU/min. The average wrist–ankle activity was 44.23 ($S = 8.43$) AU/min for males and 43.19 ($S = 11.90$) for females. The 95% confidence interval for the boys is 39.14 to 49.32 AU/min and for the girls is 36.85 to 49.53 AU/min indicating no sex effect; boys and girls appear to be equally active.

An interesting aside is that Rose and Mayer (1968) found a significant correlation between combined wrist and ankle activity and total caloric intake ($r(29) = .47, p < .01$) as well as a correlation with "extra" calories above basal requirement ($r(29) = .64, p < .0002$).

Eaton and Dureski (1986) placed actometers (Timex model-108 Motion Recorders) on both wrists and ankles of 46 infants (24 males, 22 females) aged 13.1 to 21.4 weeks ($M = 16.8$) and placed them in an infant seat inclined at 45 degrees for 15 to 52 minutes ($M = 26.8$). They reported a correlation ($r(22) = .37, p < .08$) between composite activity and recumbent length; taller infants being more active. No sex differences were reported.

Six brief comments are in order regarding the above-mentioned studies. First, activity appears to increase daily during the first few days of life. Second, being discharged home appears to inhibit activity which then increases at a much slower rate thereby requiring 6 to 7 weeks to return to levels reached by the 4th day of life. Third, evidence of further activity increases through week 10 is present for white but not black infants. Fourth, future investigators should report data separately for boys and girls. Fifth, consistent with Maccoby and Jacklin (1974), sex differences under 6 months of age have yet to be demonstrated. Sixth, site of attachment cannot be evaluated because wrist and ankle activity were averaged together.

Months 6 to 8

Chapman (1975) reports average wrist activity of 179.61 AU/min ($S = 103.36$) for boys and 136.60 AU/min ($S = 77.00$) for girls. The 95% confidence intervals for 80 boys of 156.61 to 202.61 lies entirely above that for 73 girls of 118.63 to 154.57 indicating significantly and substantially greater wrist activity for boys. Ankle activity averaged 125.99 AU/min ($S = 65.76$) for boys and 101.63 ($S = 49.17$) for girls. The corresponding 95% confidence interval for boys' ankle data ranging from 111.36 to 140.62 AU/min is sufficiently independent of that for girls ranging from 90.16 to 113.10 AU/min that the means are significantly different ($t(151) = 2.575, p < .02$) with boys again being more active than girls. Hence, activity differences are apparently established by the second half-year of life.

These data bolster Eaton and Enns's (1986) meta-analytic review (reviewed below) showing that activity in boys significantly exceeds that of girls by 0.49 standard deviations (a large effect). Because they found larger sex differences in older children and because relatively few studies were found on very young children, they were concerned that their reported sex difference might not hold up for younger children. The effect size used by Eaton and Enns was the difference between the means divided by the pooled standard deviation. The effect sizes for Chapman's (1975) wrist and ankle activity were .357 and .417 respectively. Both are substantial and consistent with Eaton and Enns's report. Kendall and Brophy (1981) reported that activity sex differences decrease with age. Eaton and Yu (1989) present data indicating that these sex differences are not due to maturity differences between boys and girls.

Chapman's (1975) wrist-ankle average of 152.8 AU/min for 6- to 8-month-old infant males and 119.12 AU/min for females are approximately 3 to 4 times as great as Rose and Mayer's (1968) measures for 4- to 6-month-old infants. Perhaps infants show a dramatic activity increase at 6 to 8 months.

Year 2.5

Pedersen and Bell (1970) placed actometers on the backs of 30 boys and 26 girls aged 2.5 years for 6 days distributed over a 1-month period while they attended nursery school. They reported significantly greater activity in boys than girls ($t(54)$ = 2.67, $p < .05$). Unfortunately, no descriptive statistics were reported.

Year 3

Buss, Block, and Block (1980) obtained nonfavored wrist actometer measurements on 65 boys and 64 girls aged 3 years for 2 hours on each of 3 days approximately 1 week apart. The conditions under which measurements were taken were not specified. The units of measure are unclear because the raw scores for both sexes were standardized with a mean of 50 and a standard deviation of 10. The boys' mean of 51.4 was not significantly greater than the girls' mean of 49.1 ($t(127)$ = 1.34, N.S.). However, the differences between the means were in the expected direction of boys being more active.

Years 4 to 5

Buss, Block, and Block (1980) retested the same 65 boys and 64 girls at age 4 but this time they aggregated over 4 rather than 3 2-hour sessions. The boys' mean of 51.3 was now significantly greater than the girls' mean of 48.6 ($t(127) = 2.33$, p < .05). The 4-year-old boys' mean of 51.3 is extremely close to the mean for 3-year-old boys of 51.4. A small activity decrease in girls' activity from 49.1 at age

3 to 48.6 at age 4 occurred. This small mean change in girls' activity explains only some of the increased t value. Probably the use of an additional 2-hour measurement period helped achieve significance. If so, then significant differences at age 3 might also have emerged had 4 rather than 3 2-hour measurements been obtained. Future investigators should base gender activity difference studies on at least $4 \times 2 = 8$ hours of activity measurement.

Eaton and Keats (1982) obtained dominant wrist and contralateral ankle actometer data from 27 girls and 42 boys aged an average of 51.1 months (4.26 years) (range = 26 to 76 months; 2.17 to 6.33 years) while they remained alone for 3 minutes and while they played for 9 minutes in same- or opposite-sex triads in a 2.3 m × 4.0 m carpeted playroom. The units of measure were unstated but probably were AU/min. A significant ($F(1,65) = 12.66$, $p < .0007$) and strong sex effect emerged where the mean for boys of 3.15 exceeded the mean for girls of 2.80 by more than three-quarters of a standard deviation ($d > 0.75$). Boys were more active than girls regardless of whether they played with other boys or with girls. Boys were no more active when they played with other boys than when they played with girls. The children were more active when placed in triads than when left alone.

Years 5 to 7

Data from Schulman, Kaspar, and Throne (1965) on eight 5- to 7-year-old boys and ten age-matched girls during free play indicates that boys are significantly more wrist active than girls. The boys' wrist averaged 48.83 AU/min ($S = 24.33$) with the 95% confidence interval ranging from 26.49 to 67.17 AU/min. The girls' wrist averaged 26.33 AU/min ($S = 15.17$) with the 95% confidence interval ranging from 15.48 to 37.18 AU/min. Despite some overlap, boys are significantly more active than girls at the wrist ($t(16) = 2.19$, $p < .05$).

The same trend exists for ankle data with boys averaging 51.50 AU/min ($S = 87.33$), and girls' averaging 40.17 AU/min ($S = 42.62$). However, excessive variability in the boys' data gave rise to an unacceptably large 95% confidence interval ranging from an impossible −21.51 to 124.51 AU/min. This enormous range completely contains the 95% confidence interval for girls of 9.68 to 70.66. Less variable data on larger samples may well show the nearly 10 AU/min mean difference to be statistically significant.

Years 7 to 8

Schulman, Kaspar, and Throne (1965) also studied 8 boys aged 7 to 8 years and 7 age-matched girls. The boys' wrist activity averaged 78.00 AU/min ($S = 36.50$) and the girls' averaged 26.67 AU/min ($S = 10.83$). The resulting 95% confidence interval for boys of 47.49 to 108.51 AU/min is independent of and larger than the corresponding interval for girls of 16.65 to 36.69 AU/min indicating that boys are significantly more wrist active than girls. The same result obtained with ankle activity data. The boys averaged 58.50 AU/min (S = 43.17) while the girls averaged 16.83 (S = 12.00). The 95% confidence interval for boys of 22.41 to 94.59 AU/min was sufficiently nonoverlapping with the corresponding interval for girls of 5.73 to 27.93 AU/min that boys were found to be significantly more ankle active than girls ($t(13)$ = 2.62, p < .05).

Years 8 to 9

Schulman, Kaspar, and Throne (1965) measured wrist and ankle activity of 11 boys aged 8 to 9 years and 7 girls of the same age. The boys' wrist activity averaged 95.50 AU/min (S = 119.50) and the girls' averaged 21.67 AU/min (S = 10.17). The excessively large 95% confidence interval for the boys ranged from 18.22 to 178.78 AU/min largely contained the corresponding interval for girls of 12.26 to 31.08 thereby indicating no significant difference in wrist activity. Less variable data on larger samples might well show a significant difference given the large difference in the means.

Ankle data averaged 76.83 AU/min for boys (S = 76.33) and 13.33 AU/min (S = 12.50) for girls. The 95% confidence interval of 25.55 to 128.11 for boys was completely independent and larger than the corresponding interval of 1.77 to 24.89 for girls indicating that boys are significantly more ankle active than girls.

Years 9 to 10

Schulman, Kaspar, and Throne (1965) measured the wrist and ankle activity of 7 boys aged 9 to 10 years and 7 age-matched girls. The wrist data averaged 56.83 AU/min (S = 57.33) for boys and 28.33 AU/min (S = 21.17) for girls. The excessively large 95% confidence interval for boys of 3.81 to 109.85 AU/min completely engulfs the corresponding interval for girls of 8.75 to 47.91 AU/min indicating no significant difference. It is likely that future studies using larger samples will find a significant difference given the nearly 2 to 1 activity level involved.

Ankle activity averaged 57.33 AU/min (S = 56.17) for boys and 18.33 (S = 17.33) for girls. The very large 95% confidence interval for boys of 5.38 to 109.28 AU/min almost entirely contains the corresponding interval for girls of 2.3 to 34.36 AU/min indicating no significant difference. Perhaps larger samples will show this difference to be significant considering the mean difference.

Years 10 to 12

Schulman, Kaspar, and Throne (1965) measured wrist and ankle activity on 7 boys aged 10 to 12 years and 7 girls of the same age. The boys' wrist data averaged

55.17 AU/min (S = 52.33) and the girls' averaged 27.33 AU/min (S = 34.50). The enormous 95% confidence interval of 6.77 to 103.57 AU/min for boys largely contains the impossible corresponding interval for girls of −4.58 to 59.24 AU/min thereby failing to find significance. Less variable larger sample results may well find a significant sex difference due to the large mean difference.

The same largely uncertain result pertains to ankle activity where the boys averaged 20.00 AU/min (S = 25.17) and the girls averaged 24.83 AU/min (S = 39.67). The boys' impossible 95% confidence interval of −3.28 to 43.28 is entirely contained within the girls' impossible interval of −11.86 to 61.52 AU/min. The very similar mean levels are particularly noteworthy given the previously large sex differences.

Years 5 to 12

The 5- to 12-year range explored above shows two consistent features. First, boys appear to be more active than girls at the wrist and ankle up until 10 to 12 years, when ankle activity appears approximately equal. Second, activity appears to increase with age at the wrist and ankle for both boys and girls. Wrist activity for boys increases from 46.83 to 78.00 to 98.50 and then decreases to 56.83 and then to 55.17 AU/min. Wrist activity for girls remains approximately the same changing from 26.33 to 26.67 to 21.67 to 28.33 to 27.33 AU/min. Ankle activity in boys shows a parallel development increasing from 51.50 to 58.50 to 76.83 and then decreasing to 57.33 and then to 20.00 AU/min. Ankle activity in girls decreases from 40.17 to 16.83 to 13.33 and then increases to 18.33 and then to 24.83 AU/min. Small behavioral samples (short measurement intervals) and small sample sizes led to large measurement uncertainty in several instances.

The following studies do not address development within the 5- to 12-year age span. They are included here because they should at least be consistent with the average developmental picture just described depending upon the proportion of the sample at each age level; a fact not presently available.

Personal communication with Russell A. Barkley reveals that the wrist actometer data for the 20 normal 5- to 12-year-old boys in Cunningham and Barkley's (1979) control group averaged 973.35 AU/30 min (S = 545.35) which we will consider as 32.45 AU/min (S = 18.18) resulting in a 95% confidence interval of 23.94 to 40.96 AU/min. This interval lies completely within the very large bottom half of Schulman *et al.*'s (1965) 95% confidence wrist interval for 8- to 9-year-old boys: below the midpoint of the 5–12 range. Ankle actometer data averaged 1008.30 AU/30 min (S = 628.11) which equals 33.61 AU/min (S = 57.10) resulting in a 95% confidence interval of 23.81 to 43.41 AU/min. This interval lies within the bottom half of Schulman *et al.*'s (1965) 95% confidence interval for 8- to 9-year-old boy's ankle activity.

Ullman, Barkley, and Brown's (1978) control group of 18 boys aged 5 to 12 years showed a wrist actometer mean of 193.77 ($S = 184.78$) AU/6 min of free play and ankle actometer mean of 95.72 ($S = 129.26$) AU/6 min of free play. Dividing by 6 to get AU/min we find a 95% confidence interval of 16.99 to 47.61 AU/min for wrist activity and 5.24 to 26.66 AU/min for ankle activity. The wrist interval lies almost entirely within the large lower half of Schulman, Kaspar, and Throne's (1965) 95% wrist confidence interval. The ankle interval is almost completely below Schulman *et al.*'s lower 95% confidence interval limit of 25 AU/min.

Pope studied a tighter age range of 19 boys aged 7–11 years. Wrist activity averaged 77.30 AU/min ($S = 43.60$) yielding a 95% confidence interval of 56.29 to 98.31 AU/min. These data are consistent with the 47.49 to 109.85 AU/min interval constructed from the lower limit of Schulman *et al.*'s (1965) 7-year-old boys and upper limit of their 10-year-old boys. Ankle activity averaged 39.30 AU/min ($S = 39.60$) resulting in a 95% confidence interval of 19.61 to 58.99 AU/min. These data are consistent with the 22.41 to 109.28 AU/min interval constructed from the lower limit of Schulman *et al.*'s (1965) 7-year-old boys and upper limit of their 10-year-old boys.

Kaspar, Millichap, Backus, Child, and Schulman (1971) studied 48 boys aged 5–8 years and 24 age-matched girls. The boys' wrist activity averaged 36.89 AU/min ($S = 11.27$) whereas the girls' averaged 13.40 AU/min ($S = 11.27$). The 95% confidence interval for boys of 33.62 to 40.16 AU/min is completely independent of and larger than that for girls' ranging from 8.64 to 18.16 AU/min and indicating that boys are significantly more active than girls at this age. These data are consistent with the 26.49 to 108.51 AU/min interval constructed from the lower limit of Schulman *et al.*'s (1965) 5-year-old boys and upper limit of their 8-year-old boys.

The same result was found for ankle activity. Boys averaged 62.10 AU/min ($S = 49.20$) and girls averaged 17.14 AU/min ($S = 14.34$). The resulting 95% confidence interval for boys of 47.81 to 76.39 was independent of and larger than that for girls of 11.08 to 23.20 indicating that boys are significantly more active at the ankle. These data are consistent with the -21.51 to 94.59 AU/min interval constructed from the lower limit of Schulman *et al.*'s (1965) 5-year-old boys and upper limit of their 8-year-old boys.

Halverson and Victor (1976) obtained actometer data from 50 boys and 50 girls in grades 1–5 (ages 6–10 years) during 1 hour of class time for 5 days. They reported a significant correlation of $r(98) = -.29$, $p < .01$ with ratings regarding 16 "minor physical anomalies" (cf. Waldrop and Halverson, 1971) for boys but not for girls ($r(98) = -.14$, N.S.).

A Review

Eaton and Enns (1986) performed a meta-analysis on 90 studies containing 127 independent sex difference results based upon sample sizes of 7 to 25,000 spanning an age range of 2 months to 30 years (median = 55.5 months). They reported that activity in boys exceeds that in girls by an average of 0.49 standard deviations, which qualifies as a large effect. Effect size [d = (boys' mean − girls' mean)/pooled SD) calculations on the Schulman, Kaspar, and Throne (1965) data indicate: d = 1.142 and 0.172 for wrist and ankle activity in 5- to 7-year-olds, d = 1.848 and 1.274 for wrist and ankle activity in 7- to 8-year-olds, d = 0.780 and 1.044 for wrist and ankle activity in 8- to 9-year-olds, d = 0.660 and 0.938 for wrist and ankle activity in 9- to 10-year-olds, and d = 0.628 and −0.145 for wrist and ankle activity in 10- to 12-year-olds. The average sex effects for wrist and ankle activity are 1.0116 and 0.6566. Both of these are substantially larger than the 0.49 average but the sample size is much smaller, which prohibits firm conclusions at this time. The implication is that measured activity may yield larger sex effects than have previously been reported.

Pedometers

The only available data on normal children wearing pedometers is that reported by Stunkard and Pestka (1962). They presented data on the activity of 15 normal girls at camp and home over a two-week period are reprinted here as Table 4.1. Their average age was 12.00 years (range = 10–13 years).

TABLE 4.1. Miles per Day Walked by 15 Normal Weight Girls over Two Weeks at Camp and Home[a]

Day	At camp	At home
1	11.8	6.3
2	9.4	–
3	11.5	12.6
4	12.0	8.2
5	7.3	—
6	9.5	3.2
7	6.3	–
8	5.7	5.0
9	4.2	1.7
10	5.3	–
11	10.0	7.6
12	7.6	5.2
13	6.1	4.3
14	7.2	5.3
15	6.5	–
Mean	8.03	5.75
SD	2.51	2.94
SE	0.65	0.89

[a]Reprinted from Stunkard and Pestka (1962).

ASSESSMENT AND TREATMENT

This section is organized around the instruments used to measure activity for several reasons. First, the operating characteristics of each device are very different thereby obviating any possibility of directly comparing results obtained with various devices even if attached to the same body part. Second, step counters and pedometers are usually attached to the waist, whereas actometers and actigraphs are usually attached to the wrist or ankle. Actigraphs have been placed at the waist and actometers on the back. Each site of attachment yields different information. Different conclusions can be reached as a function of site-of-attachment and thereby warranting separate consideration. Stabilimeters are devices that one either sits or lies on. They introduce yet further differences. Third, computerized devices such as the actigraph record activity over programmable epochs, often 1, 2, 5, 10, or 15 minutes, whereas other devices must either be read by humans at prescribed intervals throughout the day or twice daily: waking and sleeping periods. Obviously, some questions will be more accurately answered with automatic time-based devices than with instruments requiring more human intervention.

Actigraphy

We begin our review with actigraphy because it constitutes the highest quality data currently available. Porrino, Rapoport, Behar, Sceery, Ismond, and Bunney (1983) obtained 24-hour waist activity, using 1 hour epochs, for 7 days on 12 very carefully selected middle-class hyperactive boys (mean age = 8.6 years, S = 2.1 years) and 12 age- and class-matched control boys (mean age = 8.6, S = 1.9 years) using the Colburn, Smith, Guarini, and Simmons (1976) forerunner of the Ambulatory Monitoring, Inc. (Ardsley, NY) Motionlogger™. The $4 \times 6 \times 1$ cm, 75 gram actigraph, sensitive to 0.1 g (where g = 9.8 m/s/s), was placed in a pouch attached to the boy's belt. Inclusion criteria for hyperactivity were being 2 standard deviations or more above the sex-matched norms for Factor IV (hyperactivity) of the Conners' Teacher Rating Scale (Conners, 1969) and showing evidence of restlessness or inattention stemming from the home, school, or clinical examination. Exclusion criteria included hard neurological signs, major psychiatric disorder such as psychosis or depression, and full scale IQ of less than 80. It was mentioned that all children were able to function within school limits and that special living facilities were not indicated for any of the hyperactive children. Parents and children jointly completed an hourly activity diary for the entire week.

The results during the baseline week for school hours indicated significantly more activity by "hyperactive" children during reading ($p < .01$), mathematics ($p < .01$), and overall weekly mean ($p < .001$) than control children but were essentially equally active during lunch/recess and physical education. After school during baseline week, "hyperactive" children were significantly more active during outside play ($p < .05$) than were control children but equally active during inside play and while watching TV and for the average of after-school hours. However, the results for the baseline weekend indicated that the "hyperactive" children were significantly more active than control children during inside play ($p < .01$), outside play ($p < .05$), while watching TV ($p < .05$), and on average during weekend hours ($p < .01$). The "hyperactive" children were significantly more active ($p < .001$) than control children during the school nights of baseline week. Weekend nights were in the same direction but not significant. The overall baseline week night activity readings were significantly ($p < .01$) greater for "hyperactive" than control subjects. The largest activity differences between the two groups occurred during the early morning and early to midafternoon hours. Overall school activity was the best single variable for significantly discriminating (75% correct classification of cases) the two subject groups; *better than any of the attentional measures.* This result is particularly important given the emphasis DSM-III-R places on attentional rather than activity measures regarding ADHD.

The finding that "hyperactive" children were generally more active than control children in all 12 independent situations, sometimes significantly so ($F(1,21) = 6.88$, $p < .02$ for weekdays and $F(1,21) = 5.84$, $p < .025$ for weekends), other times in the predicted direction but not significant at this small sample size, plus the significantly greater sleep (0000 to 0500 hours) activity during school nights (trend on the weekend) indicate that children diagnosed as "hyperactive" are generally more active than control children. This result contrasts with the situational specificity hypothesis predicting hyperactivity only in the attentionally more demanding situations. Certainly sleep is not an attentionally demanding situation. Weekend sleep was less active for "hyperactive" children and more active for control children thereby reducing the between-group difference to a nonsignificant level. Hence, the present results are inconsistent with the view that hyperactivity is entirely derivative from short attention span. The generality of hyperactivity seems greater than was previously thought. The authors reached the following important conclusion: "In terms of diagnosis, then, motor behavior should be included as an important criterion and as a good basis on which to make diagnostic decisions." (p. 686)

Porrino, Rapoport, Behar, Ismond, and Bunney (1983) reported the effects of an individually adjusted 5- to 15-mg dose (0.23 to 0.75 mg/kg) tablet dose of dextroamphetamine or placebo administered at 0800 had on the activity of the hyperactive boys described above in an ABAB double-blind crossover design. Half of the subjects received medication during Weeks 1 and 3 and placebo during Weeks 2 and 4 whereas the other half received the opposite treatment. Waist actigraph data were collected 24 hours each day, using 1-hour epochs, for 4 weeks resulting in 672 consecutive hours of activity measurements. Activity is expressed as counts per hour where the threshold is 0.1 g: $g = 9.8$ m/s/s). A parent–child-completed activity diary regarding the child's behavior was also kept. Average 24-hour activity profiles were determined across both placebo weeks and both medication weeks for weekdays and weekends.

After discarding the first day of both medication and placebo conditions, it was found that medication significantly reduced activity in hyperactive boys during the week $(F(1,11) = 7.90, p < .02)$ but not on weekends $(F(1,11) = 0.04, N.S.)$. The activity reduction removed the significant difference from control subjects described above. The treatment effect was entirely due to activity reductions from 1000 to 1700: during school and in the afternoon after school. Weekend activity was significantly less on medication compared with placebo only at 1200 and 1300 hours.

Activity was significantly reduced under medication, compared to placebo levels, during reading $(p < .001)$, mathematics $(p < .001)$, lunch/recess $(p < .05)$, and overall school hours $(p < .001)$ but significantly increased during physical education. After school, medication significantly reduced overall activity $(p < .05)$ though no specific situations (inside play, outside play, television watching, shopping) were found. Activity under medication was significantly reduced $(p < .05)$ during outside play on the weekend. No other weekend differences emerged. Sleep activity *increased* significantly $(p < .001)$ during school nights, nonsignificantly during weekend nights, and significantly over all 12 nights $(p < .05)$. Activity reductions were not significantly below placebo levels and hence did not render them hypoactive. These analyses did not include the first day of each medication and placebo condition.

A particularly informative finding is the documentation of a drug rebound effect on weekdays. When mean placebo–mean dextroamphetamine differences were plotted for 24 hours beginning at 0900, medication was given at 0800, it became clear that therapeutic effects were present by the end of the first hour (0900), became maximum at noon (1200), and decreased irregularly during the afternoon. By about 1930, activity under medication equalled activity under placebo. The maximum rebound effect, where activity under medication was greater than under placebo, occurred at 2200 hours. This difference slowly decreased throughout the night and was present at 0800 the next morning when the next dose was administered. A similar rebound effect was observed on weekends but was slightly phase shifted later in time with the peak benefit occurring between 1400 and 1500 hours and the maximum rebound effect at 2300 hours. This biphasic drug response was reported to be clearly evident in all 12 cases. It appears to account for disruptive behavior around mealtime, during homework, and at bedtime. This rebound effect could be minimized by administering medication twice daily. The authors conclude that " . . . the use of 24-hour activity monitoring permits more careful clinically relevant monitoring of drug effects." (p. 693)

Significant improvements on teacher and parent rating scales plus the Continuous Performance Test (CPT) further support the above-mentioned activity effects.

The work of Rapoport, Buschsbaum, Weingartner, Zahn, Ludlow, and Mikkelsen (1980) regarding the behavioral effects of dextroamphetamine vs placebo, on both normal and hyperactive boys plus normal college-aged men using a double blind crossover design, extends our understanding of the above drug effects. A particular interest was to determine if medication effects are different in pre-pubescent boys than college-age men. A group of 14 normal boys (average age = 10.10 years, S = 2.10 years; average IQ = 131.0, S = 18.0) were selected from professional families. All were free from learning disabilities and none had previously taken amphetamines. Fifteen hyperactive boys (average age = 9.44 years, S = 2.12 years; average IQ = 112.0, S = 18.0) were referred by private practitioners in the local area. A total of 31 men between 18 and 30 years of age without learning disabilities, current psychiatric disorder, or regular drug use were obtained from area universities and colleges. Activity was measured with the above described actigraph for two hours (0900–1100) while subjects took a Skin-Conductance–Reaction Time Test, a Continuous Performance Test, a word game learning task, a Speech-Communication task and responded to a self-rating scale. For adults, the actigraph was placed in a pouch suspended from their belt in the middle of their back. For the boys, the actigraph was placed in a vest pocket located at the small of the back. Monday served as baseline. Subjects received drug or placebo on Wednesday and Friday in a double blind counterbalanced order. A high (0.5 mg/kg up to a maximum of 35 mg) or low (0.25 mg/kg up to a maximum of 17.5 mg) dose of dextroamphetamine sulfate elixir was given at 0830.

Hyperactive boys on medication (M = 432, S = 204) were significantly ($F(1,13)$ = 21.98, p < .0001) less active than when receiving placebo (M = 731, S = 233). Likewise, normal boys on medication (M = 284, S = 88) were significantly ($F(1,1)$ = 16.92, p < .002) less active than when receiving placebo (M = 421, S = 133). Men receiving a low dose (M = 116, S = 27) were significantly ($F(1,11)$ = 6.64, p < .03) less active than when receiving placebo (M = 134, S = 40). However, men receiving a high dose (M = 222, S = 93) were no different than when receiving placebo (M = 225, S = 88). Although 7 men and 3 normal boys responded with activity increases, all hyperactive boys responded with activity decreases.

Wren, Teicher, Baldessarini, and Lieberman (1988) obtained 64 hours of non-dominant wrist activity from a 6-year-old child diagnosed as having ADHD and a 7-year-old normal control. Pretreatment activity over 15 minute epochs revealed that daytime activity never fell below 50 counts for the ADHD child but did for the control child. Stimulant medication markedly increased the number of daytime 15-minute periods with fewer than 50 counts.

Actometers

This second section concerns actometers because the normative data reported above were largely based on them and because a substantial number of studies have used them to evaluate treatment effects.

Millichap and Boldrey (1967) obtained 24-hour pre- and post-treatment dominant wrist actometer measures from 2 boys and 2 girls receiving placebo, 4 boys receiving methylphenidate, and 3 boys and 3 girls receiving prednisone. The lack of significant results was due to two aspects of this study. First, one subject responded to medication by increasing from 26.17 to 116.13 AU/min. Such an unusual response completely dominated the results of the other four subjects. Second, the statistical power associated with such small sample sizes is so low that only an enormous positive treatment response could be detected. Hence, the null results reported here are inconclusive.

Millichap, Aymat, Sturgis, Larsen, and Egan (1968) attached actometers to the nondominant wrists of 24 boys and 4 girls aged 5 to 14 ($M = 8$) years during 45-minute periods while taking psychological tests. Measurements were taken during a no-drug baseline period, after 3 weeks of placebo, and after 3 weeks of methylphenidate at 1.5 mg/kg daily. The authors reported their results in terms of actometer hours per 45 minutes. These data were converted to AU/min by multiplying by 60 and dividing by 45. The average value of 15.05 AU/min during baseline and 15.77 AU/min during placebo conditions were not quite significantly greater than the medication average of 12.47 AU/min. No standard deviations were reported.

Millichap and Johnson (1974) seem to have re-reported the Millichap et al. (1968) results in graphical form. Reconstructing individual data values with a millimeter rule indicates an average reduction of 4.57 AU/min across the 28 subjects with the standard deviation of the difference scores being 11.27 resulting in $t(27) = 2.14, p < .05$.

Millichap (1974) apparently also re-reported the Millichap et al. (1968) data and further reported that incidence of neurologic signs correlated significantly ($r(26) = .38, p < .05$) with pretreatment activity and negatively ($r(26) = -0.59, p < .005$) with posttreatment activity showing that children with more neurologic signs benefited more from methylphenidate than did children with fewer signs.

Rapoport, Abramson, Alexander, and Lott (1971) placed a packet containing two actometers (which they mistakenly called pedometers because they cited Bell (1968) who reported exclusively on actometers), one in the horizontal and one in the vertical plane, on the backs of 19 boys aged 4.5 to 10.5 years ($M = 8.2$ years) while they played for 20 minutes in a 17' × 14' furnished playroom. They summed the two actometer readings rendering the units of measure as horizontal plus vertical per 20 minutes. Dividing the subsequent reported values by 2 × 20 = 40 yields average AU/min. Average activity during no drug of 182 was not significantly less than activity under placebo of 132 ($t(36) = -2.05$, N.S.). The mean difference of −55.58 units was substantial, and in the expected direction, but was not significant ($t(18) = 2.05\ p < .10$) with this sample size. The main difficulty probably was the extremely restricted 20 minute behavioral sample.

Rie, Rie, Steward, and Ambuel (1976) obtained wrist and ankle actometer data from 28 children (17 boys, 11 girls) aged 6 years 1 month to 9 years 1 month ($M = 7.5$ years) with a reading deficit of at least 6 months and an IQ of 85 or above. A double-blind counterbalanced design where 12 weeks of placebo was followed by 12 weeks of 5 or 10 mg per day methylphenidate (depending on size), or vice versa, was used. The duration of activity measurement and the conditions under which measurements were taken, and the units of measure were not reported. However, the results showed that arm activity went from 9.13 during pretreatment to 9.36 under placebo to 7.38 under drug ($p < .017$). Ankle activity went from 8.60 during pretreatment to 6.38 during placebo to 5.58 during drug ($p < .054$).

Barkley (1977) placed Timex Motion Recorders on the preferred wrist and ankle of 36 boys aged 5 to 12 years with IQs greater than 80 while they engaged in 6 minutes of free play, watched a 3-minute movie and received a 10-item retention test for 5 more minutes, took 25–30 minutes of structured testing (reaction time, finger tapping, and maze performance), and finally engaged in 6 minutes of restricted play where only one toy type could be used and no floor grid markings could be crossed. Half of the boys were diagnosed as hyperkinetic by pediatricians and placed on 10 to 30 mg of methylphenidate ($M = 18.6$ mg). The other 18 boys were normal children recruited from the same community. All children were tested on three separate occasions 7 to 14 days apart. The first sessions was baseline. The placebo and drug sessions were counterbalanced. Barkley did not report dividing actometer results by minutes of wearing time; hence, the units of measure appear to be AU/duration of the test interval. All significance tests were performed on the natural logarithm of the AU/recording interval data plus 1 to better normalize them. No significant differences in activity for normal children across the three situations were reported nor were their means and standard deviations reported. It was concluded that their activity remained stable across experimental conditions. The following analyses are restricted to hyperactive children.

During free play, the means (and SD) of wrist activity for the hyperactive boys were 412.89 (335.60) during baseline, 555.11 (445.98) during placebo, and 233.00 (185.00) during drug ($F(2,51) = 4.55$, $p < .05$). Only the drug vs placebo comparison was significant ($F(1,34) = 16.89$, $p < .001$). The means (and SD) for ankle activity were 389.72 (457.83) for baseline, 442.22 (626.11) for placebo, and 97.33 (105.11) ($F(2,51) = 5.85$, $p < .01$). Both the baseline vs drug ($F(1,34) = 5.13$, $p < .05$) and the drug vs placebo ($F(1,34) = 12.68$, $p < .001$) comparisons were significant.

While movie watching, the means (and SD) of wrist activity for the hyperactive boys were 107.61 (233.38) during baseline, 114.28 (76.67) during placebo, and 54.00 (38.40) during drug ($F(2,51) = 5.64$, $p < .01$). Only the drug vs placebo ($F(1,34) = 13.94$, $p < .001$) comparison was significant. The means (and SD) for ankle activity were 112.83 (242.75) for baseline, 153.50 (140.57) for placebo, and 78.22 (175.46) for drug ($F(2,51) = 11.56$, $p < .001$). Both the baseline versus placebo ($F(1,34) = 10.28$, $p < .01$) and the drug versus placebo ($F(1,34) = 17.65$, $p < .001$) comparisons were significant.

During testing, the means (and SD) of wrist activity for the hyperactive boys were 213.17 (215.17) during baseline, 242.33 (155.54) during placebo, and 143.39 (86.15) during drug ($F(2,51) = 5.23, p < .01$). Only the drug vs placebo ($F(1,34) = 13.21, p < .001$) comparison was significant. The means (and SD) for ankle activity were 260.89 (426.22) for baseline, 212.44 (178.13) for placebo, and 148.00 (286.22) for drug ($F(2,51) = 5.38, p < .01$). Only the drug versus placebo ($F(1,34) = 9.88, p < .01$) comparison was significant.

During restricted play, the means (and SD) of wrist activity for the hyperactive boys were 397.78 (261.53) during baseline, 412.83 (245.02) during placebo, and 211.83 (185.55) $F(2,51) = 5.24, p < .01$). Both the baseline versus drug ($F(1,34) = 4.43, p < .05$) and the drug vs placebo ($F(1,34) = 9.21, p < .01$) comparisons were significant. The means (and SD) for ankle activity were 215.22 (498.54) for baseline, 396.17 (355.48) for placebo, and 189.00 (245.28) for drug ($F(2,51) = 6.06, p < .01$). Only the drug versus placebo ($F(1,34) = 10.53, p < .01$) comparison was significant.

Average activity was consistently lower during drug administration than placebo or baseline given a significant difference. These results uniformly support the therapeutic effects of methylphenidate in reducing activity of hyperactive children in a variety of situations.

Millichap and Johnston (1977) obtained 45-minute nondominant wrist actigraphy measures in 24 boys and 4 girls aged 5 to 14 years pre- and post-Ritalin treatment. The pretreatment mean of 26.74 AU/min ($S = 17.15$) significantly ($t(27) = 2.14, p < .05$) reduced to 22.17 AU/min ($S = 11.27$). An associated bar graph revealed that 19 of 28 subjects showed activity decreases while the remaining 9 subjects showed activity increases.

Cunningham and Barkley (1978) reported a case study on a pair of twin boys aged 5.5 years. Activity was measured at the right dominant wrist and ankle for 15 minutes of free play and 15 minutes of structured task on four occasions. The authors reported AU/30 minutes; the data that follow have been divided by 30 to achieve the more standard unit of AU/min. The first subject's wrist measured 83.00 AU/min at baseline, dropped to 19.17 AU/min 45 minutes after receiving a 15-mg dose of methylphenidate hydrochloride (Ritalin), returned to 70.00 AU/min while receiving placebo, and dropped to 29.00 AU/min after retaking the same medication. His ankle activity measured 124.83 AU/min during baseline, 6.17 AU/min during the first medication condition, 43.00 AU/min during the placebo condition, and 39.50 during the second medication condition.

The second subject displayed less impressive results. Wrist activity was measured at 151.00 AU/min during baseline, 76.67 AU/min during the first medication condition, but dropped further to 25.50 AU/min during the placebo condition and rose to 81.33 AU/min during the second medication condition. His ankle activity followed suit. His ankle was measured at 246.33 AU/min during baseline, 76.33 AU/min during the first medication condition, 51.33 AU/min during the placebo condition, and 87.00 AU/min during the second medication condition.

Ullman, Barkley, and Brown (1978) investigated the question of whether hyperactive children on drug holiday are measurably more active than control children. They obtained preferred wrist and ankle actometer data from 18 hyperkinetic boys who responded clinically to methylphenidate and 18 control boys with no evidence of hyperactivity. Activity measurements were made during six minutes of free play after a one-day drug washout. The mean wrist activity of 412.89 AU/6 min (S = 335.60) was significantly greater ($F(1,34)$ = 4.60, $p < .05$) than the control mean of 193.77 AU/6 min (S = 184.78). The mean ankle activity of 389.72 AU/6 min (S = 457.83) was not significantly ($F(1,34)$ = 2.92, $p < .10$) different from the control mean of 95.72 AU/6 min (S = 129.26) despite the large numerical difference. Very likely, the extremely short 6-minute measurement period is responsible for the excessive standard deviations resulting in very low statistical power.

Barkley and Cunningham (1979a) studied 20 5-to 12-year-old boys for 15 minutes during free play with their mothers and 15 minutes while engaged in structured tasks with their mothers. The authors' Figure 1 plotted wrist and ankle activity for placebo and drug in AU per 30 minutes. Mean values were estimated using a millimeter rule and converted to AU/min by dividing by 30. Wrist activity was significantly ($t(19)$ = 3.44, $p < .01$) reduced from approximately 53 AU/min during the placebo condition to approximately 25 AU/min during the medication condition. Ankle activity was significantly ($t(19)$ = 4.08, $p < .01$) reduced from approximately 57 AU/min during the placebo condition to approximately 33 AU/min during the medication condition.

Barkley and Cunningham (1979b) placed Timex Model 32 Motion Recorders on the preferred wrist and ankle of 14 hyperactive boys aged 5 to 12 years with IQ of greater than 80 while they played for approximately 10 minutes in a 58 × 48 × 42-ft gym with one glass wall overlooking a tree-shaded lawn. Measurements were taken before and after stimulant medication (methylphenidate) and on placebo.

Off-drug wrist activity averaged 2160 AU per approximately 10 min (S = 956) which we will consider as M = 216.0 AU/min (S = 95.6). Placebo reduced activity to M = 1898 AU/10 min (S = 1363) or M = 189.8 AU/min (S = 136.3). Methylphenidate produced a significant ($t(26)$ = 2.05, $p < .05$) further reduction to M = 1385 AU/10 min (S = 756) or M = 138.5 AU/min (S = 75.6).

The off-drug ankle activity was 3712 AU per approximately 10 minutes (S = 1717), which we will consider as M = 371.2 and S = 171.7 AU/min. Placebo resulted in average ankle activity of 3200 (S = 2340) AU/10 minutes, which we will consider as M = 320.0 and S = 234.0 AU/min. Medication produced a nonsignificant decrease to M = 2776 (S = 1979) AU/10 min or M = 277.6 (S = 197.9) AU/min. Significant results may well have resulted from a somewhat longer measurement period.

Cunningham and Barkley (1979) placed Timex Model 32 Motion Recorders on the preferred wrist and ankle of 20 normal and 20 hyperactive boys aged 5 to 12 years with IQs of at least 80. All hyperactive children were withdrawn from their medication 24 hours before testing, which included 15 minutes of mother–child freeplay in a carpeted 4 × 6.1-m playroom and 15 minutes of structured mother–child interaction involving putting toys away, drawing increasingly complex geometric figures, doing a page of mathematic problems, and constructing two preschool puzzles. Activity was measured across the entire 30-minute session.

The mean wrist actometer score of 1982 AU/30 minutes = 60.07 AU/min for hyperactive children was significantly different from ($t(38) = 2.53$, $p < .02$), and nearly double that of the mean wrist actometer score for normal children of 973 AU/30 minutes = 32.43 AU/min. Personal communication from Russell A. Barkley indicates that the standard deviations of the hyperactive and control groups' wrist activity were 56.62 and 18.18 AU/min respectively.

The mean ankle actometer score of 2345 AU/30 minutes = 78.17 AU/min was significantly different from ($t(38) = 2.45$, $p < .02$), and more than double that of, the mean ankle actometer score for normal children of 1008 AU/30 min = 33.6 AU/min. Personal communication from Russell A. Barkley indicates that the standard deviations of the hyperactive and control groups' wrist activity were 78.72 and 20.94 AU/min respectively.

Rogers and Hughs (1981) obtained dominant wrist actometer data from nine boys aged 4 to 11 years and one 7-year-old girl from 1600 to 1800 hours five days per week for 3 weeks pre and post 6 weeks of Feingold's (1975) K-P diet or a control diet that reduced sugar intake but did not restrict substances in the K-P diet. The pretreatment mean (and standard deviation) wrist activity for the experimental subjects was 168.00 AU/min ($S = 35.22$) and for the control subjects was 155.35 AU/min ($S = 30.15$). These pretreatment means were not significantly different ($t(4) = 0.81$, N.S.). The posttreatment mean for the experimental subjects decreased 70.5 AU/min to 97.50 AU/min ($S = 21.03$) whereas the posttreatment mean for the control subjects decreased but 8.08 AU/min to 147.27 AU/min ($S = 31.72$). The difference between the posttreatment means was significant ($t(4) = 2.16$, $p < .05$).

Tilt Counters

Foster, Kupfer, Weiss, Lipponen, McPartland, and Delgado (1972) described an activity sensory constructed from a small ferromagnetic ball rolling in a wire-wrapped tube sensitive to a 5-degree tilt from the horizontal plane. Foster, McPartland, and Kupfer (1977) report their first use of this device with children. They measured the dominant and nondominant wrist plus ankle activity of 21 normal children (14 male, 7 female; 11 black, 10 white) for 20 minutes during psychological testing and for 10 minutes of free play in the playroom of the Pittsburgh child Guidance Center. The results indicated that higher ankle activity indicated more neurologic "soft" signs ($r(19) = .53$, $p < .01$), lower school achievement ($r(19) = -.67$, $p < .01$), and more self-deprecatory estimate of the child's own intelligence

$(r(19) = .46, p < .05)$. No significant correlations were obtained with either wrist activity measurement.

Williamson, Calpin, DiLorenzo, Garris, and Petti (1981) placed a mercury switch-based activity monitor (cf. Foster, McPartland, and Kupfer, 1978) on the right (nondominant) wrist of a 9-year 9-month-old white male whose hyperactivity was sufficient to cause other children to avoid him. He wore this device during all waking hours. An ankle monitor was worn on days 54–82. The research design involved baseline (A1), dexedrine (B1), baseline (A2), dexedrine (B2), dexedrine and instructions (B & C), dexedrine, instructions, and guided practice (B, C, and D), dexedrine, instructions, guided practice, feedback and reinforcement (B, C, D, and E). The results indicated that dexedrine did not noticeably alter either wrist or ankle activity. However, activity feedback and reinforcement reduced arm and leg activity from 40 to 87% below baseline levels. Feedback involved showing the subject how to check the activity monitor. His checking behavior was restricted to 4–5 times per half-hour.

Pedometers

Barkley and Ullman (1975) placed pedometers in small elastic pockets and attached them to the wrists and ankles of 16 hyperactive and 16 control boys aged 4 to 12 years just above where actometers were attached. Data were recorded during a 15-minute free-play and during a 5-minute test period; order was randomized. While wrist actometer scores significantly discriminated between the two groups, none of the pedometer results did. It should be mentioned that this was a highly unusual application of pedometers. Rapoport, Abrahamson, Alexander, and Lott (1971) also failed to find significant results.

Stabilimeters

Normal Children

The crib is the normal habitat for infants and consequently crib stabilimeters are appropriate to the study of early activity patterns. Plus, they are noninvasive and thereby unlikely to influence the behavior being measured.

Irwin (1932) presented data on 73 full-term infants from birth until day 16. One subject was followed until day 32. The infants were fed at 1400 and 1800 hours and activity was monitored from 1430 until 1745 hours; in between feedings. The data were tabulated as counts per 15-minute period. The means (and standard deviations) for the first, middle (7th), and last (13th) period are: 17.2 (20.2), 26.6 (40.4), and 49.1 (59.7) indicating a monotonic increase in activity from the end of one feeding to the beginning of the next.

The above result occurred despite a bimodal activity distribution. Activity did increase for 49 (67%) of the infants. Their first and third means (and standard deviations) were 16.2 (21.9) and 66.4 (42.6). The first and third means (and standard deviations) for the other 24 (33%) of the infants were 21.2 (22.3) and 6.9 (13.5). Hence, a minority of infants decrease activity in between feedings whereas the majority increase activity.

Campbell, Kuyek, Lang, and Partington (1971) studied infant boys and 29 infant girls 24 hours each day for the first 4 days of life. The average counts per minute for the first day were 4.07. This increased to 6.10 on the second day, 6.87 on the third day, and 8.23 on the fourth day. These results parallel the actometer data presented by the same authors (reviewed above) showing increasing activity over the first four days of life.

Sander and Julia (1966) reported 24-hour stabilimeter data on 9 infants during the first 3.5 days in hospital and for 5 subsequent days at home after discharge. Their Figure 2 shows activity increasing up until discharge as did Campbell *et al.* (1971). Activity dramatically decreased upon discharge to home and remained low for the remainder of the study. These data are also consistent with actometer data presented by Campbell *et al.* (1971).

Brackbill (1971) investigated the responsivity of infants to environmental stimuli. Twenty-four full-term clinically normal infants (9 boys, 15 girls) of median age 26.58 days ($S = 3.65$; range $= 19-33$) were stimulated in one, two, three, or all four of the following ways. Auditory stimulation was provided by an 85-dB tape-recorded heartbeat played against an ambient 65 dB background. Visual stimulation consisted of a 400-watt light versus 50-watt control condition. Proprioceptive-tactile stimulation was accomplished by tightly swaddling the child from neck to toes with long narrow strips of flannel cloth. Thermal stimulation was 31°C vs control temperature of 25.5°C.

Baseline activity in the absence of the aforementioned stimuli was 9.63 counts per minute (cpm). Infants were lying quietly in a sound-attenuated booth after having been fed. No information was given about the length of testing. Any single stimulus increased activity to approximately 10.70 cpm. Further stimulation reduced activity. Any two stimuli reduced activity to approximately 7.54 cpm, any three stimuli to 5.98 cpm, and all four stimuli further reduced activity to 2.96 cpm.

Partington, Lang, and Campbell (1971) tested stabilimetric reactivity of 136 newborn infants to pure 400-Hz 10-second tones beginning at an intensity of 65 dB and increasing in 5-dB steps until "startle was evoked." (p. 96) A correlation of $\rho = .804$, $p < .001$ was obtained between the time to settle down after startle and baseline activity. More active children took longer to settle down. The time to settle down was also directly proportional to the length of the startle response ($\rho = .311$, $p < .01$). Higher activity during startle predicted longer time to settle down ($\rho = .211$, $p < .01$). No sex differences in response by boys and girls was found. This result is consistent with previous research by Campbell (1968).

Partington, Campbell, Kuyek, and Mehlomakulu (1971) reported activity data on 5 premature infants with transient neonatal tyrosinaemia and 3 premature infants without this disorder. This common condition of premature infants fed high protein diets is characterized by elevated blood tyrosine levels and tyrosine metabolites in the urine. They twice weekly placed the infants in a stabilimetric crib for 3 hours after feeding for the duration of their hospital stay. The authors reported that tyrosinaemia decreases both the frequency and intensity of activity bursts.

Juliano (1974) measured activity in 80 normal school children aged 8.5 to 11.25 years using a stabilimetric cushion described by Sprague and Toppe (1966) while they took the Matching Familiar Figures Test (MFFT) (Kagan, 1966). Their subjects averaged 5.02 counts per minute with a standard deviation of 3.66 cpm.

Hyperkinetic Children

Juliano (1974) further reported data on 40 children aged 8.5 to 11.25 years judged to be hyperactive. The counts per minute obtained by these children while taking the MFFT was 10.04 with a standard deviation of 4.98 cpm ($t(118) = 1.21$, N.S.)

Sprague, Barnes, and Werry (1970) measured activity in 12 emotionally disturbed underachieving boys who were placed in a special education class because of hyperactivity. The subjects sat at a console on a stabilimetric cushion (Sprague and Toppe, 1966) and were reinforced with M & Ms for correctly determining if two projected images were the same or different. Two adaptation sessions were followed by the data recording session. Subjects were given methylphenidate, thioridazine, or placebo and retesting done perhaps 1.5 hours later. Each subject was given a different treatment on a different day. Results showed a significant medication effect on activity ($F(2,22) = 5.95$, $p < .01$). Their Figure 1 indicated lower activity on methylphenidate than on thioridazine or placebo.

Sykes, Douglas, Weiss, and Minde (1971) obtained stabilimetric cushion (Sprague and Toppe, 1966) data from 19 hyperactive children aged 5 to 12 years ($M = 8$ years, $S = 1$ year, 9 mo) and 19 age, sex, and IQ matched normal children. Stabilimetric cushion data were collected during the administration of the Continuous Performance Test (CPT). The hyperactive children were medicated with methylphenidate and both groups were retested 5 to 7 weeks later. The results indicated a significant groups effect for the first ($F(1,36) = 6.84$, $p < .05$) and second ($F(1,36) = 192.27$, $p < .001$) testing with the hyperactive group being more active both times. A significant groups by session effect ($F(1.36) = 7.81$, $p < .01$) indicated a greater activity *increase* from the first to the second session in hyperactive than control children. However, medication did significantly reduce errors on the CPT.

Werry and Aman (1975) obtained stabilimetric data on 20 boys and 4 girls aged 4 years 11 months to 12 years 4 months ($M = 7$ years 9 months) with IQs from 70 to 130 ($M = 100.7$) while they participated in a double-blind placebo-controlled crossover study to evaluate methylphenidate hydrochloride (0.3 mg/kg) and haloperidol (0.025 mg/kg or 0.050 mg/kg) for three weeks with 2-day washout periods in between medications. Stabilimetric counts per minute while taking a short term memory test were 147.0 under placebo, 78.9 under methylphenidate, 120.3 under low haloperidol dose and 148.8 under high haloperidol dose. These means were reported to be significantly different ($p < .05$) with the source of the effect being the superiority of methylphenidate over placebo and high haloperidol dose. No significant effects were found for stabilimetric data while taking the Continuous Performance Test.

Barkley (1977), using a stabilimetric platform (Lafayette Instrument Company) measured seat activity of 36 boys aged 5 to 12 years with IQs greater than 80 while they watched a 3-minute movie, received a 10-item retention test for 5 more minutes, and took 25–30 minutes of structured testing (reaction time, finger tapping, and maze performance). Half of the boys were diagnosed as hyperkinetic by pediatricians and placed on 10 to 30 mg of methylphenidate ($M = 18.6$ mg). The other 18 boys were normal children recruited from the same community. All children were tested on three separate occasions 7 to 14 days apart. The first session was baseline. The placebo and drug sessions were counterbalanced. All significance tests were performed on the natural logarithm of the seat counts plus 1 to better normalize them. No significant differences in activity for normal children across the three situations were reported nor were their means and standard deviations reported. It was concluded that their activity remained stable across experimental conditions. The following analyses are restricted to hyperactive children.

During movie watching, the mean (and standard deviation) of seat activity was 113.94 (145.53) during baseline, 157.67 (134.11) during placebo, and 64.72 (56.26) during drug ($F(2,51) = 9.55$, $p < .01$). Both the baseline vs placebo ($F(1,34) = 7.03$, $p < .05$) and the drug vs placebo ($F(1,34) = 30.32$, $p < .001$) comparisons were significant.

During testing, the mean (and standard deviation) of seat movement was 322.89 (361.72) during baseline, 213.00 (166.78) during placebo, and 168.78 (145.04) during drug ($F(2,51) = 2.31$, N.S.). Methylphenidate significantly reduced seat activity while watching a movie but not during test taking although the means were in the predicted direction and substantial differences were present.

Retarded Children

McConnell, Cromwell, Bialer, and Son (1964) seated 57 profoundly to mildly retarded children aged 6 years 2 months to 15 years 1 month ($M = 11$ years 9 months) in a chair placed on a ballistographic platform suspended by cables, functioning as a stabilimeter. Activity was measured over a 4-minute period while the subject was left to sit alone in a bare testing room. Subjects were divided into two groups on the basis of baseline readings taken once per week for 3 weeks. A triple-blind experimental design tested the effects of placebo, 7.5 mg dexedrine and 15 mg dexedrine for 6 consecutive days with a 1-day washout in between medications. The sequence was randomly determined for each subject and neither the subject, the rater, nor the experimenter knew which condition was in effect until the study ended.

The results for the more active subjects were 6528 counts per 4 minutes during placebo, 6999 counts per 4 minutes for 7.5 mg dexedrine, and 6838 counts per 4 minutes for 15 mg dexedrine. Opposite results were found for the less active subjects. They displayed 4095 counts per 4 minutes under placebo, 3939 counts per 4 minutes under 7.5 mg dexedrine, and 3594 counts per 4 minutes under 15 mg dexedrine. These changes were *not* found to be statistically significant.

Christensen (1975) investigated the modifiability of hyperactivity in 16 hyperactive institutionalized persons (10 males; 6 females) aged 9 to 15.8 years ($M = 11.8$) with IQs ranging from 31 to 68 ($M = 51$). Seat activity was sequentially sampled across two pairs of subjects from a stabilimetric cushion (Sprague and Toppe, 1966) resulting in 10 minutes of seat activity per subject per class period. The experimental design entailed 2 weeks of baseline, 4 weeks of behavior modification, a 2-week reversal, followed by 4 more weeks of behavior modification. Complete data were obtained from 13 subjects. The data indicated a significant effect of activity in the expected direction ($F(5,55) = 7.39, p < .001$).

Edelson and Sprague (1974) obtained stabilimetric data from 16 highly active educable mentally retarded (mean IQ = 67, mean mental age = 7.7 years) boys aged 12.7 years. After 2 days of baseline, subjects were randomly assigned to one of two experimental orders: 1, activity increase followed by activity decrease, or 2, activity decrease followed by activity increase. Reinforcement clearly influenced seat activity in the predicted direction.

SITUATIONAL VS PERVASIVE HYPERACTIVITY

Hyperactive children are said to have great difficulty learning ground rules for a new activity and then adjusting to them (Whalen, Henker, Collins, and Finck, 1979). This difficulty adapting to new situational demands is particularly apparent when changing settings. They change more readily from a formal to an informal situation than the reverse (Jacob, O'Leary, and Rosenblad, 1978).

The literature on hyperactivity supports two perspectives. First, and perhaps most popularly, hyperactive children are thought to be pervasively hyperactive meaning that they are overactive in all situations. Second, hyperactive children are thought to be hyperactive only in certain situations; ones that require them to be still, be quiet, and pay attention to another person such as a teacher. We now review the support for each position. DSM-III-R reflects both of these perspectives when discussing 314.01 Attention-Deficit Hyperactivity Disorder (ADHD): "Manifestations of the disorder usually appear in most situations, including at home, in school, at work, and in social situations but to varying degrees. Some people, however, show signs of the disorder in only one setting, such as at home or at school. Symptoms typically worsen in situations requiring sustained attention, such as listening to a teacher in a classroom, attending meetings, or doing class assignments or chores at home" (p. 50).

Situational Hyperactivity

This position holds that hyperactive children, like normal children, are more active in some situations than others and that they can behave within normal limits under certain circumstances. The most persuasive evidence that could be marshalled for this position would be to show a group-by-situation interaction showing a significant and substantial difference between hyperactive and control children in some situations and no difference in other situations. If the activity of all hyperactive children decreased by a sizable constant such that the least active hyperactive child was now very slightly more active than the most active control subject, the required interaction could be significant, yet the mean for hyperactive children would be significantly greater than the mean for control children. Such a result would show situational responsivity by hyperactive children but the person factor, relative position within the overall distribution, would remain prominent thereby implicating factors beyond current situational demands. Compelling data of these sorts is currently unavailable but perhaps will be sought by future investigators.

Zentall and Zentall (1976) demonstrated that hyperactive children are not equally active in all situations. They attached actometers to the dominant wrist and ipsilateral ankle of 16 children 7- to 11-year-olds classified as hyperactive based upon the Rating Scale for Hyperactivity (Davids, 1971) and the Conners' Teacher Rating Scale (Conners, 1969). All children were asked to wait for 10 minutes and then circle specified letters on a printed page for 10 minutes under high- and low-stimulus conditions. The low-stimulus condition involved white walls, a gray floor, and a 25-watt lamp over a desk. The high-stimulus condition involved playing Led Zeppelin's *House of the Holy* at 75 dB, a cage with 5 mice on the wall 2 m in front of the desk, and 25 colorful posters, pictures, and signs posted on the wall. Results indicated significantly less wrist ($F(1,14) = 23.24, p < .001$) and ankle ($F(1,14) = 9.88, p < .01$) activity during the high-stimulus vs low-stimulus waiting condition. Significantly less wrist ($F(1,14) = 8.96, p < .01$) but not ankle ($F(1,14) = 0.95$, N.S.) activity occurred during the high-stimulus vs low-stimulus letter circling condition. The question of whether activity was reduced to within normal limits was not considered.

Moreland (1977) demonstrated that seat activity is modifiable by contingent access to cartoons. He selected a 4-year-old hyperactive male child and measured seat activity with a stabilimeter while watching cartoons on TV once a week for 20 minutes over an 8-week baseline period. Treatment over the following 8 weeks entailed terminating a cartoon TV show when activity exceeded the median baseline activity rate during the first treatment week. The criterion was reduced by two switch-closures per second every other week thereafter. Regression results indicated a significant ($p < .005$) reduction in seat activity. The question of whether activity had been reduced to that of children not considered hyperactive was not addressed.

Pervasive Hyperactivity

Children are said to be pervasively hyperactive when they are more active than normal control children in all situations. Situational effects are allowed but subjects are expected to retain their rank order position regardless of situation. That is, the most active child during academic periods is expected to be the most active during free play. Said otherwise, most of the variance is expected to be due to person characteristics.

Pinto and Tryon (1990a) sought to help clarify whether or not hyperactive children are pervasively or situationally disordered. Four hundred and fifty boys were rated on Factor IV of the Conners' Teacher Rating Scale (CTRS) (Conners, 1969). Sixty boys were selected from this initial sample and three groups of subjects were formed. The age range of all subjects was six to twelve years ($M = 9.67$; $S = 1.62$); they were in grades one to six. The Clinically Hyperactive children ($n = 22$) scored 2 or more standard deviations above the normative mean of 0.70 ($S = 0.78$) on hyperactivity Factor IV (Goyette, Conners, and Ulrich, 1978). The Mildly Hyperactive children ($n = 7$) obtained scores of less than 2 but more than 1 standard deviations. The Normal Control children ($n = 31$) scored less than 1 standard deviation above the normative Factor IV mean on the CTRS. These selected subjects were further rated by the same teachers on the Motor Excess scale of the Revised Behavior Problem Checklist (RBPC) (Quay and Peterson, 1983) and on the Teacher Report Form (TRF) (Edelbrock and Achenbach, 1984) to confirm group assignment.

Physical activity (steps) was measured by electronic step counter (Free Style USA®; available through L. L. Bean, Inc.). This step counter was reported by the manufacturers to record walking with 97% accuracy and running with 99% accuracy.

Prior to data collection, every subject was taken on a standard one-mile walk wearing an electronic step counter. Subjects walked a measured half-mile distance away from the school in groups of two to four along with an investigator. The number of steps taken were recorded from the step counter as Walk-I. Then all subjects walked the same distance back to the school, whereupon the number of steps taken was recorded as Walk-II. These data provided a test–retest measure of person–instrument reliability plus a method of converting steps into miles walked by each subject. The conversion factor (K) is the sum of steps taken on both measured half-mile walks; the number of steps taken by the particular subject in question while walking one mile. Subsequent recorded step measures were converted into miles by dividing step totals by this K factor.

Subjects wore a digital electronic step counter at the waist for two weeks (14 days, i.e., 10 school days and two weekends = 4 days) and recorded readings at specified intervals. Readings were taken from the 8-digit LED display (LD) on the step counter. There was no need to reset counters as they were capable of counting up to 100 million steps thus allowing one to count 20,000 steps per day for 13.69 years.

Electronic step counters were worn by all subjects before they started to school. The parents recorded the steps displayed on the LCD panel as well as the time of the day, to the nearest minute, when the boys left home for school. As soon as they entered their respective classrooms (home room), their teachers recorded the number of steps taken to that point in time plus the time of the day to the nearest minute. Recordings were made by teachers before and after each specified school period required for the study, as well as just before the boys left the school to go home.

The parents/guardians recorded step counter readings and time of day to the nearest minute when the boys arrived home from school. They also made sure that their children wore the step counter before they went to school each of the 10 study days as well as on two weekends. The boys continued to wear the step counter after school hours up until bedtime, when parents/guardians again recorded the number of steps taken and the time of day to the nearest minute.

Six "in-school" situations (Mathematics, Reading, Language, Writing, Lunch hour, and Free play) and four "out-of-school" situations (Home-to-school transit, School-to-home transit, Home, and Weekends) were selected for study.

The activity data were transformed by taking their square root to better approximate a normal distribution. As expected by the situational hypothesis, activity during Reading correlated $r(58) = .37$, $p < .01$ during Week 1 and $r(58) = .53$, $p < .01$ during Week 2 with Factor IV CTRS ratings. Activity during Writing class correlated $r(58) = .38$, $p < .05$ during Week 1 and $r(58) = .34$, $p < .01$ during Week 2. However, activity during Mathematics periods was not significantly correlated ($r(58) = .23$, N.S.) with Factor IV CTRS during Week 1 but was so during Week 2 ($r(58) = .36$, $p < .01$). Measured activity significantly correlated with RBPC activity ratings in all four academic periods during both Weeks 1 and 2. Measured activity significantly correlated with TRF ratings in Language and Writing classes. These results are also expected by the pervasive-activity hypothesis.

The two hypotheses make differential predictions for the informal periods. Here the situational hypothesis presumes no significant differences thereby obviating a relationship between teacher ratings and measured activity. However, measured activity during Lunch correlated $r(58) = .30$ with Factor IV CTRS during Week 1 and $r(58) = .53$, $p < .01$ during Week 2. Activity during Free play correlated $r(58) = .78$, $p < .01$ during Week 1 and $r(58) = .29$, $p < .05$ during

Week 2. Activity during Home-to-school correlated $r(58) = .10$, N.S. during Week 1 and $r(58) = .08$, N.S. during Week 2. Activity during School-to-home correlated $r(58) = .47$, $p < .01$ during Week 1 and $r(58) = .37$, $p < .01$ during Week 2. Activity at Home correlated $r(58) = .42$, $p < .01$ during Week 1 and $r(58) = .50$, $p < .01$ during Week 2. Activity over the Weekend correlated $r(58) = .32$, $p < .01$ during Week 1 and $r(58) = .27$, $p < .05$ during Week 2. These results strongly favor the pervasive-hyperactivity hypothesis.

VALIDITY AND LIMITS OF RATING SCALES

Diagnosis of hyperactivity by means of ratings scales has a long history. The Hyperactivity Factor of the Conners' Teacher Rating Scale (CTRS) has been frequently used in studies seeking to distinguish hyperactive from normoactive children (Sprague and Sleator, 1973; Douglas, Parry, Marton and Garson, 1976). The efficacy of this scale for assessing and diagnosing hyperactive children in classroom settings has been illustrated by many investigators (e.g., Halverson and Waldrop, 1973; Douglas, Parry, Marton, and Garson, 1976; Kupeitz, Bialer, and Winsberg, 1972; Sprague, Christensen, and Werry, 1974; Sprague and Sleator, 1973; Buss, Block, and Block, 1980; Kendall and Brophy, 1981; Trites, Blouin, Ferguson, and Lynch, 1981).

Actometers

Eaton and Dureski (1986) compared measured and rated activity in two samples of infants. In Study 1 actometers (Timex Model 108 Motion Recorders) were attached to both wrists and ankles of 46 infants (24 males, 22 female) aged 13.1 to 21.4 weeks ($M = 16.8$) with velcro fasteners. Measurements were made for 30 minutes in the baby's home at a time when they were reported to be awake and alert. The correlation of composite (average) actometer measurements and the Activity scale of the Infant Behavior Questionnaire (IBQ) (Rothbart, 1981) was low and nonsignificant ($r(43) = .05$, $p = .73$). Such a result is expected 73% of the time by chance alone.

In Study 2, the IBQ Activity Scale was completed by the caregiver concerning the previous 24-hour behavior of 50 (28 males; 22 females) aged 11.9 to 20.1 weeks ($M = 15.7$ weeks) infants. Thirty-minute composite actometer scores correlated $r(48) = -.04$, N.S. with the 24-hour IBQ Activity Scale and $r(48) = .00$, N.S. with the standard IBQ Activity Scale.

The major factor limiting these relationships is probably the small behavioral sample. A full 24-hour behavioral sample or better yet a two-week behavioral sample may yield higher correlations with rated behavior.

Step Counters

Pinto and Tryon (1990b) investigated the interrelations among three activity rating scales and the correlations of each with measured activity. The rating scales were the Conners' Teacher Rating Scale (CTRS) (Conners, 1969), Revised Behavior Problem Checklist (RBPC) (Quay and Peterson, 1987) and Teacher Report Form (TRF) (Achenbach and Edelbrock, 1986). Activity was measured with Free Style USA℠ step counters obtained from L.L. Bean, Inc.. The procedures were the same as described above regarding Pinto and Tryon (1990a).

The results indicated significant and substantial relationships among all three rating scales. The hyperactivity Factor IV score on the CTRS correlated $r(58) = .89$, $p < .001$ with RBPC and $r(58) = .79$, $p < .001$ with TRF, and RBPC correlated $r(58) = .79$, $p < .001$ with TRF. These results indicate that teachers can consistently rate children.

The second purpose of the present research was to determine the extent to which rated activity correlated with measured activity. Teacher ratings on the CTRS, RBPC, and TRF are significantly and substantially correlated with measured activity during Weeks 1 and 2 (CTRS; $r(58) = .46$, $p < .01$ and $r(58) = .55$, $p < .01$: RBPC; $r(58) = .44$, $p < .01$ and $r(58) = .58$, $p < .01$: TRF: $r(58) = .32$, $p < .05$ and $r(58) = .44$, $p < .01$). A t-test for two dependent correlations (Hinkle, Wiersma, and Jurs, 1979, pp. 278–280) revealed no significant differences in the Week 1 and 2 correlations for any of the three rating scales. This is partly due to the Week 1 vs Week 2 reliability of behavioral measurements (steps per hour), which was found to be $r(58) = 0.74$, $p < .0001$.

The foregoing group data validate the use of rating scales by accepted standards. However, subject-by-subject analysis reveals the presence of substantial problems that derive from the $1 - r^2$ aspect of the above results. Two principle discrepancies were found between rated and measured data. The more important problem occurred where a child was labeled as clinically hyperactive but was not measurably so. It was found that 14 (63.6%) of the children rated as clinically hyperactive were *less* active than the most active child rated as being normal. That these mistakes are confined to the upper half of the normal distribution is supported by the finding that none of the children rated as clinically hyperactive were less active than the average child rated as normal.

The opposite discrepancy is less of a clinical problem but still disturbing. Eight (25.8%) of the children rated as normal were found to be more active than the least active child rated as clinically hyperactive. Why are these measurably active children not identified by teachers? That no child rated as normal was found to exceed the mean of children rated as clinically hyperactive shows that these discrepancies are limited to the lower half of the clinical distribution.

It is important to remember than the rating categories of normal and clinically hyperactive were not contiguous but were separated by a third group of mildly hyperactive children. This considerably augments the clinical importance of the above-mentioned discrepancies. The strong implication of these findings is that clinicians should routinely seek a "second opinion," by obtaining behavioral measurements, before rendering a firm diagnostic impression of hyperactivity. The lack of standardized norms can be circumvented by obtaining data on either another sibling or classmate for whom no question of hyperactivity exists. Practitioners can also refer to data collected on other hyperactive children they have measured.

Activity and Eating Disorders

DSM-III-R (APA, 1987) subdivides eating disorders into: 1) Anorexia Nervosa, 2) Bulimia Nervosa, 3) Pica, and 4) Rumination Disorder of Infancy. The first two disorders are considered to be related by DSM-III-R and will be treated as such below. Obesity is not even listed in the index of DSM-III-R let alone considered as an eating disorder but is covered in this chapter for two reasons. First, obesity represents an excess of energy consumption over expenditure whereas anorexia involves an excess of energy expenditure over consumption. Second, there is no better place for the topic of obesity and its relationship to activity in this book.

ANOREXIA NERVOSA

Criteria A for DSM-III-R Anorexia Nervosa (307.10) entail "Refusal to maintain body weight over a minimal normal weight for age and height, e.g., weight loss leading to maintenance of body weight 15% below that expected; or failure to make expected weight gain during period of growth, leading to body weight 15% below that expected." (p. 67) Extensive exercise is thought to supplement reduction of food intake to achieve weight loss. Activity measurements are conspicuously absent from the anorexia nervosa literature despite the central role activity is thought to play in patients' maintenance of weight loss. No published outpatient activity measurements have been located to date.

Pedometers

Blinder, Freeman, and Stunkard (1970) treated three consecutive anorexia nervosa patients on an inpatient psychiatric unit of a university hospital as part of a larger study. The ages of the three patients were 22, 15, and 20 years respectively.

Their pretreatment weights were 89.5, 91.0, and 63.5 lbs, respectively, with a mean of 81.3 lbs. Their percent weight loss was 31, 29, and 63 respectively with a mean of 41%. Unlimited passes were available during the first portion of hospitalization. The result was that all three subjects walked an average of 6.8 miles per day. Patient 1 was reported to have walked 8.5 miles per day. Stunkard (1960) reported that normal-weight women living in the nearby community walked an average of 4.9 miles per day.

Tilt Counters

Foster and Kupfer (1975) obtained nocturnal (2100–0700 hrs) wrist activity counts from a 17-year-old female during her 122-day hospitalization. They reported a significant correlation between activity and weight during an 85-day no-medication baseline ($r(83) = .77, p < .001$). Greater activity was predictive of weight gain. Administration of 200 to 800 mg/day of chlorpromazine hydrochloride changed the aforementioned positive correlation into a significant negative one ($r(33) = -.76, p < .001$). Greater activity is now predictive of weight loss. The extent to which this drug effect was mediated through appetite disturbance is unclear.

Of special clinical interest is the report by Foster and Kupfer (1975) that " . . . frequent, aperiodic, highly charged family visits produced pronounced activity changes." (p. 21)

Actometers

Falk, Halmi, and Tryon (1985) obtained 24-hour wrist and ankle activity measurements, using Timex Model 108 Motion Recorders, from 20 hospitalized female anorectics during the first two weeks (14 consecutive days) of hospitalization. Their ages ranged from 13 to 32 years with an average of 21.1 years ($S = 5.6$ years). At Day 1, subjects' weight averaged 75.38% of target weight. My first impression upon seeing low activity upon admission was that these subjects were depressed. This perception was supported by a significant negative correlation between Hamilton Depression Ratings and wrist activity on Days 2 ($r(18) = -.535$, $p < .05$) and 5 ($r(18) = -.513, p < .05$). Perhaps their inactivity was partly due to their lack of nourishment. Scrimshaw and Pollitt (1984) note that "It has long been recognized that malnourished children are apathetic and less active than well nourished children." (p. ix) Durnin (1984) further indicates that "At energy balances where body mass is either very small or very large, physical activity is usually low." (p. 101) A further reason for their inactivity is that no off-ward passes were available as was the case for Blinder, Freeman, and Stunkard (1970).

Body weight steadily increased over the two-week study period as indicated by a significant correlation ($r(12) = .991, p < .01$) between body weight and time. Wrist activity ($r(12) = .808, p < .01$) and ankle activity ($r(12) = .747, p < .01$)

also consistently increased with time. This pattern led to significant correlations between wrist ($r(12) = .811, p < .01$) and ankle ($r(12) = .760, p < .01$) activity and percent target weight. As subjects became more well nourished, they became increasingly active.

Administration of cyproheptadine hydrochloride to 7 subjects on days 8 to 14 significantly reduced activity as reflected by the correlation between a drug vs no drug code and wrist activity controlling for percent of target weight and time of $r(12) = -.878, p < .01$. The negative sign reflects coding no drug $= 0$ and drug $= 1$. Ankle activity was also suppressed by cyproheptadine hydrochloride ($r(12) = -.527, p < .06$). Amitriptyline hydrochloride suppressed neither wrist ($r(12) = -.342$, N.S.) nor ankle ($r(12) = -.016$, N.S.) activity.

The three patients reported by Blinder, Freeman, and Stunkard (1970) were about as underweight as the 14 patients studied by Falk, Halmi, and Tryon (1985). The primary difference seems to be that Blinder et al. gave unlimited access to passes allowing patients to leave the ward whereas Halmi et al. did not. Perhaps Halmi et al. did not observe hyperactivity during the initial hospitalization period because patients were restricted to the ward. Activity restriction may have produced depression that gradually reduced during their hospitalization. Second, Blinder et al. used pedometers whereas Halmi et al. used wrist and ankle pedometers. Because ankle actometers would have detected the same events as actometers, this methodological difference seems incapable of explaining the different results. Future investigators should compare activity during pass availability with pass unavailability.

Stabilimeters

Crisp and Stonehill (1971) studied nocturnal motility in 10 hospitalized (sex unspecified) patients undergoing bedrest, chlorpromazine, psychotherapy, and 3000 calorie per day "normal" diet. Their average age was 22 years ($S = 4$ years). Motility measurements were taken for the last 3 nights of the 5-night period before and after treatment. As their average weight increased from 39.9 kg to 54.4 kg ($p < .001$), their average total sleep time increased from 6 hours, 32 minutes to 7 hours, 35 minutes ($p < .01$) and total time spent awake in bed decreased from an average of 127.5 minutes to 77.5 minutes ($p < .02$).

OBESITY

Jeffrey and Katz (1977) estimate that between 40 and 80 million Americans are obese. Stewart and Brook (1983) studied 5817 Americans aged 14 to 61 years and found 10% of them to be moderately overweight and 12% to be severely overweight. Estimates of the prevalence of obesity range from 15 to 50% of adults (cf. Bray and Gray, 1988; Van Itallie, 1985).

A comprehensive discussion of obesity definitions and assessments is beyond the scope of this book and is available elsewhere (cf. Straw and Rogers, 1985; Bray, 1986; Garrow, 1986; Katch and McArdle, 1988, pp. 137–153). Bray (1976) indicates that women with more than 30% body fat and men with more than 25% body fat can be considered obese. Although height/weight charts have routinely been used, Body Mass Index (BMI), also known as Quetelet's Index, provides a better measure for reasons we shall shortly mention. It is calculated by dividing weight in kg (1 lb = .45359237 kg) by height in meters (1 in = 2.54 cm = 0.0254 m). Garrow (1981) suggested that the upper desirable limit of BMI for men and women is 25. He indicated that Grade I obesity exists between BMI of 25 and 29.9, Grade II obesity exists between BMI of 30 and 40, and Grade III obesity exists over BMI of 40. Bray (1986) indicates that overweight corresponds to BMI of from 25 to 30 kg/m^2 and obesity exists above 30 kg/m^2 where "skin-fold measures almost always confirm the presence of obesity." (p. 4) Bray reports that BMI consistently correlates between 0.7 and 0.8 with adiposity measures (Bray, 1986; p. 3). Garrow and Webster (1985) obtained an average "gold" standard of body fat from body density, total body water, and total body potassium measurements in 104 women and 24 men aged 16 to 64 years and regressed them against BMI, which they call Quetelet's Index in honor of the famous anthropometrist who observed that W/H^2 is constant across people of normal build. They reported that fat, in kilograms, (F) is highly predictable ($r(102) = .955, p < .0001$) in women using the following formula: F = $(0.713 \text{ W/H}^2 - 9.74) \text{ H}^2$. Fat in kilograms for men is also highly predictable ($r(22) = 0.943, p < .0001$) using the following formula: F = $(0.715 \text{ W/H}^2 - 12.1) \text{ H}^2$. The errors of prediction of the average body density, body water, and body potassium values from BMI is not much greater than when any one of the three gold standards is used to estimate the others. The much greater ease of calculating BMI clearly outweighs the slightly less accurate kilogram-of-fat estimates. One cautionary note: substantial errors result when predictions are made for muscular athletes and elderly persons.

Rosenbaum, Skinner, Knight, and Garrow (1985) report BMI distributions for 10,000 men and women. They report that 34% of men and 24% of women have BMI between 25.0 − 29.9; 6% of men and 8% of women have BMI between 30–40. About 0.1% of men and 0.3% of women have BMI greater than 40. By deduction, 59.9% of men and 67.7% of women have BMI less than 25.

Bray (1978) indicates that health risks associated with overweight begin as BMI exceeds 30 and continues without showing signs of leveling off. BMI greater than 40 constitutes a major risk factor for coronary disease comparable to heavy smoking, hypertension, and hypercholesterolemia.

Activity

It has long been suspected that inactivity contributes to obesity (Johnson, Burke, and Mayer, 1956; Mayer, Roy, and Mitra, 1956; Thompson, Jarvie, Lahey, and Cureton, 1962; Brownell and Stunkard, 1980; Brownell and Wadden, 1986; Stern and Lowney, 1986). Interview and self-report activity measures contain uncertain, and probably large, measurement errors thereby obscuring the true relationship between activity and percent overweight. Garrow (1978a) came to the following conclusion regarding the question of inactivity in the etiology of obesity: "For reasons explained in Section 3.4, it is technically very difficult to make the appropriate measurements with sufficient accuracy to support any firm conclusion on this matter." (p. 106) In Section 3.4 (p. 52), Garrow (1978a) indicates that approximately 200 subjects would need to be measured to statistically detect a 3% obesity-producing energy imbalance. No single study has measured activity in this size sample. The small instrumented-activity literature regarding obesity is reviewed next.

Modified Watches

Bloom and Eidex (1967) began with the observation that the knee is bent 90 degrees when sitting but is straight when standing. They inserted a weighted arm into a mechanical wrist watch such that it stopped the gears from moving when the person was sitting but allowed the gears to move while standing. The watch was attached to an aluminum holder that was attached to the leg, just above the knee, with a standard perforated rubber strap. The watch holder allowed the watch to be turned such that it did not run when sitting. They had five obese women and two obese men plus five lean women and one lean man wear this device from 2 to 35 days (84% wore them 6 days or longer). Since the devices were worn from getting up from bed until retiring to bed, a record of bedtime was also available. The major dependent variable was the amount of time spent in the upright position as this corresponds to the posture which consumes the largest number of calories.

The results indicated that obese spend 21.7 (*SE* = 4.1) percent of their day standing compared to 35.5 percent (*SE* = 2.3) for lean controls. When expressed as percent of the day out of bed on feet, the results were 36.0% (*SE* = 4.6) for the obese subjects and 53.0 percent (*SE* = 3.1) for the lean controls. Results for two obese women showed that time spent in bed plus sitting was 73% for one subject and 71% for another. Hence, these two persons spent nearly three-quarters of every day at or near basal energy level. Such inactivity undoubtedly contributes to their being overweight.

Actometers

Tryon (1987) measured wrist activity in overweight men and women (27.84 AU/min) and underweight men and women (24.57 AU/min) for two consecutive weeks and found them to be equally active ($F(1,27) = 2.20$, N.S.). He hypothesized that a rapid activity decrement might exist for men between 20 and 54% overweight and for women between 18 and 62% overweight. These ranges derive from the largest value studied by Tryon (1987) and the smallest value studied by Dorris and Stunkard (1957) and Chirico and Stunkard (1960).

Pedometers

Dorris and Stunkard (1957) reported that obese women walked significantly fewer ($t(13) = -4.13, p < .01$) miles per week (14.4) than did nonobese women (34.3). Similarly, Chirico and Stunkard (1960) reported obese women walked fewer miles per day (2.0) than did nonobese women (4.9). They also reported that obese men walked significantly fewer miles per day (3.7) than did nonobese men (6.0).

Tryon, Goldberg, and Morrison (1990) report results from two studies of the relationship between ambulatory activity and obesity. Study 1 repeated the above-mentioned Tryon (1987) actometer study of college students using pedometer (waist) measurements. Study 2 examined the missing middle portion of the full weight spectrum by examining participants in a weight reduction program and matched control subjects. Each study focused upon a different segment of the percent overweight spectrum. Their results are combined below to give the most comprehensive perspective presently available.

A total of 45 college students, 27 men (aged 19.33 years, $S = 1.02$) and 18 women (aged 18.33 years, $S = 1.08$), ranging from 21% underweight to 20% overweight participated in the first study. A total of 109 women ranging from 4% underweight to 99% overweight participated in the second study. They were either participants ($n = 79$) in Fairleigh Dickinson University weight reduction program[1] or matched control subjects ($n = 30$).

Activity was measured at the waist with a Digitron Jog-Walk pedometer set to its maximum stride length of 5 ft for maximum discrimination among activity levels. A common procedure was used for both studies. Each subject was measured for height, weight, and frame size. The 1983 Metropolitan Height and Weight Tables were used to determine the subjects' percent overweight in order to facilitate comparison with the two other relevant pedometer studies. Negative values reflect being underweight.

Subjects in Study 1 walked a level measured 0.25 mile twice to determine a personal conversion constant for translating their subsequent pedometer readings into miles. If the pedometer registered 0.4 after having walked 0.25 miles, then the conversion factor would be $0.25/0.4 = 0.625$ such that $0.625 (0.4) = 0.25$ miles. All subsequent pedometer readings for that subject–pedometer pair would be multiplied by 0.625 to obtain miles. The pedometers for subjects in Study 2 were

---

[1]I would like to thank Michael G. Perri, Ph.D., of Fairleigh Dickinson University for allowing subjects in his obesity research to participate in doctoral research conducted by Judith Goldberg under my direction.

calibrated to the subject's stride length as determined by a standard walk to provide accurate feedback regarding miles walked as part of their weight control treatment.

Subjects then wore the pedometers for 14 consecutive days. They recorded the time the pedometer was put on in the morning, the time it was taken off at night, and the mileage recorded on the three-digit display (e.g., 02.5 miles). This allowed us to calculate the wearing time in hours and activity in miles per hour.

The correlation between percent overweight (underweight) and activity (miles per hour) for $n = 109 + 18 = 127$ women was significant ($r(125) = -0.2216, p < .02$). The regression equation was MPH $= 0.252907 - 0.00078524$ (% OW); $r(125) = -.2216, p < .02$. Subjects walked $7.85254 - 10^{-4}$ miles (1.26374×10^{-3} km) per hour less for every 1% they were overweight.

Chirico and Stunkard's (1960) women averaged 63.07% overweight which predicts 0.20338103 mph (0.3273 kph). Subjects wore their pedometers for an average of 14.3738 hours per day. Personal communication with Dr. Stunkard confirms that his subjects wore their pedometers for very nearly the same average time. Hence, we predict that 2.92 miles (4.699 km) were walked per day. This value is clearly within the reported 68% confidence interval of 2.0 ± 1.2 reported by Chirico and Stunkard (1960) having an upper bound of 3.2 miles (5.1 km) per day. The upper limit of their 95% confidence limit would have been $2.0 + (1.96)(1.2) = 4.352$ miles (7.00 km) per day. Had Chirico and Stunkard's subjects worn their pedometers but 9.8338 hours per day, we would have exactly predicted their published mean of 2.0 miles (3.2 km) per day. To reach the upper limit of the 95% confidence interval of 4.352 (7.0 km) per day, Chirico and Stunkard's subjects would have had to have worn their pedometers for an unlikely *average* of 21.3983 hours per day.

Dorris and Stunkard (1957) reported that women averaging 62% overweight walked 14.4 ± 7.6 miles per week (23.2 ± 12.2 km). Using the above regression equation, we predict 0.204221252 mph times 14.3738 hours per day times 7 days per week or 20.55 miles (33.07 km) miles per week. This value is within Dorris and Stunkard's published 68% confidence interval of 14.4 ± 7.6 miles (23.2 ± 12.2 km) per week having an upper limit of 22.0 miles (35.4 km) per week. The upper limit of their 95% confidence interval would have been $14.4 + (1.96) 7.6 = 29.296$ miles (47.147 km) per week. Had Dorris and Stunkard's subjects worn their pedometers for an average of 10.0731 hours per day, we would have exactly predicted the published mean of 14.4 miles (23.2 km) per week. Their subjects would have had to have worn their pedometers for an unlikely *average* of 20.4932 hours per day to have reached the 29.296 miles (47.147 km) per week upper limit of the 95% confidence interval.

The correlation between activity (miles/hour) and percent overweight for the 27 men was not significant ($r(25) = -0.3157, p > .20$) though numerically larger than that observed for women because of the small sample size. The regression analysis revealed that MPH $= 0.350098 - 0.00532179$ (% OW) and shows that men walked 5.32179×10^{-3} miles per hour less for every 1% they were overweight.

The correlation between activity (mph) and percent overweight for all 154 subjects in the present sample (men and women) was negative, substantial, and highly significant ($r(152) = -0.3128, p < .0001$). Regression analysis showed that MPH $= 0.28167 - 0.00137461$ (% OW). Subjects walked 1.37461×10^{-3} miles (2.2122×10^{-3} km) per hour less for every 1% they were overweight.

The correlation between activity and percent overweight for all present subjects plus data published by Chirico and Stunkard (1960) is negative, substantial, and highly significant ($r(192) = -0.3151, p < .0001$). Regression analysis shows that mph $= 0.279122 - 0.00121484$ (% OW). Every 1% overweight *decreases* activity by $1.21484 - 10^{-3}$ miles ($1.9555 - 10^{-3}$ km) per hour.

The present results provide striking confirmation of the relationship between percent overweight and activity published 30 years ago by Chirico and Stunkard (1960). No evidence of a sudden change in activity was found as hypothesized by Tryon (1987). Rather, a small (1.2148×10^{-3} mph; 1.955×10^{-3} kph per 1% overweight) consistent decrement in activity appears to link subjects ranging from -21% to $+140\%$ overweight.

The present findings have implications for the etiology, diagnosis, and treatment of obesity. The calories not burned by small amounts of activity may accumulate over time causing the person to become overweight by a substantial percentage. Conversely, small activity increments over long time periods might reduce this percent overweight factor by an important amount. The slope of 1.21484 mph equals 6.414 feet (1.955 m) per hour times 14 hours a day equals 89.8 feet (27.4 m) per day times 365 days $= 32,777.4$ feet $= 6.2$ miles $= 9.98$ km per year. Therapeutic focus should be on the 2 m per hour or 28 m per day rather than on the 10 km per year per 1% reduction. A 10% reduction calls for a modest 280 m/day which accumulates to 102.2 km per year. These conclusions are consistent with Brownell and Stunkard's (1980) observations that, despite the modest weight reductions obtained, " . . . exercise may play an important role in the treatment of obesity." (p. 302)

The negative slope relating activity to percent overweight implies that activity increments are expected for underweight persons equivalent to activity decrements reported here for overweight persons. The only data found relevant to this prediction are by Blinder, Freeman, and Stunkard (1970), who reported on four patients treated for anorexia nervosa. They had a 41% average weight loss and walked an average of 6.8 miles per day. Daily mileage was reported only for Case 1 who had a 31% weight loss and walked 8.5 miles per day. The regression equation for women [mph $= 0.252907 - .000785254$ (% OW)] predicts mph $= .2851$ for % OW $= -41$, which at an estimated wearing time of 14.3738 hours per day predicts 4.1 miles walked per day vs the reported 6.8 miles. Similarly, mph $= .2772$ for % OW $= -31$ times 14.3738 predicts 4.0 miles walked per day vs the reported 8.5 miles per day. Hence, part of the hyperactivity of anorectic patients can be explained by their percentage underweight. The remaining activity seems attributable to some other aspect of their disorder. Since these patients are usually discharged at a lower than desired weight, it is predicted that they will be proportionally hyperactive. Unfortunately, no pedometer data were available at the time of discharge to determine if they were walking the predicted miles per day for their percentage underweight. It is recommended that such data be obtained in future studies.

Activity and Age

The above-mentioned data on adults clearly indicates a consistent inverse relationship between percent overweight and activity. We now ask whether this relationship exists in children as well.

Stunkard and Pestka (1962) measured the daily mileage walked in 15 obese girls and 15 age-matched control subjects for two weeks at camp and the first week home after camp. The mean and standard deviation for the obese ($M = 7.19$ miles, $S = 1.93$ miles) and control ($M = 8.03$ miles, $S = 2.51$ miles) subjects while at camp show that the obese girls were slightly less active than the control girls. This small difference is not significant on $N = 15$.

Not all subjects took activity measurements during the first week after camp, thereby decreasing the sample size as indicated. The mean and standard deviation for the obese ($M = 5.03$ miles, $S = 3.35$ miles, $n = 11$) and controls ($M = 5.75$ miles, $S = 2.94$ miles, $n = 11$) also indicates that the obese girls were slightly less active than the normal-weight girls. Again, this difference is not significant on this small sample size.

The extremely low power created primarily by the small sample size and secondarily by range restriction suggests that firm conclusions regarding activity equivalence between the two groups is unwarranted given the uncertainty associated with the 95% confidence intervals associated with the means in question. Said more directly, these data are consistent with the existence of the same small percent overweight–activity decrement noted above for adults. One method of evaluating this possibility is to use the regression equation reported above for all women to predict the activity of these girls.

Chirico and Stunkard's (1960) obese women walked only about 2.0 miles per day vs the present 7.19 and 5.03 miles per day for girls at camp and home respectively. Chirico and Stunkard's (1960) normal control women walked 4.9 miles per day vs 8.03 and 7.19 miles per day for normal weight girls at camp and home respectively. Hence, girls are somewhat more active than women.

A further test of the above-mentioned regression equation for women is to use it to predict activity in overweight girls. Because girls are more active than women, we must obtain an appropriate slope which means that we can only evaluate the slope for goodness-of-fit. Our best intercept estimate is the activity of normal girls whom we will presume are zero percent overweight. Since the regression equation refers to miles walked per hour on the basis of 14.3738 hours per day of wearing time, the normal control distance must be divided by this figure. Hence, the intercept for camp equals $8.03/14.3738 = 0.558655$ and the intercept for home equals $5.75/14.3738 = 0.400033$. The common slope remains -7.85254×10^{-4} as for adult women.

Stunkard and Pestka (1962) calculated percent overweight in two ways. The obese girls were reported to be 36.93% overweight by one method and 33.27% overweight by the other method. The prediction for obese girls at camp using the 36.93% figure is that they walk 0.52965590 mph $\times$ 14.3738 hours = 7.61 miles per day which is rather close to the observed value of 7.19 miles per day given that the 95% confidence interval for the observed mean ranges from 6.12 to 8.26 miles per day. Using the 33.27% overweight figure predicts 7.65 miles per day which is near the previous prediction and still well within the 95% confidence interval.

The prediction for obese girls at home using the 36.93% overweight figure is that they walk 5.33 miles per day, which is again rather close to the observed value of 5.03 miles per day given that the 95% confidence interval for the observed mean ranged from 2.78 to 7.28 miles per day. The 68% confidence interval (4.02 to 6.04 miles per day) also contains the predicted value. Using the 33.27% overweight figure predicts 5.37 miles per day, which again agrees quite well with the observed value and lies easily within both the 95% and 68% confidence intervals.

The conclusion drawn from these additional analyses is that obese children appear to evidence the same small but important relationship between percent overweight and activity decrement as adults but about a somewhat higher intercept value. Additional data should be gathered to confirm this deduction.

ENERGY BALANCE

Energy balance occurs when calories burned equal calories consumed resulting in constant body weight (Brownell and Lowney, 1986). Edholm (1977), Garrow (1986, 1987b), and especially Garrow (1987a) discuss the issues involved in regulating energy balance in far greater detail than present space allows. Garrow (1987b) states that " . . . the laws of thermodynamics apply to man as well as to the rest of nature. The energy stores in the human body accurately reflect the balance between energy input (from food and drink) and energy expenditure." (p. 45) Garrow (1987b) further indicates that " . . . the etiological factors, whether psychological, genetic, endocrine, or whatever ultimately must act on energy intake or output or some combination of these." (pp. 1115–1116) Obesity and anorexia are opposite ends of the energy balance spectrum. Whereas obesity represents a chronic energy reserve, anorexia represents a chronic energy debt.

Garrow (1978a; pp. 17–52) reviews methods for measuring both energy intake and output. Garrow (1978a) further reviews factors affecting energy intake in Chapter 4 (pp. 53–77) and factors influencing energy expenditure in Chapter 5 (pp. 79–112). The interdependence of body weight and activity supports the expectation that knowledge of two authorizes inference about the third.

Bomb Calorimetry

The term "energy" is used here in its strict physical sense which entails temperature. The amount of energy in food or drink is determined by bomb (direct) calorimetry as follows. The bomb calorimeter is a metal box within an insulated box separated by a water bath. The inner chamber of the bomb calorimeter contains a precisely weighed food sample, pure oxygen atmosphere, and an electrode with which to ignite and fully burn (oxidize) the food sample. The resulting heat is absorbed by a water bath surrounding the inner box. The after- minus before-combustion water temperature difference is used to determine caloric content of the sample. A "small" calorie is the amount of heat energy necessary to raise 1 g of water 1°C (from 15 to 16°C). Sometimes this smaller unit is referred to as the gram-calorie; abbreviated 'c.' A "large" calorie is 1000 times greater and is the amount of heat energy necessary to raise 1 kg of water 1°C (from 15 to 16°C). Sometimes this larger unit is referred to as the kilocalorie, abbreviated as 'kcal.'

Burning 1 g of pure carbohydrate, protein, or fat yields 4.10 kcal, 5.65 kcal, or 9.45 kcal of energy respectively. Digestion requires energy leaving 4.0 kcal, 4.0 kcal, and 9.0 kcal net energy available for carbohydrate, protein, and fat, respectively, making protein the most "costly" to digest. Katch and McArdle (1988, p. 94) estimate that a 4 oz (113.5 g) piece of apple pie yields 350 kcal of heat when completely burned. This equals 3.5×100 kcal meaning that 3.5 kg of water can be raised 100°C which is the equivalent of bringing 3.5 kg (7.7 lbs) of ice water to the boiling point!

Caloric Intake

Direct Method

The best method for determining caloric intake is to carefully prepare and weigh all food and drink taking care to keep careful records. Unfortunately, the effort and inconvenience required limits its applicability, especially for longitudinal studies. Compromises made to augment compliance can be expected to diminish accuracy.

Indirect Method

Sopko, Jacobs, and Taylor (1984), reviewed below under diet under indirect calorimetry, presents evidence that activity level can be estimated from a knowledge of weight and diet (caloric intake). The basis of this approach is that energy balance requires covariation among weight, caloric intake, and energy expenditure; especially when controlling for variation in basal or resting metabolism through knowledge of height, age, and sex, in addition to weight.

The same reasoning can be reversed. Ravussin and Bogardus (1989) indicate that changes in body weight, given nearly constant activity level, strongly implicate corresponding changes in caloric intake once associated BMR changes have been considered. This can be done using the regression equations cited above which require only a knowledge of weight, height, age, and sex. Estimates of caloric intake can probably be improved by correcting for variation in activity.

Energy Expenditure

Estimating caloric intake is more straightforward than estimating energy expenditure. The uncertainty associated with estimates of caloric intake is probably much less than the uncertainty associated with estimates of energy expenditure for at least two reasons. First, eating typically occurs at breakfast, lunch, and supper. Perhaps a snack or two are added. Energy expenditure through activity occurs all day long. Efforts to keep a minute by minute activity log are impractically time consuming and probably not very accurate. Second, the caloric content of food is not influenced by the topography of eating. Taking small bites does not reduce the number of calories in a hamburger. "Wolfing" food down may make it disappear quicker but doesn't reduce caloric content, either. However, energy expenditure varies directly with the rate of activity as evidenced by all charts used to estimate caloric expenditure from activity (cf. Katch and McArdle, 1988).

Basal and Resting Metabolic Rate

The concept of Basal Metabolic Rate (BMR) pertains to the minimum energy required to sustain quiet consciousness. It is determined under the following conditions: the person is without food for 12 to 18 hours, is in a neutral thermal environment, and is both bodily and mentally at rest. Oxygen consumption is measured for 6 to 10 minutes after the person has been lying quietly in bed for 30 to 60 minutes (cf. Katch and McArdle, 1988, pp. 101–102).

Resting Metabolic Rate (RMR) is a somewhat less stringent concept and requires that oxygen consumption be measured for 1 hour prior to breakfast beginning at 0800 hours in a thermally neutral environment while the subject rests quietly in bed (Garrow, 1986).

Geissler, Miller, and Shah (1987) calculated BMR using the following formula originally published by Harris and Benedict (1919): BMR for women = 655 + 9.56 (Weight in kg) + 1.85 (Height in cm) − 4.68 (Age in years). The exact formulas published by Harris and Benedict (1919, p. 227) are: Calories/24 hours for men =

66.4730 + 13.7516 (Weight in kg) + 5.0033 (Height in cm) − 6.7550 (Age in years) and calories/24 hours for women = 655.0955 + 9.5634 (Weight in kg) + 1.8496 (Height in cm) − 4.6756 (Age in years). Table 75 on page 192 of Harris and Benedict (1919) indicates that the root-mean-square (RMS) deviation between predicted and measured BMR is 101.7 calories = 6.23% for men and 106.3 calories = 7.88% for women. Table 74 of Harris and Benedict (1919) indicates that the average deviation between predicted and measured BMR is 81.2 calories = 4.98% for men and 84.6 calories = 6.27% for women. On page 195, Harris and Benedict indicate that athletes' BMR is 1 to 189 cal/day (0.1 to 9.8%) greater than predicted; the average being 56.37 cal/day = 3.03% more than predicted. On page 247 Harris and Benedict indicate that vegetarian men have BMR expenditures of 21 to 404 cal/day (1.4 to 28.7%) more than predicted with an average of 11.55% greater than predicted. BMR for vegetarian women ranges from 39 to 229 cal/day (3.4 to 19.8%) greater than predicted with an average of 10.78%. The vegetarian analyses are based upon 19 men and 4 women. Harris and Benedict (1919; p 195) report that one man fasted for 31 days and reduced his BMR by 28%.

Harris and Benedict (1919; p. 194) provide equations for predicting BMR in babies. Boy babies = −22.104 + 31.050 (Weight in kg) + 1.162 (Height in cm). Girl babies = −44.901 + 27.836 (Weight in kg) + 1.842 (Height in cm). The RMS deviation between predicted and measured BMR for boys was 13.78 cal/24 hrs and 13.53 cal/24 hrs for girls. The average deviation between predicted and measured BMR for boys was 11.02 cal/24 h and 10.84 cal/24 h for girls. No age limits were provided for switching to the above-mentioned equations.

Weight and Activity

Knowing that BMR is highly correlated with body weight allows one to track changes in BMR by tracking changes in body weight given an initial BMR measurement. The importance of this information is underscored by Ravussin and Bogardus (1989), who report that BMR can account for up to 80% of daily energy expenditure. Further changes in body weight, given nearly constant activity level, strongly implicate corresponding changes in caloric intake once associated BMR changes have been considered.

Resting Metabolism Resets

Garrow (1987b) reported that body weight is highly correlated ($r = .96$) with body fat because each pound of body weight is composed of approximately 75% fat and 25% lean tissue called Fat Free Mass (FFM). The 95% confidence limits reported for fat range from 70% to 78% and 22% to 30% for FFM. Resting Metabolic Rate (RMR) is largely a function of FFM thereby allowing Garrow and Webster (1985) to predict body fat from body weight and thereby deduce FFM and

RMR. Because every pound gained or lost is 25% FFM, every pound gained will increase RMR and every one lost will decrease RMR causing the breakeven point for quiet consciousness to be reset in accordance with body weight. Garrow (1987b) reports that changes in RMR are symmetrical for weight gains and losses.

RMR Increases. Overfeeding increases body weight which increases energy expenditure (Garrow, 1978a; pp. 91–93). Approximately 75% of excess calories become fat while 25% become FFM and increase RMR proportionally. Garrow (1987b) reported that RMR increases exceed body weight predictions by approximately 10% probably because of unknown endocrine changes. These increases occur similarly in persons who claim to be easy and difficult weight gainers (cf. Webb and Annis, 1983; Daniels, Katzeff, Ravussin, Garrow, and Danforth, 1982). Such metabolic inefficiency facilitates weight reduction and is a natural form of weight regulation.

RMR Decreases. RMR decreases normally with age as indicated by the Harris and Benedict (1919) regression equations discussed above. Garrow (1987a) reports that the RMR of a child of 5 ranges from 55 to 60 kcal/m²/hr. By age 20, the RMR range has decreased to between 35 and 40 kcal/m²/hr and by age 70 reduced further to between 30 and 33 kcal/m²/hr. Developmental changes in growth were cited as the reason for this effect.

Garrow (1987b) measured the metabolic rate (ml O_2/min) upon admission and at discharge in 111 women admitted for 3 weeks to a metabolic ward where they were maintained on an 800-kcal/day diet. The average decrease in RMR was 14% despite a body weight decrease of just 6%. Garrow (1978a; p. 90) reports data from Benedict, Miles, Roth, and Smith (1919) showing decreases in BMR, resting pulse rate, and body weight in response to underfeeding for approximately 150 days. Hence, RMR decreased by more than twice the reduction in body weight. This makes weight reduction exclusively through dieting especially difficult.

Durnin (1984) reported an extension of a previously reported study by Ghali and Durnin (1977) wherein a middle-aged woman's daily caloric intake was modified by adding or subtracting, more or less randomly, 1000 kcal per day from her normal intake of approximately 2000 kcal per day during 4-week (1-month) periods over approximately 90 weeks. They observed (as did Keys, Brozek, Henschel, Mickelsen, and Taylor, 1950; Grande, Anderson, and Keys, 1958; Garrow, 1987b; and Geissler, Miller, and Shah, 1987), that Basal Metabolic Rate (BMR) decreased as body weight decreased in response to caloric restriction and increased as body weight increased in response to overeating.

During (1984) unexpectedly found that repeated periods of undereating reduced BMR to progressively lower levels resulting in a final reduction of 15% from normal during the approximately 20-month study interval. This finding is especially important for at least two reasons. First, the metabolic efficiency brought about through caloric restriction appears to increase with repeated trials thereby giving the appearance of learning. Second, it is possible to lower one's BMR by 15% through repeated dieting thereby subsequently increasing body weight to 15% above normal given return to previous eating habits. It is curious that definitions of obesity begin at 15% overweight.

Geissler, Miller, and Shah (1987) carefully matched 16 post-obese women with 16 normally lean women. No significant differences in age, weight, height, BMI (kg/m^2), or percent body fat were found. The post-obese women had 2.1 kg less lean body fat than did the controls ($p < .05$). They found that the metabolic rates of the post-obese during the night and day were significantly less than for control subjects. Post-obese women engaged in sedentary, normal, or normal plus aerobic activity expended just 83%, 85%, and 86% of the calories consumed by lean controls respectively. When post-obese subjects slept at the end of a day of sedentary, normal, or normal plus aerobic activity they expended but 89%, 89%, and 92% of the calories burned by lean control subjects.

Hirsch and Leibel (1988) has recently questioned the extent to which BMR remains depressed.

Underfeeding reduces RMR because it reduces body weight and thereby reduces FFM. The resulting lowered energy requirements reduces the initial effects of underfeeding. This mechanism serves to conserve body weight in the presence of underfeeding. Reduction of RMR in response to lowered caloric intake makes biological sense given that famine results in caloric restriction. Increased metabolic efficiency partly compensates for food restriction.

Direct Calorimetry

This method requires that all of the heat energy associated with energy expenditure be collected and measured. The person lives inside an insulated room lined with water coils that absorb heat. Caloric expenditure is calculated from changes in this water temperature. Oxygen must be carefully supplied to the room and CO_2 in exhausted air may be analyzed. See Garrow (1987a) and Katch and McArdle (1988) for additional details.

Indirect Calorimetry

Oxygen Consumption. Katch and McArdle (1988) indicate that metabolism (oxidation) requires oxygen and that approximately 1 liter of oxygen is required to produce 4.82 kcal of heat energy. Hence, caloric expenditure can be calculated oxygen consumption is known. The authors illustrate the use of a portable spirometer for ambulatory oxygen measurements (pp. 98–100). Geissler, Miller, and Shah (1987) confined subjects to a 3.3-m long by 2.5-m wide room with a volume of 21,000 L furnished with a desk and chair, arm chair, wash basin, toilet, telephone, television, heater, exercise step, and a bicycle. Air was collected and analyzed for oxygen content using a Servomex OA 272 oxygen analyzer (Taylor Servomex Ltd., Crowborough, Sussex, England).

Tilt Counters. LaPorte, Kuller, Kupfer, McPartland, Matthews, and Caspersen (1979) placed an activity sensor (GMM Electronics Inc., 1200 Riverview Drive, Verona, PA 15147) at the waist and wrist of 10 Physical Education majors and 10 control students (9 Psychology and 1 English majors). Data were recorded four times each day (0930, 1300, 1630, and 2000 hours) for two days. All 20 subjects self-rated energy expenditure. The correlation between average waist activity counts per hour and average energy expenditure was $r(18) = .69$, $p < .001$. A lesser correlation was observed between ankle activity counts per hour and energy expenditure ($r(18) = .43$, $p < .07$). The trunk is more highly correlated with energy expenditure because it approximates the center of gravity.

McGowan, Bulik, Epstein, Kupfer, and Robertson (1984) estimated caloric expenditure in three nonobese, nonsmoking young adult males using large-scale integrated sensor (LSI) mercury-switch-based tilt sensors at the nondominant ankle and ipsilateral hip. The first step in caloric estimation was to measure heart rate while pedaling a cycle ergometer for 3 minutes at each of the following work loads: 0, 300, 600, and 900 kg/min. Caloric expenditure was determined using a pulmonary pneumotachometer and O_2 and CO_2 gas analyzers for measuring VO_2 uptake resulting in respiratory quotients. A regression equation was calculated for each subject predicting caloric expenditure due to work from heart rate; all correlation coefficients were greater than .98. The second step was to measure heart rate plus hip and ankle activity while taking a 1- and 2-mile walk around a 0.25-mile track. Separate regression equations were calculated for predicting energy expenditure from ankle and hip activity. The correlations for the three subjects for the hip regressions for the three subjects were .999, .980, and .999. The corresponding three ankle correlation were .999, .995, and .901.

Two qualifying comments are in order. First, heart rate is known to be linearly related to energy expenditure for activities such as moderate continuous movement, as was studied here, but nonlinearly related to energy expenditure at low and high activity levels. Second, the regression equations were calculated on very few points where high correlations occur by chance. The top panel of their Figure 1 is based on 4 points or 2 degrees of freedom where r must exceed .9501 to be significant at the 5% level. The bottom panel is based based on 3 points or 1 degree of freedom where r must exceed .9969 to be significant at the 5% level.

Accelerometers. Wong, Webster, Montoye, and Washburn (1981) described the use of a portable accelerometer device for measuring energy expenditure in humans. They begin by indicating that such devices should exclude the contribution of gravity (0 Hz = DC) meaning that a 0.21-Hz high pass filter should be used. They did not expect significant human activity above 10 Hz and therefore recommended a 11.8-Hz low pass filter. They began by attaching a 255-mg ball bearing to the tip of a Calectro S2–294 (GC Electronics, Rockford, IL) piezoelectric monaural phonocartridge. This accelerometer was attached to the trunk of 15 subjects while walking on a motor-driven treadmill with 0% grade for 3 minutes at 2, 3, and 4 mph; running for 3 minutes at 6 and 8 mph; and stepping up onto an 8-inch bench and down again for 3 minutes at the rate of 80, 120, and 140 repetitions per minute. Evaluation of the relationship between vertical acceleration and normalized oxygen consumption (ml of VO_2/kg/min) was restricted to graphical presentation but clearly indicated a strong linear relationship. Simultaneous pedometer readings also indicated a strong linear relationship with oxygen consumption.

Wong, Webster, Montoye, and Washburn (1981) cite a Yugoslavian symposium presentation by Reswick, Perry, Antoneilli, Su, and Freeborn (1978) showing that both vertical acceleration, and its integration over time, correlate well with oxygen consumption. Although their results were limited to graphical presentation, Wong et al. estimated that their figure represented at least $r = .90$. Brouha (1960) reported a correlation of $r = .83$ between the temporal integral of vertical platform acceleration and oxygen consumption by office and industrial workers.

Montoye, Washburn, Servais, Ertl, Webster, and Nagle (1983) attached the 400 gram $14 \times 8 \times 4$ cm accelerometer developed by Wong et al. (1981) to the waist, at the back, of 21 healthy subjects aged 20 to 60 years. Subjects performed each of the following 14 exercises, 4 minutes each, on two separate days while oxygen uptake (ml VO_2/kg/min) was monitored: walking on a motor-driven treadmill at 2 mph at 0%, 6%, and 12% grades; walking on the same treadmill at 4 mph at the same grades; running on the treadmill at 6 mph at 0% and 6% grades; stepping up on and down from an 8-inch bench 20 and 35 times per minute; half knee-bends at 28 and 48 repetitions per minute; and floor touches while bending knees at the rate of 24 and 36 touches per minute.

The results indicated that first and second trial accelerometer readings (integrals over time) taken from 4 subjects during each of the 14 activities ($N = 56$) correlated $r(54) = .94$, $p < .0001$. Correlation of all $N = 14 \times 21 = 294$ acceleration and oxygen readings was $r(294) = .74$, $p < .0001$. The average within subject correlation over 14 data points was $r(12) = .79$, $p < .001$.

Servais, Webster, and Montoye's (1984) Figure 1 is a block diagram of the human energy system and shows various ways in which energy is consumed including dynamic physical activity. Work (W) in joules, as defined by physicists, equals one-half mass (M) in kg times the square of velocity (V) in meters/second. Velocity equals the integral of acceleration over time.

$$W = \frac{M \, V^2}{2} \qquad V = \int_{0}^{t} a \, dt$$

On this basis they integrated absolute acceleration (vertical at the waist) values over an unspecified time interval (perhaps 1 minute) to get velocity which they squared, multiplied by body weight in kilograms and divided in half to get joules of kinetic energy (work). Knowing that 4.183 joules equals 1 calorie allows one to calculate calories per minute expended. That the waist is the approximate center of gravity of the body supports vertical acceleration of body weight as a proper index of work.

The authors demonstrated that a graph of vertical acceleration at the waist is highly similar to force platform output during half-kneebend exercise and that loose physical coupling of the device to the waist does not alter the results in any important way. It was further demonstrated that accelerometer-estimated calories expended while walking at 2, 3, and 4 mph are extremely close to accepted energy expenditure values for these activities. Accelerometer-estimated calories were somewhat overestimated when running at 5, 6, and 7 mph.

The Actillume™ (Ambulatory Monitoring, Inc., Ardsley, NY 10502) measures acceleration with 8-bit (1/256) resolution over programmable epochs (cf. Chapter 2). It could be used to measure caloric expenditure due to activity if worn at the waist to sense vertical acceleration.

Hemokinetics, Inc. (1987) (3102 Watford Way, Madison, WI 53713) manufactures an accelerometer-based microprocessor-controlled calorie expenditure counter called CALTRAC™ described previously (see Chapter 2) in greater detail. Personal communication with Hemokinetics (May 4, 1990) indicates that CALTRAC™ has improved correspondence between estimated and accepted calorie values by incorporating a microprocessor running proprietary software. An added feature of CALTRAC™ is that it will calculate basal (resting) metabolism if programmed with height, weight, age, and sex information and not moved for one hour. The following equations are used:

$$\text{Male (kcal/min)} = \frac{473 \text{ (lb)} + 982 \text{ (in)} - 531 \text{ (yr)} + 4686}{100,000}$$

$$\text{Female (kcal/min)} = \frac{331 \text{ (lb)} + 251 \text{ (in)} - 352 \text{ (yr)} + 49854}{100,000}$$

An integrated activity value can be obtained by entering weight = 85 pounds, height = 8 inches, age = 99 years, and sex = male rather than personally relevant information.

A report entitled "CALTRAC study in obese and non-obese individuals confined into a respiration chamber" made by Dr. Yves Schutz (Physiologie Clinique, 7, rue du Bugnon, CH-1011, Lausanne-CHUV, Switzerland) to Hemokinetics, Inc. (available on request from Hemokinetics) compared energy expenditure estimated by CALTRAC™ with direct calorimetry. Subjects were 29 "obese" women whose BMI ranged from 17.3 to 40.7 kg/m^2 (BMI under 25 are not considered obese). One group of 17 women were not asked to perform specific exercises; their activity was considered spontaneous. The remaining 12 women were asked to walk at 2 mph on a 10% grade for 30 minutes twice during their 24-hour confinement.

CALTRAC™ estimated an average (and standard deviation) 24-hour energy expenditure of 1564 (118) calories for the $n = 17$ spontaneous-activity women compared to direct calorimetry measurements of 1822 (171). The CALTRAC™ result was 14% less than the direct calorimetry figure. The regression equation for predicting direct calorimetry (DC) from CALTRAC™ (C) was: DC = .780 C + .410 ($r(15) = .5366, p < .05$). This correlation is low primarily because of restricted range in energy expenditure.

CALTRAC™ estimated an average 24-hour energy expenditure of 1907 (307) in the $n = 12$) women walking on the treadmill compared to direct calorimetry measurements of 2254 (433). The CALTRAC™ result was 15% less than the direct calorimetry value. The corresponding regression equation was: DC = 1.344 C − .214 ($r(10) = .9511, p < .001$).

The average CALTRAC™ energy expenditure for all 29 subjects was 1706 (272) vs direct calorimetry values of 2000 (370), the CALTRAC™ estimate being 15% less than the direct calorimetry value. The corresponding regression equation was: DC = 1.253 C − 0.95 ($r(27) = .9203, p < .001$).

Basal metabolism was measured between 0700 and 0800 by CALTRAC™ and direct calorimetry. The average (and standard deviation) for CALTRAC™ was 1535 (174) calories compared to direct calorimetry of 1450 (177). CALTRAC™ was 6% greater than the direct calorimetry value. The corresponding regression equation was: DC = 0.800 C − .155 ($r(27) = .7863, p < .001$).

Heart Rate. Bradfield, Paulos, and Grossman (1971) and Goldsmith, Miller, Mumford, and Stock (1976) discussed the use of heart rate to measure energy expenditure. Chapter 2 discusses several problems with using heart rate measures to evaluate activity. It is expected that many of the same problems extend to estimating caloric expenditure from heart rate.

Diet. An interesting twist on the relationship between diet, weight, and activity is suggested by Sopko, Jacobs, and Taylor (1984). They suggest that adjusting caloric intake for body weight provides a "long-term measure of habitual physical activity." (p. 900) They obtained anthropometric data from free-living volunteer participants in two feeding studies where food intake was carefully monitored. The primary findings of Study 1 were that kcal/kg of food intake was correlated $r(19) = -.79, p < .001$ with percent body fat, $r(19) = -.75, p < .001$ with body weight (kg), and $r(19) = .76, p < .001$ with VO_2 max (ml/kg × min) in 21 healthy men aged 20 to 44 years.

Study 2 revealed that kcal/kg of food intake was correlated $r(53) = -.51, p < .0001$ with percent body fat and $r(53) = -.73, p < .0001$ with body weight (kg) in 55 active-duty soldiers. In both studies, calories per kilogram of body weight ingested was negatively related to adiposity and positively related to ability to perform work which is maintained by being physically active. Hence, the authors conclude that physical activity can be monitored through dietary measurements.

Antonetti (1973) has argued that knowledge of food input enables one to calculate energy expenditure on the basis of changes in both body weight and fat.

These above-mentioned correlations, and their implied regression equations, can be reversed to argue that kcal/kg of caloric consumption can be predicted from a knowledge of activity. This argument is based on the fact that caloric consumption, activity, and body weight are interdependent such that knowledge of any two constrains the third.

COROLLARY ISSUES

Activity and Caloric Intake

A concern about prescribing activity increase to facilitate weight decrease is that increased caloric intake will result and prevent weight reduction. The literature on this issue is divided. Studies supportive of this position will be reviewed first and then opposite findings will be presented.

Activity May Increase Caloric Intake

Mayer, Marshall, Vitale, Christensen, Mashayekhi, and Stare (1954) demonstrated that mice initially increase food intake in response to activity, then decrease food intake as activity increases through what is called the "sedentary range," and then increase their food intake linearly with further activity increases throughout what is called the "normal activity range" resulting in a constant body weight (cf. Brownell and Stunkard, 1980; Thompson, Jarvie, Lahey, and Cureton, 1982).

Regarding humans, both Mayer, Roy, and Mitra (1956) plus Durin and Brockway (1959) reported that caloric intake does in fact increase along with activity resulting in stable body weight. These studies appear to apply to the normal activity range.

Epstein, Wing, and Thompson (1978) reported a pair of studies, one replicating the other, supporting a positive relationship between activity and caloric intake. Study I involved 17 nonobese female college students who participated in daily aerobic exercise classes for 5 weeks. The first 3 days were used for instruction and initial conditioning. Then the time to run (jog) 1 or 2 miles around an indoor 1/5-mile track was determined. Body weight was obtained daily along with self-reported caloric intake. The correlation between running time and caloric intake was $r(15) = -.69$, $p < .01$; faster pace was associated with greater caloric intake. Apparently running time for those completing 1 mile was doubled to be comparable to those running 2 miles or the time for those running 2 miles was halved to be comparable to those running 1 mile. Body weight remained constant across running rates ($r(15)$ = .08, N.S.).

Study II involved 16 nonobese female college students. Daily activity logs and digital pedometer readings were self-recorded for one week prior to beginning the above-mentioned aerobic condition. The relationship between running rate (number of $\frac{1}{8}$-mile laps in 12 minutes) and caloric intake was $r(14) = 0.48$, $p < .06$. As before, average weight and average running rate were independent ($r(14) = -0.07$, N.S.).

An important note regarding both Epstein, Wing, and Thompson studies is that the average running time over all five weeks was correlated with average body weight thereby removing within- and between-subject changes over time. Hence, subjects who on average ran faster ate more but retained their body weight.

Activity Does Not Necessarily Increase Appetite

Mayer and Bullen (1974; p. 270) recognized that moderate activity does not increase caloric intake by referring to such as the "nonresponsive range" of activity.

Woo, Garrow, and Pi-Sunyer (1982a,b) reported that the spontaneous caloric intake of obese women living on a metabolic ward did not change in response to short- and long-term moderate treadmill exercise. The explanation given was that compensatory caloric intake might not occur until fat reserves were expended.

McGowan, Epstein, Kupfer, Bulik, and Robertson (1986) investigated the effects of no exercise, regular exercise, and double exercise on the self-reported caloric intake of 7 male joggers aged 22 to 27 years ($M = 24.7$, $S = 1.9$). Regular exercise involved jogging 2.5 to 4 miles per day ($M = 3.5$, $S = 0.7$ miles per day) 5 days per week for the previous 3 to 6 months. No exercise was calculated to produce an 18% reduction in energy expenditure whereas double exercise was calculated to produce a 13% increase in energy expenditure. Average (and standard deviation) of calories consumed during regular exercise was 2534.7 (768.5). Nearly the same caloric intake was found for no exercise ($M = 2,529.0$, $S = 845.6$) and for double exercise ($M = 2.695.3$, $S = 980.1$). These negligible differences were nonsignificant.

Thompson, Jarvie, Lahey, and Cureton (1982) indicate that light exercise of long duration produces little change in caloric intake (p. 61).

Activity May Reduce Caloric Intake

Thompson, Jarvie, Lahey, and Cureton (1982) report that studies by Ahrens, Bishop, and Berdanier (1972), Crews, Fuge, Oscai, Holloszy, and Shank (1969), Katch, Martin, and Martin (1979), Nance, Bromley, Barnard, and Gorski (1977), Oscai and Holloszy (1969), Oscai, Mole, Brei, and Holloszy (1971), Premack and

Premack (1963), and Stevenson, Box, Feleki, and Beaton (1966) as demonstrating that exercise generally decreases caloric intake in male and female rats. Thompson *et al.* (1982) indicate that moderate exercise for 20 minutes to 1 hour significantly reduced food intake (p. 61). Their Table 2 reveals that 5 of 7 human studies reported decreases in caloric intake as a result of exercise. They further report that intense exercise for a short period is most likely to reduce caloric intake in rats (p. 61).

Activity and Adiposity

Greene (1939) reported that activity reductions accompanied weight gains in 67.5% of his adult patients. Keys (1970) reported that men with sedentary occupations had higher obesity rates than men whose occupation required regular exercise. Approximately 70% of the sedentary men were obese. Bray (1976) reported that animals given palatable food gain 50% more weight than similar subjects on the same diet but engage regularly in exercise.

Ingle (1949) demonstrated that forced inactivity causes obesity in the rat; a fact long known to farmers who restrict activity in animals they wish to fatten for market. Mayer (1953) demonstrated that spontaneous inactivity is how hereditary obesity–diabetes mice become obese.

Stern and Johnson (1977) reported that preweaning activity in genetically obese and normal rats is equivalent. The postweaning activity of genetically obese rats remains at the low preweaning level whereas the postweaning activity of lean littermate control animals increases linearly with time over the first 2 months of life. By 8 weeks of age, obese animals were only half as active as controls. Food intake was significantly greater in obese than control animals. Activity decreases were observed only after the onset of hyperphagia and corresponding increased body weight. It could either be that activity is a consequence of obesity as in genetics produces hyperphagia produces obesity produces inactivity or quite possibly genetics produced both hyperphagia and inactivity with phase delay sufficient to allow weight gain to be observed prior to inactivity.

Weight and Caloric Intake

Having demonstrated that obesity is associated with decreased activity, it is important to ask whether or not obese persons eat more than normal-weight persons. Equivalent or reduced caloric intake by obese vs normal controls is reported by Rose and Mayer (1968) regarding infants, Epstein, Parker, McCoy, and McGee (1976) regarding young children, Stefanik, Heald, and Mayer (1959), and Johnson, Burke, and Mayer (1956) regarding adolescents, and Mayer, Roy, and Mitra (1956), Dodd, Birky, and Stalling (1976), and Hill and McCutcheon (1975), Maxfield and Konishi (1966), and Meyer and Pudel (1972) regarding adults.

Wilkinson, Parkin, Pearlson, Strong, and Sykes (1977) obtained a single-day pedometer reading for 10 obese boys, 10 control boys, 10 obese girls, and 10 control girls within 3 months after evaluating their caloric intake over one weekend (Friday teatime through Monday breakfast). Caloric intake was reported in MJ (mega-joules) where 1 MJ = 239 kcal. Over the weekend, the obese boys (M = 31.4 MJ; range = 20.3 − 46.9 MJ) ingested slightly, but not significantly ($t(28)$ = 0.18, N.S.), more food than did control boys (M = 30.8 MJ; range = 17 − 39.8 MJ). Obese girls ingested (M = 27.0 MJ; range = 21.3 − 35.0 MJ) slightly, but not significantly ($t(28)$ = 1.4, N.S.), *less* food than did control girls (M = 31.3 MJ; range = 22.1 − 46.6 MJ).

The stride index of the pedometers were all set to the same value but no attempt was made to convert the readings to distance walked. Hence, the activity measures have unknown and arbitrary units. Obese boys walked (M = 7.2; range = 3.6 − 12.6) slightly, but not significantly ($t(28)$ = 1.2, N.S.), *less* than control boys (M = 9.0; range = 4.1 − 17.6). However, obese girls walked (M = 8.7; range = 4.2 − 16.2) slightly, but not significantly ($t(28)$ = 0.2, N.S.), more than did control girls (M = 8.4; range = 5.3 − 13.6). The work of Tryon, Goldberg, and Morrison (1990) indicates that these nonsignificant effects are probably due to insufficient sample size to detect small real differences.

Durnin (1984) reported that the fattest 10% of 14-year-old girls consumed 1690 kcal/day whereas the thinnest 10% of 14-year-old girls consumed 2207 kcal/day. The fattest 10% of 3-month-old to 2-year-old infant girls were reported to consume 867 kcal/day vs 946 kcal/day for the thinnest 10% of the same-aged infant girls.

Weight Loss Maintenance

Short-term weight loss, if achieved, is usually modest and maintenance is rare (Stunkard and McLaren-Hume, 1958; Perri, Shapiro, Ludwig, and Twentyman, 1984). Consequently, investigators are especially interested in factors contributing to maintenance.

Marston and Criss (1984) tracked 47 formerly overweight persons by questionnaire every 3–4 months for one year. They had been 32.7% overweight prior to treatment and now 94% remained below 15% overweight. The total score in connection with 8 questionnaire items correctly predicted 95% of those persons who relapsed and 79% of those maintaining the weight reduction. One of these items referred to exercising "several" times per week.

Colvin and Olson (1983) interviewed 41 carefully selected men and women from 112 responses to radio, television, and newspaper publicity regarding how they lost weight and how they were able to maintain their weight loss. Eligibility requirements included: a) being at least 21 years of age, b) having lost at least 25% of one's body weight, c) regained less than 5 lbs from lowest weight during the next 2 years.

The 13 men ranged in age from 21 to 70 years (Mean = 45.5 yrs) and had maintained an average weight loss of 76.2 lbs for 5.8 years. Eleven men used a personalized combination of vigorous exercise for at least 30 minutes per day and diet to both lose and maintain weight loss. One man used diet alone and the other used exercise alone.

The 41 women ranged in age from 21 to 69 years (Mean = 40.0 yr) and had maintained an average weight loss of 53.2 lbs for 6.0 years. Diet was the method of choice followed by 38 women. Two women combined diet and exercise while one woman reported losing 61 lbs through exercise alone.

Hoiberg, Bernard, Watten, and Caine (1984) studied 531 Navy women and 155 Navy men reporting average weight losses of 22 lbs and 28 lbs respectively for 1 year after weight loss. Correlates of weight-loss included participation in physical exercise. However, activity was not significantly correlated with maintenance. They indicated that moderate exercise tends to suppress appetite and partially offsets decreases in metabolic rate caused by reduced caloric intake.

A review by Westover and Lanyon (1990) indicates that Graham, Taylor, Hovell, and Siegel (1983), Jeffery, Bjornson-Benson, Rosenthal, Kurth, and Dunn (1984), Katahn, Pleas, Thackrey, and Wallston (1982), Perri, Shapiro, Ludwig, Twentyman, and McAdoo (1984), and Wing, Epstein, Marcus, and Koeske (1984) have all reported significant weight reduction maintenance effects associated with activity. Objective ambulatory measuring devices (cf. Chapter 2) are strongly recommended to track daily activity in between fitness tests as they can serve to enhance personal motivation for activity both by rewarding its presence and documenting its absence.

Health Improvement

Generalized health benefits also appear related to activity increases. The initial benefit of weight reduction is the reduction of risk for a wide variety of disease discussed by Bray (1986). More specifically, Paffenbarger and Hale (1975) and Kannel and Sorlie (1979) reported that activity was prophylactic against heart disease. Gerhardsson, Norell, Kiviranta, Pedersen, and Ahlbom's (1986) 19-year follow-up study of 1.1 million Swedish men reported the relative risk of colon cancer to be 1.3 times as great for men with sedentary as active jobs (90% confidence interval = 1.2 − 1.5).

Slattery, Schumacher, Smith, West, and Abd-Elgahny (1988) report that "Total physical activity was protective against the development of colon cancer for both males (odds ratio (OR) = 0.70) and females (OR = 0.48) when high and low quartiles of activity were compared." (p. 989) Slattery, Jacobs, and Nichaman (1989) indicate that modest exercise significantly reduces mortality from *all* causes. When activity is divided into quintiles (five levels), escaping the most sedentary (1st quintile) category substantially reduces mortality risk. Hence, positive physical benefits of small activity increases extend well beyond maintaining weight reductions which have their own physical benefits.

Oscai, Spirakis, Wolff, and Beck (1972) reported that male rats given daily swimming had smaller epididymal fat pads with lesser lipid content than did control subjects whose diet was restricted such that their weight gain matched that of experimental subjects. "The carcasses of the sedentary food-restricted controls contained roughly twice as much fat as those of the exercisers" (p. 590).

6

Activity and Sleep

Sleep research can be divided into two eras around the work of Aserinsky and Kleitman (1953, 1955), and Dement and Kleitman (1957), who discovered rapid eye movement during sleep, now referred to as REM sleep, which revitalized research in this area.

Sleep stages are defined in terms of electroencephalograph (EEG: scalp above ear), electrooculogram (EOG: beside the eye), and electromyogram (EMG: muscle below chin) recordings (Mendelson, 1987; pp. 4–5) and therefore constitute the de facto standard measurement of when sleep is occurring and how deep sleep is. Rechtschaffen and Kales (1968) published a manual of terminology, techniques, and scoring criteria for human sleep that is still used today.

Polysomnography extends the above measurements to include leg EMG (anterior tibialis), nasal and oral air flow by thermistors near nose and mouth, blood oxygen saturation with an oximeter passing a light beam through either the finger or ear lobe, chest and abdominal movement with mercury-filled strain gauge, and electrocardiogram (EKG) (Mendelson, 1987; pp. 5–6).

Investigators studying sleep and/or the effects of medications and other variables on sleep as well as clinicians evaluating sleep complaints presently must use the facilities of a sleep laboratory or retain the services of a polysomnographer to make a home visit. Several major problems are associated with this approach. First, limited research and clinical resources restrict both the number of persons who can be studied and the number of repeated measurements that can be made. The extensive data collected during just one night often require considerable time to analyze which further adds to the overall cost associated with this approach.

The decision to prescribe expensive tests must increasingly be balanced by the information gained and whether substantially equivalent information can be obtained by less expensive and/or intrusive methods. The purpose of this chapter is to describe behavioral research on body motility that provides a cost effective method for conducting even extended sleep evaluations.

Behavioral measurements during sleep, leg actigraphy, can be the primary method of choice in cases such as Restless-Leg Syndrome where the clinical and/or research focus is upon when and how long leg movements occur during sleep. We will see below that sleep apnea, a potentially life-threatening condition, can readily be detected using abdominal actigraphy.

A more economical and less invasive method for measuring sleep has broad clinical relevance. Carson, Butcher, and Coleman (1988) discuss sleep disorders in connection with: adjustment disorders, alcohol and drug abuse, anxiety-based disorders, brain disorders, childhood disorders, deprivation, grief, mood disorders, plus posttraumatic stress after rape and suicide attempts.

ARCHITECTURE OF SLEEP

Snyder and Scott (1972), Davies and Horne (1975), and Mendelson (1987) provide a concise and informative overview of human sleep. The electroencephalogram (EEG) is divided into four primary frequency bands. Alpha frequencies range from 8 to 12 (or 14) Hz with an amplitude of 25 to 100 microvolts (μV). Beta frequencies range from 14 to 30 (or 35) Hz with amplitudes below 20 μV. Theta frequencies range from 4 to 7 Hz with an amplitude of approximately 30 μV. Delta frequencies range from 0.5 to 3.5 Hz with amplitudes up to 150 μV. Jasper (1958) describes the International 10/20 system for EEG electrode placement.

Waking with eyes closed produces alpha waves, fairly high muscle tone, and irregular eye movement. Stage 1 sleep is associated with decreased alpha waves and increased beta and theta waves, somewhat reduced muscle tone (EMG), and slow eye rolling. Blake, Gerard, and Kleitman (1939) reported that subjects drop hand-held objects seconds after alpha waves disappear. Stage 2 sleep is characterized by theta waves, sleep spindles (0.5-second bursts of 12–14 Hz), and K complexes (burst of negative followed by positive voltage). Muscle tone is reduced from that shown in Stage 1. Stages 3 and 4 are referred to as slow-wave or delta sleep. Stage 3 is scored when delta waves constitute 20 to 50% of the record. Muscle tone equals that of Stage 2. Stage 4 is scored when delta waves constitute more than 50% of the record. Muscle tone is lower than Stage 3 but higher than REM sleep. Coleman (1986) describes REM sleep as "an active brain in a paralyzed body." (p. 104) EEG returns to a nearly wakeful state, muscle tone (EMG) decreases to very low levels, and rapid eye movements (EOG) occur. Respiration and heart rate become irregular (Oswald, Berger, Jaramillo, Keddie, Olley, and Plunkett (1963). This stage has a sudden onset and offset. In sum, sleep Stages 1–4 show progressive EEG frequency and EMG (muscle tone) declination. REM sleep results in brain activation in unison with muscle "paralysis."

Other physiological changes also occur during sleep (Davies and Horne, 1975; pp. 47–51). Body (rectal) temperature decreases to a minimum about half way through sleep and then gradually increases until two hours before becoming awake. Heart rate decreases progressively until approximately the seventh hour of sleep whereupon it increases to near daytime levels shortly before awakening. Changes in heart rate are not related to body motility. Respiration decreases through sleep Stages 1–4 resulting in increased CO_2 levels. Hodes and Dement (1964) reported the absence of reflex contractions during REM sleep. Penile erection is associated with 90% of REM periods (Fisher, Gross, and Zuch, 1965), snoring occurs most at the beginning of sleep (Albert and Ballas, 1973), and bruxism (tooth grinding) occurs most frequently in Stages 1 and 2, rarely in Stage 4 and almost never during REM sleep (Satoh and Haroda, 1973).

Approximately 20 to 60 position changes occur during sleep with poor sleepers showing more motility than good sleepers, though considerable individual differences exist (Monroe, 1967). Hobson, Spagna, and Malenka (1978) photographed 50 sleepers at 15-minute intervals and calculated a consolidation index equal to the percent of adjacent frames showing no major postural shifts; higher scores reflect less activity. Their Figure 2 reports that the consolidation index of the 6 best self-described sleepers ranged from approximately 47 to 64 compared to approximately 23 to 44 for the 6 worst self-described sleepers.

Hobson, Spagna, and Malenka (1978) reported that postural immobility was associated with descending NREM sleep Stages 1–4. Oswald, Berger, Jamarillo, Keddie, Olley, and Plunkett (1963) have reported that body motility is more likely in Stages 1 and 2 than in Stages 3 and 4 indicating that the body becomes increasingly quiescent as sleep deepens. Dement and Kleitman (1957) reported that body movement occurred before and after but not during REM periods. It appears that REM sleep reduces muscle tone to where large movements are not possible. However, Wolpert (1960) reported micromovements of the wrist and legs during REM sleep.

Wolpert (1960) obtained all-night EEG and wrist EMG on 8 male subjects aged 9 to 31 years. The wrist EMG electrode was placed over the flexor tendon for the third and fourth digits proximal to the wrist joint. Correct placement was visually verified by instructing the subject to move their fingers. The amplifier was set such that minute movements were not recorded but slightly larger movements were recorded. Their Figure 1 shows that wrist movements did not appear in the leg EMG lead or eye lead thereby verifying independence. The incidence of wrist activity during REM and NREM periods was determined. Wolpert reports that in 24 of 25 records the incidence of isolated wrist activity was greater while dreaming than in other sleep stages. The average number of movements per minute during REM was 0.30 compared to 0.01 during NREM.

Baldridge, Whitman, and Kramer (1965) used a very sensitive semiconductor strain gauge described by Baldridge, Whitman, and Kramer (1963) to measure minute movements of the eye, throat, wrist and ankle of 10 paid adult volunteers who slept overnight in a private hospital room. These devices attach to the eyelid, throat, wrist, and ankle with a small piece of adhesive tape. The eyelid sensor is capable of detecting movements as small as 2 degrees. Wrist and eye movements were separately averaged over 10-minute epochs and correlated for each of the 10 subjects. The resulting correlation coefficients in descending order of magnitude (with degrees of freedom) are: .84 (35), .83 (38), .80 (36), .79 (46), .78 (39), .76 (33), .62 (35), .60 (38), .56 (41), .55 (41). All correlations are significant $p < .0001$ except the lowest correlation which is significant $p < .01$. An average (Fisher-Z transformation) of these correlations is $r(38) = .73$, $p < .0001$.

Total sleep time decreases from birth to approximately 40 years of age, where it remains essentially constant until age 80, when a slight further decline begins (Feinberg and Carlson, 1968). The number of wakenings after going to sleep increases steadily with age across the lifespan (Feinberg and Carlson, 1968).

Mendelson (1987, pp. 33–79) discusses the effects of drugs and neurotransmitters on sleep along with an extensive discussion of the benzodiazepine receptor and sleep (pp. 107–179).

SELF-REPORT AND BEHAVIORAL OBSERVATION

Montgomery, Perkin, and Wise (1975), Carskadon, Dement, Mitler, Guilleminault, Zarcone, and Spiegle (1976), Knapp, Downs, and Alperson (1976), and Ribordy and Denney (1977) all concluded that self-reported sleep is inaccurate when compared with EEG measures. Kupfer, Wyatt, and Snyder (1970), and Weiss, McPartland, and Kupfer (1973) reported that nurses ratings of sleep do not correlate well with either activity or EEG sleep estimates.

Andersen, Keenan, and Carson (1989) had the parents of 30 children, aged 6 months to 6 years, complete a rest–activity questionnaire and a rest–activity log for one 24-hour period regarding their children's behavior. The children also wore a wrist actigraph (Ambulatory Monitoring Inc., Ardsley, NY). The reported correlation between measured activity and rest–activity questionnaire data of $r(28) = .21$ was not significant. The correlation between measured activity and rest–activity log data of $r(28) = .42$ was significant ($p < .05$).

BED STABILIMETERS

Kleitman (1963, pp. 81–91) reviews the early work on body motility in more detail than present space permits. He indicates that Maclay reported that people changed position while sleeping without awakening and that Szymanski (1922) first described a device for measuring body motility through bed spring movement. Cox and Marley (1959) described a simple apparatus that attaches to bed springs for measuring body motility. Using a related device, Kleitman (1963, pp. 85–86) reported 30 seconds of motility per hour of sleep typically accumulating from 3 to 5 minutes of activity produced by 20 to 60 movements per night. Motility was reported to be greater during the second than first half of sleep by a ratio of from 2:1 to 3:2. Activity cycles appear to have 50- to 60-minute periods in infants, 60 to 70 minute periods in preschool children, and 85- to 90-minute periods in adults.

Stonehill and Crisp (1971) reported the curious finding that motility during sleep is positively related to body weight. They report the following regression equation based on 37 subjects: Motility Score = 8.20 + 0.42 (weight in lbs). Although they do not report a correlation coefficient, their Figure 3 indicates a sizable relationship between these two variables.

ACTIGRAPHY

Motility Detection

Devices such as the Motionlogger™ and Actillume™ (cf. Ambulatory Monitoring, Inc.) were designed to measure wrist, leg, and waist activity. The sensitivity of these devices to movement makes it difficult to move them without the motion being detected. Their onboard clock and programmable epoch allows the user to select the temporal resolution by which presence of movement is detectable. It has become standard to use a 1-minute epoch thereby identifying activity onset to an accuracy of within 1 minute.

Tzischinsky, Epstein, Zomer, Varak, and Lavie (1987) reported that sleep motility decreases with age in healthy children aged 5 to 18 years with no sleep complaints. They placed an actigraph (Ambulatory Monitoring Inc., Ardsley, NY) on the nondominant wrist of 13 female and 24 male children for one night using either a 5-second, 20-second, or 40-second epoch. Sleep activity (standard error) counts for three age groups were: children 5–8 years = 19.5 (1.77), children 9–10 years = 12.1 (6.05), children 11 to 18 years = 4.91 (1.54). Hence, elevated sleep motility is normal for 5- to 8-year-old children but steadily decreases through age 18.

Sleep Detection

Sleep is associated with prolonged inactivity. Therefore, sleep can be indirectly behaviorally studied using a time-based recording system such as the Ambulatory Monitoring, Inc. Motionlogger™ or Actillume™ (Borbely, 1986; Mullaney, Kripke, and Messin, 1980; Kripke, Mullaney, Messin, and Wyborney, 1978; Webster, Kripke, Messin, Mullaney, and Wyborney, 1982). Figure 6.1 was taken from the wrist of a college student between the hours of 22:09:00 of Day 289 and 09:44:10 of Day 290 of 1989. The Actigraph was programmed for a 1-minute epoch in threshold mode. The indication of a 00:01:09 epoch is the result of software compression to graph the requested interval in the available space as indicated by the compression ratio (Comp) of 1:16. The maximum vertical display is 250 counts. The horizontal tic marks are at 30 minute intervals. Notice that activity during sleep is clearly less than during wake as expected. Notice also that activity is periodically present throughout sleep.

Figure 6.2 is an exploded presentation of the sleep onset portion of Figure 6.1. Each 1-minute epoch is now clearly separated. The primary feature of these data is that activity declines rapidly with sleep onset. Figure 6.3 is an exploded presentation of the sleep offset portion of Figure 6.1. The primary feature of these data is that activity rapidly increases upon awakening.

Hand Scoring

Ferromagnetic Ball Sensor. Kupfer, Detre, Foster, Tucker, and Delgado (1972) used a sensor containing a 3.0-mm ferromagnetic ball rolling within a small coil to sense activity and transmit a signal to a nearby receiver indicating the presence of activity. This light-weight (50-g) device was strapped to the wrist of the nondominant hand of 8 hospitalized patients (6 females, 2 males) aged 21 to 70 years (mean = 51.6 years) suffering from manic depression, recurrent depression, schizoaffective schizophrenia, or hypochrondrical neurosis, for two consecutive nights. The authors reported correlations of $r = .76$, $p < .001$ to $r = .96$, $p < .001$

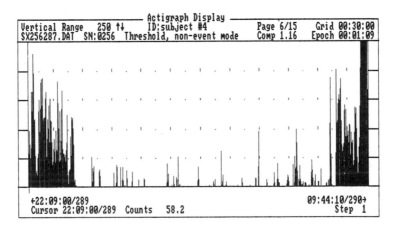

FIGURE 6.1. Sample wrist actigraph sleep record.

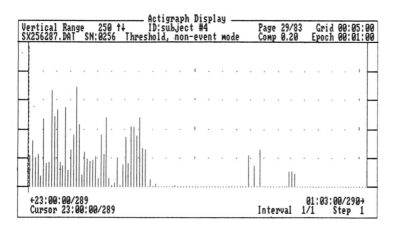

FIGURE 6.2. Sleep onset portion of Fig. 6.1.

(average $r = .88$, $p < .001$) between activity counts and simultaneously EEG measured movement time. EEG determined wakefulness was correlated $r = .84$, $p < .001$ with wrist activity.

Weiss, Kupfer, Foster, and Delgado (1974) measured wrist activity, using the Kupfer *et al.* (1972) device described above, in 11 patients (7 females, 4 males) aged 25 to 63 years (mean = 48.4 years). They reported a significant negative correlation between nighttime (midnight to 0700) activity and EMG-determined time-spent-asleep ($r = -.65$, $p < .05$). A curious aside is the significant relationship between daytime activity (0700–2100) and intermittent nocturnal awakening ($r = .66$, $p < .05$).

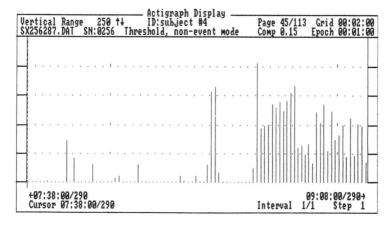

FIGURE 6.3. Sleep offset portion of Fig. 6.1.

Kupfer and Foster (1973) detailed a case study of a 54-year-old black female suffering from psychotic depression. Longitudinal sleep EEG and 24-hour wrist activity using the Kupfer *et al.* (1972) device revealed a correlation of $r = -.88$, $p < .001$ between nighttime activity (midnight–0700) and time-spent-asleep. Periods of insomnia were associated with nocturnal activity increases whereas periods of hypersomnia were associated with activity decreases. A curious aside was the significant negative correlation ($r = -.63$, $p < .01$) between 24-hour activity and time-spent-asleep, and time-spent-asleep with activity during the preceding day ($r = -.53$, $p < .05$).

Reich, Kupfer, Weiss, McPartland, Foster, Detre, and Delgado (1974) analyzed activity counts for the first 120 minutes of bedtime and all-night EEG, EOG, and EMG in 26 (11 male, 15 female) psychiatric patients aged 15 to 55 years (mean = 27.7). Ten patients were depressed (2 psychotic; 8 nonpsychotic), 7 were schizophrenic, and 9 had neurotic or personality disorders. All were drug free for at least 14 days prior to this study. Polygraphic sleep latency correlated $r(24) = .85$, $p < .001$ with activity counts over the first 120 minutes of bedtime. Time spent asleep correlated $r(24) = -.80$, $p < .001$ with activity counts during the first 120 minutes of bedtime.

Accelerometers. Kripke, Mullaney, Messin, and Wyborney (1978) measured wrist activity of five subjects with a custom-made piezo-ceramic accelerometer-based device (Webster, Messin, Mullaney, and Kripke, 1982) whose output was recorded onto C-120 cassette tapes over a 24-hour period using a Medilog tape recorder. Simultaneous EEG channels were recorded during sleep. They reported a correlation of $r(3) = .954$, $p < .01$ between EEG (using Rechtschaffen and Kales, 1968, criteria) and activity estimates of Total Sleep Period (TSP). The EEG–activity data pairs for the five subjects were 436 vs 433, 442 vs 446, 497 vs 485, 466 vs 454, and 512 vs 528 minutes. The associated differences of -3, -4, 12, 12, and -16 minutes equal -0.69%, -0.9%, 2.4%, 2.6%, and -3.1% respectively of the average TSP estimates. These discrepancies are all quite small and average out to be 0.062% which is less than 0.1% error.

Kripke *et al.* (1978) reported a correlation of $r(3) = .982$, $p < .01$ between EEG and activity estimates of Total Sleep Time. The EEG–activity (TST) data pairs for the five subjects were 434 vs 410, 348 vs 345, 442 vs 439, 462 vs 453, and 502 vs 473 minutes. The associated differences of 24, 13, 3, 9, and 29 minutes equal 5.7%, 3.8%, 0.7%, 2.0%, and 5.9% respectively of the average TST estimates. Though somewhat larger than TSP errors, the TST errors average to be just 3.62%.

EEG and activity Wake Time Within Sleep (WTWS) was reported by Kripke *et al.* (1978) to correlate $r(3) = .851$, $p < .10$. The EEG–activity WTWS data pairs for the five subjects were 94 vs 100, 54 vs 46, 4 vs 1, 10 vs 55, and 2 vs 23 minutes. The first three pairs correspond quite well with differences of but -6, 9, and 3 minutes respectively. However, the final two pairs had discrepancies of -45 and -21 minutes. The actigraph results indicate greater wakefulness in the latter two subjects compared to EEG data.

The section below entitled EEG Uncertainty demonstrates that subjects are behaviorally awake until the beginning of Stage 2 sleep. Hence, EEG will categorize subjects as in Stage 1 sleep while they can still respond to auditory signals by pressing a hand-held microswitch. This would account for the slightly greater EEG TST and two discrepant WTWS estimates just reported. In these cases, the actigraph is consistent with operant sleep data discussed below.

Actigraph. Mullaney, Kripke, and Messin (1980) continued the above research with 58 males and 27 females aged 18 to 66 years ($M = 33.6$, $S = 13.5$). Sixteen subjects were recorded twice and one subject was recorded three times. Of the resulting 102 recordings, 39 were from 32 patients with psychiatric disorder, alcoholism, or chronic pain. The remaining 63 recordings were from 53 normal controls including college students and hospital staff. Data collection was the same as described above (cf. Kripke, Mullaney, Messin, and Wyborney, 1978). A correlation coefficient of $r(100) = 0.89$, $p < .0001$ was found between EEG and actigraphic (Ambulatory Monitoring Inc., Ardsley, NY) estimates of Total Sleep Time (TST). However, actigraphic estimates of TST (about 402 min) averaged 15.33 minutes longer than EEG estimates (about 386 min) ($t(101) = 3.82$, $p < .0001$). The problem appears to be with persons who are awake but lie still. In a subsequent section entitled EEG Uncertainty, we will discuss the position that sleep onset is gradual rather than abrupt. Perhaps lying still is an even earlier stage in the sleep onset process.

EEG and actigraphic Total Sleep Period (TSP) correlated $r(100) = .90$, $p < .0001$. EEG and actigraphic Wake After Sleep Onset (WASO) correlated $r(100) = 0.70$, $p < .0001$. EEG and actigraphic Mean Sleep Awakenings (MSA) correlated $r(100) = .25$, $p < .01$.

Stradling, Warley, and Sharpley (1987) studied time of sleep onset, prolonged arousals during sleep, and time of awakening, in 14 subjects aged 21–45 years (12 normal, 1 with REM-sleep obstructive apnea, 1 with REM-sleep hypoventilation) using conventional (EEG, EMG, EOG) and wrist actigraphy (Ambulatory Monitoring, Inc.) measures. Sleep onset was defined for the conventional measures as entering Stage 2 or below for three or more minutes. Actigraph criteria for sleep onset was the beginning of a period with no activity for 10 minutes. Prolonged arousals during sleep were defined for conventional measures as 10 minutes or more of Stage W (wakening) or MT (movement) with no more than 5 minutes of Stage 1 and 1 minute of Stage 2 during this 10 minute period. Actigraph criteria for prolonged arousal was 5 minutes or more of 5 activity counts within any 10-minute period. Awakenings were conventionally defined as beginning a period scored waking or movement lasting 2 minutes with no lapses below Stage 1 for more than 1 minute or by the subject's signaling with an event marker that sleep terminated.

The results were that the average time of sleep onset for actigraph minus conventional measurements was 0.9 ($S = 9.0$) minutes. Only 8 subjects evidenced prolonged arousals. The same 8 periods of prolonged arousal were detected by both procedures but no timing information was provided except to say that much less temporal agreement was noted. The average time of awakening for actigraph minus conventional measurements was 1.1 ($S = 7$) minutes. Again we find evidence that motility decreases prior to satisfying EEG Stage 1 sleep criteria though one precedes the other by approximately 54 seconds, a very small fraction of the entire night.

Newman, Stampi, Dunham, and Broughton (1988) compared actigraphic (Ambulatory Monitoring, Inc., Ardsley, NY) and polysomnographic (PSG) measures of Total Sleep Time (TST) and Total Wake Time (TWT) in 3 male narcolepsy-cataplexy patients aged 21–59 years (mean = 42.0) withdrawn from tricyclics for at least 3 weeks and from methylphenidate for at least 1 week and 4 control (1 male, 3 female) subjects aged 43–72 years (mean = 51.8). Sleep onset was defined in the actigraphic record to start at the first of 3 successive (probably 1-minute) epochs containing 20 or fewer activity counts each. The beginning of the waking state was defined as the first of 3 successive epochs containing more than 20 activity counts each. Sleep and wake were defined by Rechtshaffen and Kales (1968) criteria. Continuous data collection proceeded over a 24-hour period using a 4-channel Medilog (Oxford Medical Systems) recorder.

The PSG data found the 3 narcoleptic subjects to be asleep for an average of 604.7 minutes whereas actigraphy produced an average of 602.0 minutes. The difference of 2.7 minutes is but 0.4% of the average of both measurements. The PSG data indicated that the 4 control subjects slept an average of 422.2 minutes whereas actigraphy produced an average of 441.5 minutes. The difference of -19.3 minutes is 4.5% of the average of both measurements. The between-group to within-group variance ratios (t-tests; $F = t^2$) are about equal for both data sets. For PSG $t(5) = 5.22$, $p < .002$. For actigraphy $t(5) = 4.59$, $p < .006$. A Pearson product moment correlation coefficient found the two data sets to be highly correlated $r(5) = .91$, $p < .002$. This study indicates that motility decreases can precede EEG Stage 1 sleep by as much as 19.3 minutes indicating that this possibly earliest sleep stage can be of substantial length though it may be as short as the 54 seconds noted above.

The PSG data found the 3 narcoleptic subjects to be awake for an average of 775.8 minutes while actigraphy indicated they were awake on average for 764.9 minutes. This difference of 10.9 minutes is but 1.4% of the average of both measurements. The PSG data indicated that the 4 control subjects were awake for an average of 957.2 minutes as compared with the actigraph measurement of 971.8 minutes. The difference of -14.6 minutes is but 1.5% of the average of both measurements. The actigraphic measures gave slightly better between- vs within-group ratios (*t*-tests). For PSG $t(5) = 4.12$, $p < .01$. For actigraphy $t(5) = 6.12$, $p < .002$). Normal sleep onset appears to involve a period of immobility followed by EEG Stage 1 sleep; a feature seemingly absent in narcoleptic subjects.

Stampi and Broughton (1989) compared polygraphic and actigraphic measurements of Total Sleep Time (TST) in 4 male subjects during baseline, ultrashort sleep (anchor sleep plus ultrashort sleep vs ultrashort sleep only), and recovery conditions equated for 8 hours of sleep per 24-hour period. The baseline and recovery phases involved one 8-hour sleep period. Two forms of ultrashort sleep were studied. In the first condition, 4 hours of anchor sleep from 01.00 to 05.00 was followed by three 80-minute naps equally spaced over the remaining 20 hours. This condition continued for 3 consecutive 24-hour periods, followed by a 2-week "washout" followed by another 3 consecutive 24-hour periods of ultrashort sleep. In the second condition, the 8 hours of sleep were obtained through 80-, 50-, or 20-minute naps spread over each 24-hour period for 12 consecutive days. Wrist actigraphic (Ambulatory Monitoring, Ardsley, NY) measurements were taken using 1-minute epochs. Ambulatory EEG, EOG, EMG, EKG, and core body temperature were recorded using an 8-channel Oxford Medilog.

During baseline, polygraphic TST was measured to be 396 minutes whereas actigraphic TST was measured at 397 minutes yielding 99.7% agreement. During all forms of ultrasleep, polygraphic TST equalled 383 minutes whereas actigraphic TST was 486 minutes for 78.8% agreement. The discrepancies were explained by quiet wakefulness and stage 1 sleep without movement. During recovery, polysomnographic TST equalled 370 minutes and actigraphic TST measured 385 minutes for 96.1% agreement. The multistage sleep onset process discussed below in the EEG Uncertainty section is consistent with these data. EEG Stage 1 sleep appears to quickly follow motility reduction in normal sleep but not during ultrasleep which seems to involve protracted immobility prior to EEG State 1 sleep.

Levine, Moyles, Roehrs, Fortier, and Roth (1986) used a Vitalog 6 (Redwood City, CA) mercury-switch-based actigraph using a 15-second epoch and polygraphic (undefined) measurements to identify sleep vs wake periods in 7 young college students during an 8-hour nocturnal sleep period and a sleep latency (MSLT) test the following day. Waking was scored for each epoch containing 1 or more activity counts. Sleep was scored only when no activity was measured. The polygraphic record was scored using standard Rechtschaffen and Kales (1968) criteria for wake and sleep over 30-second epochs. Agreement between the two methods was reported over 5-minute and 2.5-minute epochs.

Using 5-minute epochs, polygraphic measurement of Total Sleep Time (TST) during the 8 nocturnal hours averaged 455.0 minutes whereas actigraphic measurements averaged 440.0 minutes. The difference of 15 minutes equals 3.4% of the average of both measurements. The percent agreement was listed as 92.6. Using 2.5-minute epochs, polygraphic TST measurements averaged 454.3 minutes whereas actigraphic TST measurements averaged 430.4 minutes. The difference of 23.9 minutes longer EEG defined TST equals 5.4% of the average of both measurements.

Using 5-minute epochs during the subsequent sleep latency test, polygraphic measurements indicated 15.7 minutes of sleep whereas the actigraphic records suggested 35.0 minutes of sleep; 2.23 times as great. This raises questions about how awake subjects really were during this test. Further comments pertinent to this matter appear in the "EEG Uncertainty" section later in this chapter.

Ancoli-Israel, Kripke, Mason, and Messin (1981) studied 24 older adults (11 recruited men aged 63–79 years; $M = 72.5$ years; 13 recruited women aged 58–79 years; $M = 68.5$ years; 3 referred senior males aged 60–61 years; 9 middle-aged referred males aged 31–55 years; $M = 48.5$ years). One night of home recording was accomplished as follows. Thorax and abdominal respiration were measured using Respitrace™ (Ambulatory Monitoring Inc., Ardsley, NY) sensors. One channel of wrist activity and another channel of tibialis EMG summed from both legs were all recorded on a 4-channel portable analog Medilog recorder. A second night of recording was done in a sleep laboratory using a Grass model 78 polygraph to record EEG, EOG, Chin EMG, EKG, tibialis EMG summed from both legs, and three channels of respiration including nasal airway temperature, thorax, and abdominal Respitrace™ expansion. The portable apparatus was also worn while the subject slept in the laboratory to allow simultaneous comparison between portable and laboratory instrumentation. All sleep scoring was accomplished with Rechtschaffen and Kales (1968) criteria using two trained personnel.

Total sleep period measures, as determined by portable and laboratory equipment, correlated $r(22) = .82, p < .0001$. Total sleep period between home and laboratory correlated $r(22) = .53, p < .01$. This correlation coefficient underestimates the true correlation by the amount of night-to-night variation in total sleep period. Analysis of variance revealed no significant mean differences in total sleep period across methods.

Total sleep time measurements obtained by portable and laboratory equipment correlated $r(22) = .69, p < .0002$. The corresponding attenuated home vs laboratory correlation was $r(22) = .44, p < .05$. Analysis of variance revealed no significant mean differences in total sleep time across methods.

Wake after sleep onset measures were significantly correlated between devices ($r(22) = .61, p < .002$) during the same night and between nights ($r(22) = .40, p < 05$). Analysis of variance revealed no significant mean differences in wake after sleep onset across methods.

The number of apneas lasting more than 10 seconds during both REM and NREM sleep were divided by the number of hours of sleep. The correlation between the portable and laboratory apnea indices in the laboratory was $r(22) = .80, p < .0001$. The between-nights correlation was $r(22) = .68, p < 001$). Analysis of variance revealed no significant differences between the mean number of apneas determined at home and in the sleep laboratory.

Urbach, Lavie, and Alster (1989) reported a very interesting synthetic approach. Polysomnography was used to determine waking and sleeping in 7 normals during each 1-minute epoch. Dominant wrist actigraphy (Ambulatory Monitoring Inc., Ardsley, NY) counts were then plotted for polysomnographically defined "wake" and "sleep" periods on the same graph. The point of their intersection, approximately 25 counts/minute, was taken as the empirically determined sleep–wake threshold. Counts equal to or greater than this threshold defined wake; lesser activity counts defined sleep. Sleep ratios were defined as the number of 1-minute sleep epochs as a percentage of all sleep plus wake epochs. The 7 normals had an average (SE mean?) sleep ratio of 84.3 (2.8). The 12 sleep apnea patients averaged 62.4 (15.6) while the 6 insomniacs averaged 67.5 (15.3). Fifteen of the 18 (85%) patients were beyond the normal mean minus two standard deviations and were reported to be significantly ($p < .01$) different from the normal group.

Computer Scoring

In Experiment I, Webster, Kripke, Messin, Mullaney, and Wyborney (1982) continuously stored wrist activity to a waist-worn Medilog recorder as described by Kripke, Mullaney, Messin, and Wyborney (1978). Seven subjects wore this device from the early morning, through the night, until some time the following morning. To remove 60-Hz artifact (from electric blankets) from the analogue activity signal, it was digitized with an analog-to-digital (A/D) converter at $4 \times 60 = 240$ Hz so that four data points would be obtained during each of the 60 cycles per second of artifact. Summing over the four data points gave 60 artifact-free data points per second or 120 such data points over the desired 2-second epoch. Ten transformations were performed on these data and the best one (algorithm 5) chosen for further study. Letting X = the sum of the four A/D conversions, algorithm 5 is presented here as Equation (1):

$$
\begin{aligned}
f[X(i)] = 10 \times X(i) - [X(i - 5) + X(i - 4) + X(i - 3) \\
+ X(i - 2) + X(i - 1) + X(i + 1) + X(i + 2) + X(i + 3) \\
+ X(i + 4) + X(i + 5)]
\end{aligned} \tag{1}
$$

where i represents the current minute.

Experiment II began by collecting 20 overnight data sets from 17 subjects; three subjects were tested twice. Seventeen data sets were used to calculate weights for Equation 1 resulting in Equation (2):

$$
\begin{aligned}
D = 0.25X[(.15T(i - 4) + .15T(i - 3) + .15T(i - 2) \\
+ .08T(i - 1) + .21T(i) + .12T(i + 1) + .13T(i + 2)]
\end{aligned} \tag{2}
$$

where i represents the current minute and T equals the maximum 2-second epoch value in the designated 1-minute interval. If D is equal to or greater than 1 then wake is scored; otherwise sleep is scored.

A retrospective analysis over the 17 records upon which these weights were developed revealed a 94.46% agreement between wrist actigraphic and EEG sleep–wake discriminations. A prospective analysis of the remaining three subjects revealed 96.02% agreement. The conditional probability of misscoring wake as sleep was .062 whereas the conditional probability of misscoring sleep as wake was .039.

The following rules slightly improved retrospective agreement to 94.74%: "(a) after at least 4 min scored wake, the first period of 1 min scored sleep is rescored wake; (b) after at least 10 min scored wake, the first 3 min scored sleep are rescored wake; (c) after at least 15 min scored wake, the first 4 min scored sleep are rescored wake; (d) 6 min or less scored sleep surrounded by at least 10 min (before and after) scored wake are rescored wake; and (e) 10 min or less scored sleep surrounded by at least 20 min (before and after) scored wake are rescored wake." (p. 396) No mention was made of improvement to prospectively scored records.

In Experiment III, wrist activity was measured in 14 healthy college students along with EMG, EOG, and EMG using a modified Vitalog Corporation (Redwood City, CA) PMS-8 monitor and digitized as described in Experiment II. Optimal weights were calculated and are presented as Equation (3):

$$D = .036X[.07T(i - 5) + .08T(i - 4) + .10T(i - 3)$$
$$+ .11T(i - 2) + .12T(i - 1) + .14T(i) + .09T(i + 1)$$
$$+ .09T(i + 2) + .09T(i + 3) + .10T(i + 4)] \qquad (3)$$

where i represents the current minute and T equals the maximum 2-second epoch value in the designated 1-minute interval. If D is equal to or greater than 1 then wake is scored; otherwise sleep is scored.

Overall sleep–wake agreement with polygraphic data on these 14 data sets equalled 93.88%. The actigraphic and polygraphic data sets correlated $r(12) = .9724, p < .0001$.

Prospective analysis of 14 additional data sets from 12 healthy college men and two patients with sleep complaints undergoing clinical evaluation yielded 93.04% agreement between actigraphic and polygraphic sleep–wake measurements. The two data sets correlated $r(12) = .9692, p < .0001$.

The authors concluded that the slight discrepancies associated with actigraphic data could be more than compensated for by collecting data over multiple nights. The noninvasive and relatively inexpensive characteristics of actigraphy make longitudinal sleep study practical. Moreover, the authors indicate that " . . . we suspect that where the two methods are discrepant, behavioral criteria would on some occasions favor activity scoring." (p. 399) The subsequent section on EEG Uncertainty strongly supports this contention.

Zomer, Pollack, Tzischinsky, Epstein, Alster, and Lavie (1987) compared wrist actigraph (Ambulatory Monitoring Inc., Ardsley, NY) and polygraph (EEG, EOG, ECK, and EMG, plus Leg Movements, respiration, and ear oximetry as needed) measures of sleep time and latency in 2 normal healthy males and 13 patients: 5 with sleep apnea, 4 with sleep maintenance insomnia, 1 with periodic leg movements in sleep, 1 with paroxysmal awakening from sleep, plus 2 persons referred for penile erection during sleep (probably to evaluate impotence complaint). The actigraph was programmed for a 5-second epoch (12 subjects) or for 1 minute (3 subjects) and placed on the nondominant wrist. Polygraphic sleep latency was defined as the time from lights off until the beginning of the first occurrence of 3 continuous minutes of Stage 2 sleep. Polygraphic sleep time was defined as total bed time minus sleep latency minus wake and movement time within sleep.

Sleep vs waking was determined with the actigraph record as follows. The mean and standard deviation associated with lights out were calculated. For the 5-second epoch, wake was scored whenever activity exceeded the mean plus two standard deviations in three consecutive epochs; sleep was scored otherwise. For the 1-minute epoch, wake was scored whenever activity exceeded the mean plus two standard deviations in any epoch; sleep was scored otherwise. Sleep latency was calculated as lights off until first sleep. Total sleep time was calculated as bed time with lights out minus sleep latency.

Polygraphic total sleep time averaged 364.8 ($S = 54.1$) minutes. Actigraphic total sleep time averaged 376.7 ($S = 45.0$) min. These total sleep time measurements are correlated $r(13) = .82, p < .0002$. The absolute error was under 10% for all subjects except one who obtained a sleep latency of 80 minutes by lying "almost motionless" in bed. The total sleep time correlation increases to $r(12) = .94, p < .0001$ when this one data pair is removed. No data were provided on sleep latency.

It was mentioned that the actigraph record clearly revealed periodic leg movements and repetitive brief body movements. Movements associated with sleep apnea were also captured by the actigraph record though no formal analysis of these associations were presented.

Sadeh, Alster, Urbach, and Lavie (1989) describe a two-phase research effort. Phase 1 was devoted to developing an algorithm for determining sleep and wakefulness from actigraph records and comparing these results with polygraphic data. Phase 2 evaluated the validity of using the actigraph as a sleep disorder screening device by testing its ability to discriminate between a normal and two patient groups.

A total of 67 subjects (13 normals and 54 patients including 13 children) participated in the Phase 1 by spending one night in a sleep laboratory with an actigraph (Ambulatory Monitoring, Inc., Ardsley, NY), programmed for 1-minute epochs, attached to their nondominant wrist. Concurrent polygraphic data were scored according to the Rechtschaffen and Kales (1968) criteria. Sleep was defined as Stages 1, 2, 3–4, and REM. Wake was defined as Stage 0 and movement time

(MT). A sleep–wake discriminant function was calculated using data from the first 9 subjects and an unspecified number of predictors using a stepwise procedure until the 5 best predictors were selected. They write, "The input parameters for this procedure include activity level, minimum value and standard deviation during all combinations of up to 10 minutes before and after the given minute." (p. 210) Equation (4) presents the obtained sleep–wake discriminant function:

$$PS = 4.532 - [.06828\ X_0 - .0385\ S_{-5} - .038\ S_{+9}$$
$$+ .0298\ M_{+2} - .0299\ S_{-2}] \tag{4}$$

where X_0 is the number of zero crossings (activity count) associated with the classified minute, S_{-5} is the standard deviation of the activity counts during the previous 5 minutes, S_{+9} is the standard deviation of the activity counts in the following 9 minutes, M_{+2} is the minimum value of activity during the following 2 minutes and S_{-2} is the standard deviation during the prior 2 minutes. Sleep is scored if PS is greater than or equal to zero; else wake is scored.

This discriminant function correctly identified 95.49% of the 2692 (91.91%) polysomnographically defined sleep periods and 63.54% of the 237 (8.09%) waking periods in the 9 normal "calibration" subjects for a total of 91.76% correct identification of all 2929 episodes (see section later in this chapter on base rates for additional comments).

Equation (4) was validated against the remaining 4 normals and 54 patients. This function correctly identified 88.25% of the 969 (84.63%) polygraphically defined sleep periods and 76.19% of the 176 (15.37%) waking periods in the 4 normal validation subjects for a total of 86.16% correct identification of all 1145 episodes.

Equation (4) was further validated against 13 child patients where it correctly identified 92.91% of the 4430 (91.68%) polygraphically defined sleep periods and 66.01% of the 402 (8.32%) waking periods for a total of 89.86% correct identification of all 4832 episodes.

Further validation of Equation (4) was against 16 insomnia patients yielded 95.43% correct identification of the 3320 (77.30%) polygraphically defined sleep periods and 48.48% of the 975 (22.70%) waking periods for a total of 78.23% correct identification of all 4295 episodes.

Validation against 25 sleep apnea syndrome patients yielded 92.06% correct identification of the 7486 (88.27%) polygraphically defined sleep periods and 56.47% of the 995 (11.73%) waking periods for a total of 85.72% correct identification of all 8481 episodes. Examination of individual sleep apnea syndrome subject records revealed that "polysomnographic scoring was insensitive to the multiple micro-arousals which accompanied the periodic terminations of the apneas." (p. 212) The question of EEG inaccuracy is discussed further below.

Phase 2 began by testing 28 additional adults (10 normals, 7 insomniacs, and 11 sleep apnea syndrome) having a mean age of 39.8 years. The 13 children were dropped because they were not clinically homogeneous. The resulting sample 67 + 28 − 13 = 82 adults was divided into three groups on the basis of interview and polysomnographic data: normals, insomniacs, and sleep apnea syndrome. A new discriminant function using fourteen unspecified actigraph variables was developed on 34 randomly chosen (from the 82) subjects and validated on the remaining 48 subjects.

Discriminant Equations (5), (6), and (7) give the probability of normal (*PN*), insomnia (*PI*) and sleep apnea syndrome (*PA*) group membership. The subject was classified as belonging to the group associated with the largest probability.

$$PN = -87.90 - .310 \, TBT + 6.39 \, TRS + 25.05 \, MD$$
$$+ 1.53 \, STABR + .808 \, STAB + .507 \, SDS \tag{5}$$

$$PI = -92.15 - .339 \, TBT + 6.99 \, TRS + 23.64 \, MD$$
$$+ 1.43 \, STABR + .842 \, STAB + .628 \, SDS \tag{6}$$

$$PA = -98.52 - .273 \, TBT + 6.29 \, TRS + 29.19 \, MD$$
$$+ 1.34 \, STABR + .799 \, STAB + .557 \, SDS \tag{7}$$

Where *TBT* equals Total Bed Time, *TRS* equals sleep–wake transitions as a proportion of *TBT, MD* equals Movement Density as movements per minute, *STABR* equals the number of transitions from one 10-minute sleep or wake state to another, *STAB* equals the number of minutes that follow 10 minutes of wake or 10 minutes of sleep, and *SDS* equals the standard deviation of activity during sleep.

An overall "hit" rate of 64.6% (of 48 subjects) was achieved which is significantly better than, and nearly double, the 33.3% chance expectation. Of 15 normals, 9 (60%) were correctly identified as Normal, 3 as Insomnia, and 3 as Apnea. Of 13 insomnia patients, 7 (53.8%) were identified as Insomnia, 4 as Apnea, and 2 as Normal. Of 20 sleep apnea syndrome patients, 15 (75%) were identified as Apnea, 3 as Insomnia, and 2 as Normal. The authors comment that "*post-hoc* analysis of the misclassified cases revealed that their diagnosis based on polysomnographic data itself was marginal." (p. 214) The importance of base rates in connection with the proper interpretation of these results is addressed below.

Stepwise regression of actigraphic variables on number of sleep apneas identified movement density and number of successive sleep minutes as significant predictors [$R(17) = .5481$, $p < .005$]. Movement density was the better predictor [$r(18) = .448$, $p < .01$].

Cole and Kripke (1989) published an interim report on their progress in constructing an automatic sleep–wake actigraphic scoring system. Twenty adults (12 men, 8 women aged 30–72) served as subjects. Six were normal controls, 4 had sleep disorders, 6 were either depressed or schizophrenic, and 3 were bereaved widows. Each minute of the polygraphic records was scored as sleep (Stages 1–4 + REM) or wake (including movement time). Actigraphs (Ambulatory Monitoring, Inc., Ardsley, NY) were programmed with 2-second epochs.

Actigraph records were scored in a unique way. For each minute, a 16-second (8-point) window was imposed at the beginning and activity counts summed. The window was moved to the right by one 2-second interval (1 data point) and the sum of the next 8 points determined. Twenty-three such sums were created for each minute and the largest sum was recorded as the score for that minute. Activity during the present minute (A_0), activity during the previous 5 minutes (A_{-1} to A_{-5}) and activity during the following 2 minutes (A_{+1}, A_{+2}) were used in the linear prediction of sleep-wake resulting in Equation (8).

$$S = -.001\, A_{-5} - .001\, A_{-4} - .001\, A_{-3} - .001\, A_{-2}$$
$$- .003\, A_{-1} + .001\, A_{+2} + 1.004 \qquad (8)$$

Sleep is scored when S is less than or equal to 0.5; else wake is scored. This equation correctly predicted 88.3% of the sleep/wake episodes in the 10 training subjects and 87.8 of the 4409 sleep/wake episodes in the 10 validation subjects. Rescoring with the Webster, Kripke, Messin, Mullaney, and Wyborney (1982) rules described above increased correct sleep/wake identification to 88.5%. This function correctly identified 95.9% of the 3278 (74.35%) polygraphically defined sleep periods and 67.3% of the 1131 (25.65%) waking periods of all 4409 episodes for all subjects.

Prediction by subgroup revealed substantial differences. For 3 normals, 91.7% of 1197 polygraphic defined sleep/wake episodes were consistently scored by actigraphy. For 3 psychiatric patients 90.7% of 1225 episodes were consistently scored by actigraphy. For 2 sleep-disorder patients 88.9% of 824 episodes were correctly scored. For 2 bereaved widows 79.6% of 658 episodes were correctly scored.

Discriminant Function Comment

Multiple regression attempts to predict a single quantitative dependent variable (Y) using data on multiple independent or predictor variables (X). Cohen and Cohen (1983) describe discriminant analysis as an extension of multiple regression to where membership in two or more groups is predicted from the same set of independent (X) variables. The group membership dependent variable is represented using the same dummy coding scheme as would be used if it were employed as a predictor variable (cf. Cohen and Cohen, 1988; Chapter 5). The degrees of freedom (df) equal $N - k - 1$ where N is the number of subjects and k is the number of predictors (Cohen and Cohen, 1985, pp. 103–105). The standard error of the regression (discrimination) weights is inversely proportional to df. Small df results in large error of prediction weights. Hence, the probability increases that the prediction weights do not differ from random chance expectation, which implies that they will not be well replicated in subsequent samples.

Usually, the data for each subject involve one value for the dependent variable and one value for each of the independent variables. In this context textbooks on multivariate statistics (cf. Harris, 1985, p. 64) typically recommend a minimum of 10 subjects for each variable or that the number of subjects minus the number of variables exceed 50, in order to obtain stable statistically significant results. Had each night's actigraph record yielded this set of scores for each subject, Webster, Kripke, Messin, Mullaney, and Wyborney (1982), and Sadeh, Alster, Urbach, and Lavie (1989), reviewed above, would have calculated their sleep–wake discriminant functions using many variables and few subjects: the reverse of what is recommended. Because multiple instances of waking and sleeping occur for each subject during one night, subjects repeatedly, and probably unequally, contribute to the data set upon which the above investigators calculated their discriminant function. Psychometric theory requires that each contribution to the data set be independent of every other. This assumption is called into question when subjects repeatedly contribute to the data set. This problem is compounded in complex ways when the contributions across subjects differ; some subjects therefore influence the final discriminant weights more than others.

This problem aside, the degrees of freedom become $N - k - 1$ where N equals the number of sleep and wake contributions across all subjects and k equals the number of predictor variables. In the Sadeh, Alster, Urbach, and Lavie (1989) study, 2692 sleep episodes and 237 wake episodes occurred for a grand total of $N = 2929$ episodes. Such information should be routinely provided in all future studies of this kind.

It is advisable to equalize the contributions by each subject in one of two ways. Either randomly delete contributions from more prolific subjects to equal the number of contributions made by the least productive subject or drop the least productive subject and equalize against the next most prolific subject by random deletion. Random deletion is accomplished by consecutively numbering each subject's contributions and choosing entries within this range from a random number table. Delete those contributions corresponding to chosen random numbers.

EEG Uncertainty

Attenuation of the correlations between EEG and actigraphic sleep measures has been discussed from the perspective that EEG measurement and sleep scoring is a perfectly reliable and valid "gold standard" by which all other sleep measures are to be judged. Evidence presented below seriously questions this position.

Reliability Issues. The reliability coefficients for the Rechtschaffen and Kales (1968) scoring criteria were reported by Ogilvie and Wilkinson (1988) to range from 80% to 98%; a 4-month test–retest reliability of $r = .875$ was specifically cited. The square of this correlation equals .7656 indicating a 76.56% concordance. Since the square of the reliability coefficient indicates the percentage of variance accounted for, one minus the squared correlation coefficient yield the percentage error. Accordingly, we find that error in EEG sleep scoring associated with $r = .875$ is $1 - .7656 = .2344$ or 23.44%. This value is close to the 80% agreement (20% error) figure cited above.

Computer scored actigraph data for sleep/wake typically agrees 95% of the time with EEG scoring. The remaining 5% is well within the 10% to 20% uncertainty (unreliability) associated with EEG scoring and therefore can be entirely explained away in this manner. Computer scored protocols are perfectly reliable in the sense that they give the same results when analyzed twice by the same computer or by two different computers running the same software. This leaves uncertainty in EEG scoring to account for the observed discrepancies. Webster, Kripke, Messin, Mullaney and Wyborney (1982) concur with my EEG criticism: "Given the known unreliability in hand scoring, some of the small discrepancies between activity and EEG scoring in the present study are undoubtedly due to inaccuracies in EEG scoring." (p. 399) Snyder and Scott (1972) identify between subject differences in alpha waves as partly responsible for uncertainty in EEG scoring, since a reduction in alpha is considered to herald the approach of sleep.

Validity Issues. Figure 6.4, reprinted from Sadeh, Alster, Urbach, and Lavie (1989), indicates that the actigraph revealed various microarousals during normal sleep not detected by polysomnography. Figure 6.5, reprinted from Sadeh, Alster, Urbach, and Lavie (1989), indicates that the actigraph revealed numerous microarousals associated with the termination of apneas during sleep not detected by polysomnography. Figure 6.6, also reprinted from Sadeh, Alster, Urbach, and Lavie (1989), indicates that the actigraph revealed numerous microarousals associated with insomnia not detected by polysomnography. Though these differences were all scored against actigraphy, they should have been scored against polysomnography.

Initial attempts to validate EEG as capable of discriminating sleep from wake were done against behavioral criteria of wakefulness (cf. Blake and Gerard, 1937; Snyder and Scott, 1972), including dropping of hand-held objects, which then served as the "gold" standard for sleep. That EEG sleep criteria (cf. Rechtschaffen and Kales, 1968) could be developed in no way detracts from the soundness of the original behavioral criteria. Hence, actigraphy can no more be faulted for disagreeing with EEG than EEG can be faulted for disagreeing with behavioral sleep criteria. Whether or not to entirely supplant one gold standard with another or to retain two such standards is largely a theoretical matter that has yet to be widely discussed.

A behavioral definition of sleep is that point beyond which the person becomes totally unresponsive to otherwise perceptible environmental stimuli. Such a view accords well with everyday experience. We do not expect sleeping people to follow even simple commands or respond meaningfully to stimuli. Behaving under stimulus control is theoretically reserved for waking states.

Several investigations have been conducted to determine changes in auditory threshold from waking through complete sleep (Rechtschaffen, Hauri, and Zeitlin,

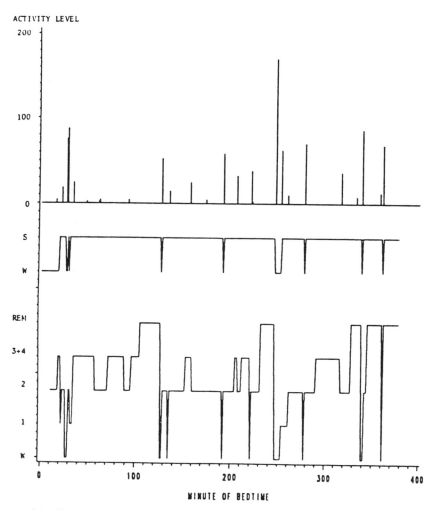

FIGURE 6.4. Microarousals during normal sleep detected by actigraphy (top graph) and not detected by polysomnography (bottom graph).

1966; Bonnet and Johnson, 1978; Bonnet and Moore, 1982). They have consistently shown substantial increases in auditory threshold when asleep. Coleman, Gray, and Watanabe (1959), Wilkinson (1968, 1970), and Ogilvie and Wilkinson (1984) have demonstrated that reaction time can be used to assess drowsiness and sleep. All of these investigators relied upon the subject's behavioral response to determine wakefulness. They notably did not use EEG sleep–wake criteria and this includes Dr. Rechtschaffen, who is senior author on the landmark publication defining EEG sleep stage criteria (cf. Rechtschaffen and Kales, 1968).

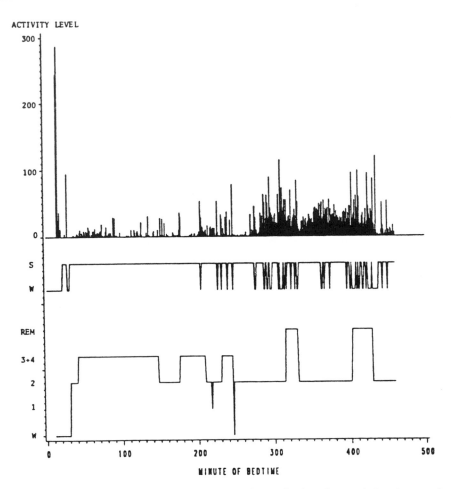

FIGURE 6.5. Microarousals (top graph) associated with the termination of apnea during sleep not detected by polysomnography.

Lindsley (1957) had subjects press a microswitch with the thumb of their preferred hand to reduce the intensity of a 30-dB 2-kHz tone delivered through ear phones sewn into a soft aviator's helmet worn by the subject while sleeping. Microswitch closures registered on a cumulative recorder. The above literature on auditory threshold indicates that such a soft tone was well below the auditory threshold of sleeping persons and consequently was insufficient to waken subjects once asleep. Two adult males aged 20 and 34 years served as subjects.

The results for 15 hours of sleep deprivation, one normal day, was 24 minutes until responding noticeably decreased, called sleep latency, and 40 minutes until the

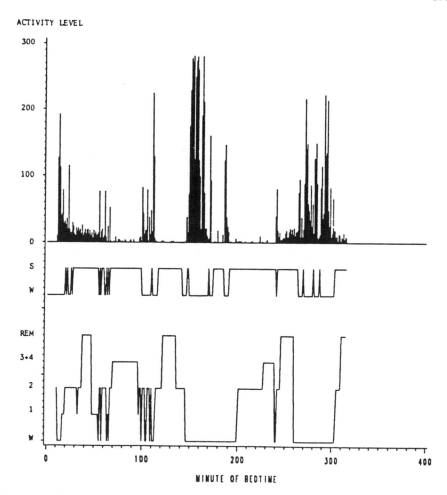

FIGURE 6.6. Microarousals (top graph) associated with insomnia not detected by polysomnography.

rate dropped to zero, called sleep onset. Taking 1.5 grains of seconal 5 minutes before retiring reduced sleep latency to 13 minutes and sleep onset to 16 minutes. Seconal doubled the sleep period to 4 hours. Thirty-eight hours of sleep deprivation produced a sleep latency of 7 minutes and sleep onset of 12 minutes.

Kelley and Lichstein (1980) compared behavioral and EEG sleep measures in three subjects (24-year-old female, 20- and 21-year-old male) without sleep complaints. The subjects slept in a laboratory where a Grass model 7B polygraph was used to collect EEG data and a portable device, designed for home use, was used to obtain the behavioral data. A timer turned on a standard portable tape recorder and emitted a soft tone every 10 minutes 30 seconds. The intensity of the tone and duration of the timer could be altered with a screw adjustment. The timer range is 5 to 25 minutes. A second timer shut the tape recorder off 10 seconds later. This interval could be from 5 to 30 seconds depending upon another screw setting. The subject was instructed to say "I'm awake" in response to the tone. The entire device is contained by an ordinary attaché case and is meant to be set on a chair approximately 1 m from the head of the bed. Data retrieval was simple and short. The stimulus tone was recorded and provided a clearly marked interval in which the reply "I'm awake" either occurred or not. Only about 1 minute of tape was used for each hour in bed.

Both behavioral and EEG data were divided into comparable intervals called "points." The average percent agreements between "points" scored sleep both behaviorally and by EEG were 68.3, 91.1, 95.1, 90.0, and 94.3 for Subject A resulting in a 5-night mean of 87.8%. The first-night discrepancy was explained by an air-conditioning failure necessitating an open door to a noisy corridor. For Subject B, the percentage agreements over 4 nights were 91.8, 96.4, 85.1, and 90.2 resulting in a 4-night mean of 90.9. For Subject C, the percentage agreements were 92.9, 97.3, and 93.6 for a 3-night average of 95.6%. The grand mean was 91.1%.

The initial behavioral sleep latency for Subject A was 0:31:40. The EEG latency to enter sleep Stages 1 and 2 was 0:17:08 and 0:30:38 respectively. Hence, the subject was behaviorally awake through all of Stage 1 sleep and for about the first minute of Stage 2 sleep. The initial behavioral sleep latency for Subject B was 0:21:49 and the EEG latencies to enter Stages 1 and 2 were 0:17:00 and 0:24:23 respectively. Hence, this subject was behaviorally asleep about 2.5 minutes prior to EEG Stage 2. The initial behavioral sleep latency for Subject C was 0:23:20 and the EEG latencies to enter Stages 1 and 2 were 0:17:30 and 0:27:20 respectively. This subject was behaviorally asleep approximately 4 minutes before Stage 2.

These data "validate" the new sleep-recording machine. The term validate is in quotes because these data actually validate EEG since the behavioral sleep recorder is an operational definition of the theoretical state of sleep.

Especially important is an analysis of the "points" where disagreement between the two approaches occurred. The percentage disagreement statistic gives the percentage of these disagreements where subjects were behaviorally awake but in an EEG sleep stage. The percentage disagreement values for Subject A were: 100, 75, 100, 100, and 100 for an average of 95.0%. Percentage disagreements for Subject B were 25, 100, 71.4, and 50.0 for an average of 61.6%. Percentage disagreements for Subject C were 33.3, 100, and 0 for an average of 44.4%. The grand mean was 67%. These data strongly indicate that subjects are meaningfully awake throughout EEG sleep Stage 1 and during the beginning of sleep Stage 2.

Lichstein, Nickel, Hoelscher, and Kelley (1981) compared the Somtrak Sleep Assessment Device (SSAD; available from Farrall Instruments, Inc., P.O. Box 1037, Grand Island, NE 68802) and polysomnographic measures of sleep latency, total sleep time, and sleep efficiency in two men (ages 32 and 61) and three women (ages 54, 64, and 37) seeking treatment for insomnia over 4 consecutive nights. Mean reliability for SAAD scoring was 98% (range = 90.9 to 100%). Mean reliability for sleep scoring according to Rechtschaffen and Kales (1968) criteria was 95.1% (range = 87.6 to 99.2%). All analyses were over 19 nights as the experimenter forgot to turn on the SAAD one night for one subject. Mean percentage agreement between SAAD and point scored EEG was 92.2%. Fifty-four percent of the remaining 7.8% "errors" were due to the subject saying "I'm awake" during either Stage 1 or 2 sleep. Lichstein, Hoelscher, Eakin, and Nickel (1983) reported that use of a standard intertone interval by the SAAD does not have sleep-inducing properties.

Birrell (1983) compared EEG and behavioral sleep onset measurements in 17 (8 male and 9 female) first-year psychology students aged 18 to 23 years while they slept in a laboratory on a Monday, Wednesday, and Friday night for approximately 4 hours each night. Because of debate over the definition of sleep onset (cf. Dement and Kleitman, 1957; Agnew and Webb, 1972; Williams and Karacan, 1976), Birrell used both a liberal and conservative definition. The liberal criterion scored sleep onset at the first occurrence of Stage 1, even though transitory awakening occurred thereafter, while the conservative criterion scored sleep onset when Stage 1 criteria were met and transient awakening did not occur before entering Stage 2. Behavioral sleep onset latency (SOL) was evaluated by sounding a 50-dB chime 2 feet from the subject's head on either a 2-minute, 5-minute, or random (1, 3, 5, 7, and 10 min) interstimulus interval. All three schedules were used with each subject; each on a different night. The tone was described as "loud enough to be heard but not so loud as to be sleep disturbing." (p. 182) Subjects were awakened twice each night and the latency to go back to sleep was obtained. The EEG sleep stage during the 30 seconds preceding each tone onset was determined and occurrence/nonoccurrence of response to the tone was also noted.

The EEG results for the first awakening indicated an average "liberal" and "conservative" Stage 1 SOL of 10.0 and 20.4 minutes respectively and a Stage 2 SOL of 31.7 minutes. The behavioral sleep monitor gave SOL as 32.6 minutes. Hence, subjects were in Stage 2 for approximately 0.9 minutes = 54 seconds before being behaviorally asleep. The EEG results for the second awakening indicated an average "liberal" and "conservative" Stage 1 SOL of 4.6 and 11.0 minutes respectively and a Stage 2 SOL of 19.6 minutes. The behavioral sleep monitor gave SOL as 20.2 minutes. Hence, subjects were in Stage 2 for approximately 0.6 minutes = 36 seconds before being behaviorally asleep. Two important conclusions to be drawn from these results are: 1) subjects are not behaviorally asleep until shortly after EEG Stage 2 begins, and 2) subjects went to sleep sooner after the second than first awakening.

Ogilvie and Wilkinson (1984) measured sleep onset in 5 male and 7 female paid volunteers aged 18 to 55 years ($M = 37.5$, $S = 15.3$ years) using a device that delivered a 30-dB 1000-Hz tone at random intervals of between 1 and 10 seconds 0.5 m above the subject's pillow as they slept in an experimental chamber. Ambient room noise was 25 dB. This procedure falls below the 15-dB change threshold that Rechtschaffen, Hauri, and Zeitlin (1966) determined would cause awakening. The subject was instructed to signal hearing these tones by pressing a switch located in a $9 \times 5 \times 2.5$-cm box held comfortably in one hand and to keep pressing as long as they remained awake. Polygraphic sleep data were also collected. Subjects were awakened 4 to 12 times per night to obtain repeated instances of sleep onset.

The polygraph records were divided into 10-second epochs and scored for sleep stages using the Rechtschaffen and Kales (1968) criteria. The failed response percentages as a function of sleep stage were: 0.7% for Stage W (waking), 27.8% for Stage 1, 76.0% for Stage 2, and 94.7% for Stage 3. This means that 99.3% of the tones were responded to during Stage W (waking), 72.2% during Stage 1 sleep, 24% during Stage 2 sleep, and 5.3% during Stage 3 sleep.

Ogilvie and Wilkinson (1988) examined 5 male and 6 female healthy normal-hearing volunteers without sleep problems aged 25 to 45 ($M = 32.5$, $S = 6.5$) who slept for two nights in a sleep laboratory. Data were analyzed only for the second night; the first night served to adapt subjects to the new environment. Sleep recordings followed recommendations by Rechtschaffen and Kales (1968). All subjects were videotaped with an infrared camera. An Apple IIe computer was programmed to present a 7.5-second 250-Hz tone at 5 to 10 dB above the ambient 32-dB(A) noise present during the night. This procedure falls below the 15-dB change threshold that Rechtschaffen, Hauri, and Zeitlin (1966) determined would cause awakening. The tone could be terminated by lightly squeezing (125 g of pressure over a 2-mm distance) a microswitch sewn into a squash ball held in the palm of the preferred hand with a Velcro strap. The intertone interval varied randomly between 1 and 32 seconds ($M = 16.2$ seconds, $S = 7.3$ seconds) plus response time. The authors carefully distinguish their behavioral response (BR) time from reaction time (RT) in that readiness is absent. Subjects were instructed to get as good a night's sleep as possible and not to listen for the next tone. They were to continue pressing in response to the tone until overcome by sleep. Upon awakening, they were to press in response to the tone until they went back to sleep.

A "point scoring" approach was taken wherein the sleep stage at the time of every tone onset was determined. One to five seconds of antecedent EEG could be consulted if necessary to decide which sleep stage was present. The upper portion of Table 6.1 presents the probability of responding to the tone as a function of point-scored sleep stage.

Only one subject (LS) was completely awake, in the sense of responding to every tone. Ten of eleven (91%) of the subjects were not completely behaviorally awake when EEG data indicated that they were awake. Subject MST only responded to 79.6% of the tones during the time that EEG scored him/her as awake. This subject appears to have been asleep 20.4% of the time that the EEG was scored awake. On average, 94.3% of the tones were responded to, which means that 5.7%

TABLE 6.1. Probability of Responding (PR) as a Function of EEG S/W Stage*

Subject	W	1	2	3	4	REM
		"Point" scoring of EEG stage at each tone onset.				
JG	0.922	0.250	0.035	0.000	0.000	0.000
RM	0.980	0.029	0.000	0.000	0.000	0.000
LS	1.000	0.667	0.000	0.000	0.000	0.000
KW	0.922	0.143	0.018	0.000	0.000	0.000
MH	0.968	0.350	0.009	0.000	0.000	0.000
RH	0.962	0.402	0.028	0.011[a]	0.000	0.004[a]
MSW	0.961	0.240	0.000	0.000	0.000	0.000
PG	0.979	0.167	0.028	0.000	0.000	0.000
AW	0.909	0.208	0.017	0.000	0.000	0.000
MST	0.796	0.123	0.007	0.000	–	0.000
JM	0.971	0.010	0.035	0.000	0.000	0.000
		PR using 40-second S/W scoring epochs				
Mean	0.943	0.235	0.016	0.001	0.000	0.004
SD	0.056	0.186	0.014	0.003	0.000	0.001
Mean	0.879	0.394	0.029	0.008	0.001	0.007
SD	0.101	0.212	0.026	0.026	0.003	0.010
Mean No tones	245.0	71.3	413.0	95.1	118.1	216.5
SD	106.3	47.0	120.4	65.1	73.4	55.4

*Reprinted from Ogilvie and Wilkinson (1988).
[a]In one instance, a subject responded during her first epoch of Stage 3. She also responded once in the middle of an REM period, but at a point where her EEG was ambiguous, the latter being as consistent with stage W as with REM.

of the time subjects were behaviorally asleep when considered EEG awake. This 5.7% discrepancy is almost exactly equal to the difference between computer-scored actigraph and EEG sleep/wake scoring reviewed above.

When sleep is scored in 40-second epochs (lower portion of Table 6.1) subjects are judged to be behaviorally awake only 87.9% of the time their EEG's are scored wake (Stage W), which means that 12.1% of the time subjects were behaviorally asleep when considered EEG awake. This very substantial discrepancy is larger than all computer-scored actigraphy vs EEG deviations thereby completely explaining away these differences in favor of actigraphy. Since behavioral criteria were used to validate EEG sleep scoring, nonresponding to tones audible only when awake raises serious question about how wakeful subjects necessarily are during EEG Stage W.

Examination of the disagreements between EEG and behavioral sleep/wake scoring revealed that most of them occurred during the transition from clearly awake to clearly asleep. This is exactly the point where actigraphy and EEG sleep/wake scoring disagreements occur.

These findings imply that what was previously reported as actigraphic overestimates of sleep in people lying "quietly awake" (cf. Zomer, Pollack, Tzischinsky, Epstein, Alster, and Lavie, 1987) may actually be EEG overestimates of wake. Future research should combine polysomnography, actigraphy, and behavioral response to determine whether the implied greater agreement between actigraphy and behavioral response than between EEG and behavioral response occurs.

Discrepancies of the opposite kind, where EEG indicates sleep and behavioral response indicates wake, are revealed in Sleep Stage 1 where on average, 23.5% of the tones were correctly responded to under point scoring and 39.4% of the tones were correctly responded to under 40-second epoch scoring. How can people who are truly asleep hear and purposively respond to randomly occurring tones that are below the auditory threshold of truly sleeping people? Either one admits that sleeping people are capable of conscious mental activity and purposeful responding or one concludes that people who behave this way are not truly asleep. The latter alternative seems more reasonable. It therefore appears that people in Sleep Stage 1 are not completely asleep. We shall soon see that EEG Stage 1 "Sleep" is actually a transitional state rather than a true sleep state.

Table 6.1 further indicates that subjects correctly respond to the tone 1.6% of the time under point scoring and 2.9% of the time under 40-second epoch scoring during Stage 2. A Wilcoxon nonparametric t-test indicated significantly greater response rates in Stage 2 than in Stages 3, 4, or REM ($p < .001$). Further analysis revealed that correct responses during Sleep Stage 2 occurred within the first 5 minutes of entering this stage. Correct responding during the first 5 minutes occurred more than seven times as often as correct responding during the remainder of Stage 2 sleep. It therefore appears that "true" sleep begins after EEG Stage 2 sleep has been scored for at least 5 minutes.

Subjects appear uniformly unresponsive during Sleep Stages 3, 4 and REM. Footnote a to Table 6.1 indicates that EEG may arguably have been scored W at the time subject RH correctly responded during Sleep Stage 3 and REM.

To obviate the criticism that the behavioral data are an artifact of peculiar sleep patterns, Ogilvie and Wilkinson (1988) compare their percentages of Stages W, 1, 2, 3, 4, REM, and MT (movement time) to those of Agnew and Webb (1968) to demonstrate that their subjects slept normally.

Ogilvie, Wilkinson, and Allison (1989) investigated sleep onset in 9 female and 3 male volunteers aged 20 to 46 years ($M = 26.9$, $S = 9.1$ years). In addition to electroencephalographic recordings, 1-kHz tones were presented 5 dB(A) above an ambient background of 27 dB(A) through a 6-cm diameter speaker located 1 m above the subject's head by an Apple IIe microcomputer for a maximum of 5 seconds at intertone intervals ranging from 10 to 30 seconds ($M = 21.2$, $S = 5.6$ seconds). The subject was instructed to respond to these tones by pressing a small switch sewn into a squash ball weighing 125 g and requiring a 2-mm excursion for closure. A "deadman" switch requiring 90 grams of pressure to maintain closure was to be held constantly closed while awake. This device was patterned after Blake, Gerard, and Kleitman (1939), who observed falling of hand-held objects during sleep onset.

The response time to tone data averaged 1371 milliseconds (ms) during sleep stage W (awake), 3073 ms during sleep Stage 1, and 4804 ms during sleep Stage 2. These changes are statistically significant ($F(2,22) = 144.43$, $p < .001$). The primary importance of these data lies in demonstrating wakefulness during the first two stages of sleep as determined by EEG criteria.

The "deadman" data were analyzed by constructing individual 2×2 χ^2 tables for each subject on the basis of deadman sleep–wake vs EEG Stage W (awake) plus Stage 1 vs Stage 2. These tables were statistically significant for 9 of the 10 subjects with an overall χ^2 (10, $N = 10$) $= 224.27$, $p < .001$. Again we find evidence of wakefulness during what would otherwise be characterized by EEG as Stage 1 sleep. An advantage of the deadman switch is that it provides a continuous record of wakefulness whereas presenting tones randomly from 10 to 30 seconds produces a similar uncertainty regarding the time of sleep onset.

Bonato and Ogilvie (1989) describe an Apple IIe-based home sleep-onset assessment device and data regarding its use on 15 male and 3 male students aged 18 to 39 years ($M = 21.1$ years) who slept with this device for three consecutive nights. Evidence of its validity was finding the expected "first night" effect. Significantly fewer microarousals were found on Night 3 vs 1 ($F(2,34) = 4.08$, $p < .05$), more macroarousals on Night 1 than Nights 2 or 3 ($F(2,34) = 6.49$, $p < .01$). Fair sleepers required two nights to adapt to the device whereas good sleepers required but one night to adapt.

Sleep Onset Spectrum. Ogilvie and Wilkinson (1988) argue that sleep onset is a gradual process beginning during EEG Stage W continuing completely through EEG Stage 1 into the first 5 minutes of EEG Stage 2. Their behavioral definition of sleep was nonresponse to 6 consecutive tones. I assume they ascribed sleep onset to the time when the first of these 6 tones began. Support for the progressive sleep onset hypothesis is provided by a gradual lengthening of response times as sleep develops from wakefulness. The authors refer to this as the Sleep Onset Period (SOP).

The term Sleep Onset Spectrum (SOS) has been adopted here to refer to the fact that sleep onset is a gradual rather than discrete event. Initial efforts to sleep involve activity reduction. People start to sleep by lying still. EEG Stage 1 sleep follows but auditory threshold remains near waking level which allows one to discriminate quiet tones from background noise and respond by closing a micro-switch with the hand. Zomer, Pollack, Tzischinsky, Epstein, Alster, and Lavie (1987) report that up to 80 minutes of quiet waking can occur before EEG Stage 1 occurs. Perhaps this unusual person would have been discovered to be awake had micromovements been monitored (cf. Wolpert, 1960; Baldridge, Whitman, and

Kraemer, 1965). After the first 5 minutes of Stage 2 sleep, auditory thresholds increase to where the tones can no longer be heard and the person is now completely asleep.

Because subjects are still behaviorally awake during EEG Stage 1 and through the first 5 minutes of Stage 2, as operant data have shown, activity may be detectable during these same EEG sleep periods. This is especially true if micromovements are being assessed.

It is important to stress that motility is subject to an important amplification or scale factor that EEG and operant data are not. Operant responses are amplified to where they are clearly visible and capable of incrementing cumulative recorders. EEG signals are amplified by standard factors that render brain waves discernible. No such conventions have yet been adopted regarding activity (motility). The Ambulatory Monitoring actigraph described by Redmond and Hegge (1985) has a zero crossing and threshold detection mode; the former being more sensitive than the latter. Sleep activity studies typically use the more sensitive zero crossing mode and somewhat different results would no doubt be obtained using the less-sensitive threshold mode. The use of even greater amplification factors, as were apparently used by Wolpert (1960) and Baldridge, Whitman, and Kraemer (1965) in their micromovement studies, very likely reveals activity where none was previously observed much as a higher-power microscope is capable of revealing phenomena undetected at lower magnifications. Similarly, the new Hubble space telescope will, from time to time, be focused upon areas of the heavens currently thought to be totally dark and may reveal the presence of previously undetected matter.

Another issue peculiar to activity (motility) monitoring is the site of attachment. Actigraphs are typically attached to the wrist and ankle but perhaps finger or toe movements would reveal different findings. Site of electrode attachment issues has already been standardized for EEG recording.

A primary result of endorsing the Sleep Onset Spectrum is to reject the concept of a "gold sleep standard" which arbitrarily elevates one aspect of sleep to a theoretically superior position. Emphasis is placed upon developing standard activity and operant sleep stages as has previously done with sleep. This objective can best be accomplished by examining activity and operant behavior during many sleep onset periods and attempting to describe them quantitatively in their own right. One approach to the behavioral data would be to calculate interresponse times and calculate their tendency to increase as a function of time since beginning of SOP. This same approach could be used with activity measurements where the length of the recording epoch would provide the lower limit of temporal resolution. Another approach to activity data is to fit a curve to the counts per epoch as they decrease throughout the SOP.

When the SOS has been well characterized from the activity and operant perspectives, research should simultaneously compare both of them with EEG sleep stages to determine the phase relationships among these three aspects of sleep onset.

The presence of a SOS makes good biological and evolutionary sense. It would

be dangerous for the brain to loose all consciousness while the person was ambulat-
ing at normal levels for they would fall down and possibly become seriously injured. Hence, activity decreases to a low level before consciousness is impaired.
The ability to rest the frontal lobes while retaining a reasonably normal auditory
threshold allows one quiet repose without losing complete contact with the environment. This ability undoubtedly allowed hunters and warriors of the past to rest while
remaining aware of predators and enemies. It also serves today's subway and other
mass-transit riders who spend some of their early morning and evening rush hours in
a semiconscious state while listening for their stop.

The Sleep Onset Spectrum view is consonant with recent theories of sleep
emphasizing diffuse central nervous system control of sleep/wake transition (cf.
McGinty, 1985).

Base Rate Issues

Not unexpectedly, the 2692 sleep episodes reported by Sadeh, Alster, Urbach,
and Lavie (1989) equal 91.91% of the 2929 total record. It is therefore possible to
be 91.91% accurate by scoring all episodes as sleep. It follows that statistical
significance must be judged against this high rate of chance agreement which is
asking a great deal. Statistical tests usually have their greatest power when base
rates are 50% (cf. Meehl and Rosen, 1955).

The clinical utility of the discriminate functions, and all psychological tests,
biochemical assays, and other such tests, signs, and indicators is also a function of
the base rates of the disease or target classes in question. The following comments
serve only to introduce the basic issues and refer the reader to more detailed
sources. It is deemed necessary to treat this topic here because obviously, from the
above research, it has escaped the attention of investigators in this field.

Rorer and Dawes (1982) present the basic issue in two parts. The first aspect of
the matter is that tests, psychological and biomedical, are validated by documenting
that the clinic or disorder group scores significantly higher or lower than the control
group. The conditional probability of having a high (or low) score given the presence of disease (disorder) is shown to be significantly greater than the probability of
having a high (or low) score given the absence of the same disease (disorder). The
same reasoning is true of all other signs and indicators. Their probability in subjects
with the disease (disorder) must be greater than in subjects without the disease
(disorder) if they are to be statistically and clinically important. Symbolically,
validation establishes $p(+/D)$ where $+$ refers to the presence of a sign, indicator, or
test score above or below established cutting scores indicating the presence of a
disorder, and D refers to actually having the disorder in question.

The necessary, and therefore unavoidable, connection with base rates comes
from the fact that diagnosis requires information about the inverse probability of

having the disorder given a positive test sign: $p(D/+)$. The version of Bayes' theorem presented in Equation (9) indicates that the required probability can be calculated from the validity information plus a knowledge of the disorders base rate $[p(D)]$ and the probability of getting a positive test score by chance $[p(+)]$:

$$p(D/+) = \frac{p(+/D)\ p(D)}{p(+)} \tag{9}$$

The reader is referred to Meehl and Rosen (1955), Dawes (1962), Rimm (1963), Cronbach and Gleser (1965), and Rorer, Hoffman, LaForge, and Hsieh (1966) for a further discussion of these issues.

The above dialogue focuses upon groups of subjects. Glaros and Kline (1988) concern themselves with the clinical relevance of tests results for individuals. Their work stems from efforts to evaluate the use of laboratory tests as screening procedures. They present the concept of Sensitivity (Se) as per Equation (10):

$$\text{Se} = \frac{\text{Diseased Persons with (+)Results}}{\text{All Diseased Persons}} \tag{10}$$

The numerator refers to joint occurrences where diseased persons have the expected positive test score or sign and the denominator refers to all persons with the disorder in question. The resulting fraction is the proportion of disordered persons having the expected positive sign; the proportion of *true positives*.

Glaros and Kline (1988) define Specificity (Si) as per Equation (11):

$$\text{Si} = \frac{\text{Nondiseased Persons with (−)Results}}{\text{All Nondiseased Persons}} \tag{11}$$

The numerator refers to the opposite joint occurrences where nondiseased persons have the expected negative (−) score or sign and the denominator refers to the population of disease-free people. The resulting fraction is the proportion of normal persons having the expected negative sign; the proportion of *true negatives*.

Both positive and negative signs (test scores above or below cutoff scores indicating diagnostic status) have predictive value regarding possible diagnosis. Positive and negative predictive value (PPV and NPV) are defined by Glaros and Klein (1988) as per Equations (12) and (13):

$$\text{PPV} = \frac{\text{Diseased Persons with (+)Sign}}{\text{All Persons with (+)Sign}} = p(D+/T+) \tag{12}$$

$$\text{NNV} = \frac{\text{Nondiseased Persons with (−)Sign}}{\text{All Persons with (−)Sign}} = p(D-/T-) \tag{13}$$

Equations (14) and (15) connect the concepts of PPV and NNV with the base rate of the positive sign $[p(D+)]$, test sensitivity $[p(T+/D+)]$, and $1 -$ test specificity $[p(T+/D-)]$:

$$p(D+/T+) = \frac{p(D+) \, p(T+/D+)}{[p(D+) \, p(T+/D+)] + [p(D-) \, p(T+/D-)]} \tag{14}$$

$$p(D-/T-) = \frac{p(D-) \, p(T-/D-)}{[p(D-) \, p(T-/D-)] + [p(D+) \, p(T-/D+)]} \tag{15}$$

All of the above information stems from a 2×2 table where rows are positive and negative test results and columns are attribute present and absent. The row marginal entries of this table give the total $+$ and $-$ scores whereas the column marginal entries give the total diseased and nondiseased subjects.

The relevance of the above-mentioned discussion for sleep motility research will now be addressed. As expected, the base rate for scoring nocturnal minutes as Sleep is high. Sadeh, Alster, Urbach, and Lavie (1989) reported that approximately 92% of bedtime 1-minute epochs are scored Sleep. Improving on this hit rate is restricted to a maximum of 8%. More room for improvement would exist with insomniacs who spend rather less of their bedtime asleep. See related arguments and examples are presented by Glaros and Klein (1988).

Second, and probably more importantly, the central issue of the sleep–wake studies reviewed above is the extent to which actigraphy is *sensitive* to polysomnographically defined sleep. If we substitute Sleep for Disease, epoch for persons, and epoch-scored sleep by actigraphy as $+$, then Equation (10) indicates that the sensitivity of actigraphy for detecting polysomnographically defined sleep equals the number of epochs that were jointly scored sleep by polysomnography and actigraphy (agreements) by the number of polysomnographically defined sleep epochs since that is our "gold standard" of sleep. What was done instead is to divide the agreements by agreements plus disagreements, which is to say, total epochs. Since some epochs were spent awake, the number of epochs scored as Sleep by polysomnography is less than the total number of epochs. Hence, sensitivity of actigraphy to polysomnographically defined sleep is higher than previously reported. The degree of underestimation is directly proportional to the extent to which total epochs exceed polysomnographically defined sleep epochs. Time spent awake in bed before sleep is a major cause of underestimation of actigraphy sensitivity to polysomnographically defined sleep. Time spent awake during the night further underestimates actigraphy sensitivity to polysomnographically defined sleep.

SLEEP EFFICIENCY

Sleep efficiency is defined as the percentage of minutes the person is actually asleep while in bed. It is typically defined as the time from lights out until awakening in the morning minus sleep latency and awakenings during the night. Sleep latency is defined as the time from lights out until the beginning of the first period scored Sleep.

Tilt Sensors

Reich, Kupfer, Weiss, McPartland, Foster, Detre, and Delgado (1974), using a mercury switch sensor, reported that activity counts recorded during the first 120 minutes of bedtime correlated $r(24) = -.56$, $p < .01$ with a polygraphically determined sleep efficiency index.

Weiss, Kupfer, Foster, and Delgado (1974) studied 11 hospitalized depressed patients (7 females, 4 males) aged 25 to 63 years (Mean = 48.4) with continuous 14-hr telemetric activity sensors (described by Kupfer, Detre, Foster, Tucker, and Delgado, 1972). The average sleep efficiency of all patients was 74.3% ($S = 4.0$). Sleep efficiency was significantly and negatively correlated [$r(9) = -.61, p < .05$] with activity from between midnight and 0700 as required by the definition of sleep efficiency. That this correlation is not substantially larger is explained by the low coefficient of variation (CV = SD/Mean $\times$ 100) of 14.89% for activity and extremely low CV of 5.38% for sleep efficiency.

Time-Based Actigraphy

Levine, Roehrs, Zorick, and Roth (1988) measured sleep efficiency on the basis of minutes of active and inactive time during the entire sleep period using an algorithm described by Levine, Moyles, Roehrs, Fortier, and Roth (1986).

Motionlogger™ data like those shown above enable one to compute sleep efficiency in the subject's natural environment (outside of the sleep laboratory). Sadeh, Alster, Urbach, and Lavie (1989) computed sleep efficiency indices during Phase 1 of their research, described above, in conjunction with computer-scored sleep/wake measures. The average sleep efficiency estimates obtained by polysomnography and actigraphy for 13 normals were 87.07 and 85.65 minutes respectively resulting in a correlation of $r(11) = .905$, $p < .0001$. The discrepancy of 1.42 is but 1.64% of the average sleep efficiencies. The average sleep efficiency estimates for 13 children were 88.85 and 86.48 minutes respectively resulting in a correlation of $r(11) = .813$, $p < .001$. The difference of 2.37 between sleep efficiency estimates is just 2.70% of their average. The average sleep efficiency estimates for 16 insomniacs were 63.30 and 78.56 minutes respectively resulting in a correlation of $r(11) = .785$, $p < .0005$. The difference of 15.26 in sleep efficiency estimates is 21.51% of their average. The average sleep efficiency estimates for 25 sleep apnea syndrome patients were 82.15 and 83.52 minutes respectively resulting in a correlation of $r(11) = .630$, $p < .001$. The difference of 1.37 in sleep efficiency scores is just 1.37% of their combined average. With the exception of insomnia, sleep efficiencies calculated on the basis of actigraphy are both highly correlated with and nearly equal to sleep efficiency values calculated by polysomnography.

Hauri (1989a) calculated average sleep efficiency scores for 16 insomniacs aged 25 to 67 years (mean = 43) over three consecutive nights using polysomnography and actigraphy. Patients had to have had insomnia three times per week for the past six months or more, experienced daytime fatigue as a result, not have chronic pain or other obvious diseases, and have a normal Minnesota Multiphasic Personality Inventory.

In seven patients sleep time estimated by actigraphy exceeded that estimated by polysomnography from 9 to 51 minutes. For the patient with the 9-minute discrepancy in sleep time polysomnography yielded a sleep efficiency of 82.1% whereas actigraphy indicated 84.3%. For the patient with the 51-minute sleep time discrepancy, polysomnography yielded a sleep efficiency of 73.8% whereas actigraphy reported 85.5%. Notice that the actigraphy estimates are much more consistent with each other than are the polysomnography estimates. No comment was made as to whether this subgroup of insomniacs was as clinically homogeneous as actigraphy indicates or as heterogeneous as polysomnography indicates in connection with their sleep behavior. It is interesting to note that all 6 patients whose insomnia derived from psychophysiologic or psychiatric issues had their sleep time overestimated by actigraphy.

In the remaining 9 patients, sleep time estimated by polysomnography exceeded that estimated by actigraphy from 2 to 266 minutes. For the patient with the 2-minute discrepancy, polysomnography yielded a sleep efficiency of 96.5% whereas actigraphy estimated 95.8%. For the patient with the 266-minute discrepancy, polysomnography estimated sleep efficiency at 64.4% vs actigraphy at 10.2%. The polygraph/actigraphy sleep efficiencies for the 98-minute discrepant patient were 95.6% and 74.2% respectively. For the patient with 53 minutes of discrepancy (essentially the opposite of the −51-minute patient), polysomnography estimated sleep efficiency at 90.4% whereas actigraphy indicated 77.9%. The four most discrepant patients had sleep time differences of 60, 78, 98, and 266 minutes. It is curious that the actigraph sleep efficiency evaluations of these four patients agreed closely with the patient's subjective evaluation of their sleep. Had actigraphy not been available, the discrepancy between subjective ratings and objective polysomnography would probably have been explained in terms of the unreliability and invalidity of subjective reports. That these ratings agree better with the objective actigraphic method than with the objective polysomnographic method is to actigraphy's advantage and credit and suggests that actigraphy might be more psychologically relevant than polysomnography.

Hauri (1989b) obtained 7 consecutive 24-hour home actigraph recordings on 9 of the 16 insomniacs reported above (cf. Hauri, 1989a). Six of the insomniacs slept better at home on average over 7 days than in the laboratory by 12, 33, 38, 42, 65, and 65 minutes respectively; up to just over an hour more. Three other insomniacs slept better in the laboratory by 30, 52, and 77 minutes respectively. Unusually short sleep times were more often seen at home than in the laboratory. Both of these findings indicate that home recording may be more behaviorally representative, and therefore clinically useful, than laboratory estimates. Those patients with large sleep variations due to particularly short sleep periods on some nights were seen as in need of treatment, which they would not have received if assessment were based exclusively upon their prior sleep lab data. A combined analysis was recommended: one night in the sleep lab with concurrent actigraphy to obtain standard information and to "calibrate" the actigraph followed by one week at home to better assess total sleep time and sleep time variability.

DSM-III-R SLEEP DISORDERS

DSM-III-R indicates (p. 297) that a sleep complaint must exist for at least one month to be diagnosable. This requirement strongly suggests that longitudinal measurements over a one-month period be used to document the nature of the sleep disorder prior to treatment. Such an individual work-up is possible with wrist actigraphy as discussed below. Section II of Mendelson (1987) discusses "pathology of sleep" including sleep-related breathing disorders (pp. 183–219), narcolepsy, and disorders of excessive sleepiness (pp. 221–245), alcohol, alcoholism and the problem of dependence (pp. 247–268), affective disorders (269–294), circadian rhythms and sleep (pp. 295–314), nocturnal myoclonus and the restless legs syndrome (pp. 315–322), and chronic insomnia (323–342). The purpose of the following sections is to comment upon the role of activity measurement (motility) in the diagnosis and assessment of DSM-III-R sleep disorders rather than to provide a comprehensive discussion of all sleep disorders.

Dyssomnias

DSM-III-R defines dyssomnias as a disturbance in "the amount, quality, or timing of sleep." (p. 297)

Insomnia Disorder

The three primary criteria for diagnosing Insomnia Disorders are: "A. The predominant complaint is of difficulty in initiating or maintaining sleep, or of nonrestorative sleep (sleep that is apparently adequate in amount, but leaves the person feeling unrested). B. The disturbance in A occurs at least three times a week for at least one month and is sufficiently severe to result in either a complaint of significant daytime fatigue or the observation by others of some symptom that is attributable to the sleep disturbance, e.g., irritability or impaired daytime functioning. C. Occurrence not exclusively during the course of Sleep-Wake Schedule Disorder or a Parasomnia." (pp. 299–300)

Complaints about sleep onset are more frequent in younger than older people. Sleep onset almost certainly occurs after motility ceases. Because the Motionlogger™ and Actillume™ actigraphs allow data to be collected for at least one week using a 1-minute epoch, one can reasonably determine the time before which the subject was not asleep to within one minute. DSM-III-R indicates that "For the vast majority of people, sleep begins within 30 minutes of creating an environment that encourages sleep ("going to bed") and lasts from four to ten hours." (p. 298) Wrist activity declines very substantially as one lies in bed preparing to sleep. Measuring the duration of such reduced activity to be more than 30 minutes in duration is one index that insomnia is present.

Older people more frequently complain about repeatedly awakening throughout the night. Because these conscious episodes very likely involve some tossing and turning before going back to sleep, they should be easily discernible in the actigraph record. Both the duration of these nighttime activity periods and their intensity, number of counts, can be measured.

Still other people indicate that they go to sleep easily and stay asleep but wake up tired. If one equates such nonrestorative sleep with inefficient sleep, then 15-second actigraph epochs can be scored using the Levine, Moyles, Roehrs, Fortier, and Roth (1986) algorithm described above to evaluate whether behavioral evidence for inefficient sleep is present in a particular case.

Documenting at least three incidences of insomnia per week for one month is more reasonably accomplished with outpatient actigraphy than through a sleep laboratory. The sleep–wake studies comparing actigraphy and polysomnography reviewed above indicate that home activity measurements can be a useful adjunct to sleep laboratory evaluation, especially when an actigraph is worn in the sleep lab thereby allowing an empirical "calibration" of actigraph data against sleep polysomnographic criteria. Actigraphy can then be used for extended sleep–wake assessments in the patient's home.

Differential diagnosis of insomnia from Sleep–Wake Schedule Disorder is achieved by allowing the person to sleep when they want to and demonstrating the absence of the above-mentioned difficulties.

Mendelson (1987, pp. 81–105) provides an extensive discussion of pharmacological treatments of insomnia. The major point to be made here is that actigraphy can be used to evaluate treatment effects in addition to the nature and severity of the disorder prior to intervention. Chapter 7 of this volume reviews the effects of drugs on sleep as measured by actigraphy.

Espie, Lindsay, and Espie (1989) used the Sleep Assessment Device (SAD), described by Kelley and Lichstein (1980), to investigate the extent to which insomniacs overreport sleep problems. The subjects were 20 physician-referred chronic insomniacs randomly drawn from a larger study. The sample contained 12 women and 8 men averaging 43.2 years ($S = 13.9$) with a mean insomnia duration of 11.4 years ($S = 10.7$). Subjects slept with the SAD in their own home for 2 to 10 nights (median $= 6$) using a 12-minute intertone interval and a 10-second response interval; intensity was set to each subject's preference. A total of 110 subject nights of data were collected. Self-report data were recorded on the Daily Sleep Questionnaire (DSQ) (Monroe, 1967) regarding how many minutes they took to fall asleep, hours and minutes of sleep time, plus how many times they awoke and had trouble getting back to sleep.

The results showed that self-report significantly ($t(109) = -3.30, p < .001$) overestimates sleep-onset latency (SOL) by approximately 10 minutes due to the greater difficulty of estimating lengthy ($41 - 300$; $M = 89.9$ min) vs shorter ($5 - 40$; $M = 23.6$ min) periods. Insomniacs also significantly ($t(109) = -2.05, p < .05$) overestimated total sleep duration due to the greater difficulty of estimating longer (> 6 hr; $M = 6.84$ hr) vs shorter (< 6 hr; $M = 4.6$ hr) sleep periods. Insomniacs substantially and significantly ($t(107) = 7.15, p < .001$) underestimated waking after sleep onset. They reported 63% arousal-free nights vs 33% measured arousal-free nights.

Carskadon, Dement, Mitler, Guilleminault, Zarcone, and Spiegel (1976) compared self-reports and polysomnographic measures of sleep in 122 insomniac patients screened for sleep apnea and nocturnal myoclonus and found that they overestimated the amount of time it took them to fall asleep and underestimated their total sleep time. However, these data were collected for one night in a sleep laboratory, where sleep may not be representative of nights at home. Espie, Lindsay, and Espie (1989) show that multiple nights of sleep at home show the same finding. Their interpretation contrasts with the usual hypochondrical explanation (cf. Mendelson, 1987, pp. 330–332) by indicating that it is simply more difficult to estimate longer intervals accurately.

Insomnia Related to Another Mental Disorder (307.42). Axis I disorders associated with insomnia include Depressive Disorders, Anxiety Disorders, and Adjustment Disorders with Anxious Mood such as might be associated with a myocardial infarction or other severe physical complication. Early morning awakening is sometimes associated with Depressive Disorders (see Chapters 3 and 4 for pertinent studies). Axis II disorders associated with insomnia include Obsessive Compulsive Personality Disorder.

Insomnia Related to a Known Organic Factor (780.50). Organic factors include diseases such as arthritis, Parkinson's disease, and angina all of which disturb sleep. Sleep apnea plus periodic leg twitches associated with nocturnal myoclonus and restless legs syndrome can also disturb sleep. Amphetamines, steroids, bronchodilators, and alcohol can also disrupt sleep.

Milk Allergy. Kahn, Mozin, Rebuffat, Blum, Casimir, and Duchateau (1986) obtained actigraphic data from 20 infants with chronic insomnia, 18 infants with digestive manifestations of milk allergy, and 20 normal infants matched for sex and age. The average age of all subjects was 15.3, $S = 9.8$ weeks. Milk protein allergy was diagnosed in all 38 clinic children. Sleep was evaluated using "home ambulatory accelerometry monitoring." The clinic children had from 2 to 6 arousals during their medial 5.2 hours of sleep before treatment. The control children had less than 2 arousals per night during their median of 10 hours of sleep. Two to three weeks of a milk-free diet resulted in the normalization of sleep of all 38 clinic children.

Restless Legs Syndrome. This condition involves a dysesthesia of the legs resulting in prickling sensations when the legs are at rest which are relieved by movement (Frankel, Patten, and Gillin, 1974). These symptoms of partial anesthesia often begin when lying down to sleep and consequently interfere with going to sleep. They also produce brief arousal from sleep (cf. Coleman, 1982). This clinical condition is also referred to as Periodic Leg Movements in Sleep (PLMS) (Kovacevic-Ristanovic, Cartwright, and Lloyd, 1989).

Downey, Bonnet, Lin, and Dexter (1989) report that leg movements greater than 4 mm separated by at least 5 seconds can be reliably scored from polygraphic records. Data from a group of 10 subjects shows that the reliability of leg movements frequency was $r(8) = .86, p < .01$ and the reliability of arousals was $r(8) = .92, p < .01$ over two consecutive nights. Some investigators believe that leg movements cause EEG arousals while others argue that a common CNS mechanism produces both EEG arousals and leg movements. Data from another group of 11 subjects using test–retest intervals of 2-, 3-, 10-, and 365-nights were used to evaluate the stability of EEG arousals and leg movements over time. The EEG arousals demonstrated good temporal stability. The 2-, 3-, 10-, and 365-night EEG arousal stability coefficients were: $r(9) = .86, p < .01, r(7) = .80, p < .01, r(9) = .80, p < .01$, and $r(7) = .37$, N.S.). Leg movements demonstrated substantially less temporal stability. The 2, 3, 10, and 365 night leg movement stability coefficients were: $r(9) = .55, p < .05, r(7) = .64, p < .05, r(9) = .50$, N.S., $r(7) = 0.00$, N.S.). These data were said to favor the common CNS mechanism on the basis that leg movements would have to be as consistent as EEG arousals to be their cause. However, a common CNS cause of both EEG arousals and leg movements implies that they both occur with equal temporal stability. A more empirically consistent conclusion is that EEG and Leg arousals have separate causes that gradually become desynchronized over time. This could occur if each were governed by a biological process with a slightly different period.

Poceta, Hajdukovic, Menn, Ruddy, and Mitler (1989) selected three groups of patients from the charts of 250 patients who underwent full nocturnal polysomnography: Sleep Apnea Syndrome only (SAS: $n = 153$), Sleep Apnea Syndrome with Periodic Leg Movements in Sleep (SAS + PLMS: $n = 77$), and a subset of the second group who were awakened by their leg movements (SAS + aPLMS: $n =$ 37). All three groups were matched for age (mean = 53.4, 55.9, and 56.2 years, respectively).

The Movement Index (MI) was defined as the number of muscle contractions of greater than one-half of the calibration signal for 0.5 to 10.0 seconds per hour of sleep. The MI for normals was 0. The average (and S) MI for SAS + PLMS was 24.0 (20.6) and for SAS + aPLMS was 28.0 (21.0). The average (S) MI for the subset of this group awakened by leg movements (SAS + aPLMS) was 28.0 (21.0). The Movement Arousal Index (MAI) was defined as the number of arousals associated with anterior tibialis contractions. The average normal MAI was 0. For SAS + PLMS the average (S) MAI was 7.5 (7.2) and for SAS + aPLMS was 11.5 (38.7). Hence, about one-third of patients with SAS experience periodic leg movements and nearly half of patients with periodic leg movements will awaken because of them. These results were reported as consistent with those of Coleman, Pollak, and Weitzman (1979), and Hartman and Scrima (1986).

Kovacevic-Ristanovic, Cartwright, and Lloyd (1989) indicated that efficacious treatments for PLMS include L-dopa, opioids, and clonazepam but have adverse side effects including tolerance and high addictive potential. They report effects 30-minute treatment before bedtime of the bilateral dorsiflexor of the ankle plus extensors of the toes using an EMS-250 (Electronic Medical Sciences, Inc., San Antonio, TX) neuromuscular stimulator on three male and two female PLMS patients aged 33 to 66 years. Mean leg movements per hour were reduced from a baseline value of 39.36 to 15.06 ($p < .05$). Movements per hour resulting in arousal were reduced from 28.14 to 6.68 ($p < .10$). These changes were largely due to a reduction of movements in non-REM sleep from 145.2 per night to 52.8 per night ($p < .05$). The substantial reductions in movements per hour resulting in arousal would be significant on just a slightly larger sample.

Nocturnal Myoclonus. Smith (1985) reports that Nocturnal Myoclonus results in dorsiflexion of the ankle and toes plus flexion of the knee and hip. The comments above pertinent to Restless Legs Syndrome indicate that ankle actigraphy is also capable of documenting Nocturnal Myoclonus.

Sleep Apnea. Lavie (1983) selected 78 men from a population of 1502 healthy working men for polysomnography. Workers with more than 10 apneas per hour also demonstrated hypermotility during sleep and complained of excessive daytime sleepiness.

Ancoli-Israel, Kripke, Mason, and Kaplan (1985) used wrist actigraphy and polysomnography to identify sleep apnea (18%), periodic movements in sleep (myoclonus index greater than 5) (34%) and both (10%) in a sample of 145 volunteers 65 years of age and older. These figures are consistent with those published by Carskadon and Dement (1981).

Reitman, Tryon, and Gruen (1990) report a case where abdominal actigraphy was used to detect sleep apnea. The actigraph, programmed for a 10-second recording epoch, was placed under a Respitrace™ abdominal respiratory transducer, an elastic belt several inches wide that fits snugly around the abdomen and expands and contracts with each breath. A typical apnea lasts for about 30 seconds. The initial portion of the cycle contains little behavior. As each episode progresses, the respiratory effort increases ending in violent gasps for air followed by a microarousal that once again enables breathing. Sleep is restored and another 30-second cycle begins. This repetitive stereotypical pattern is characteristic of patients with severe Obstructive Sleep Apnea (OSA).

Continuous Positive Air Pressure (CPAP) of approximately 5–15 cm H_2O (cf. Mendelson, 1987, pp. 204, 211) has been shown to consistently and substantially decrease apnea. The results of an ABAB design, where A is baseline and B is 10 cm H_2O of CPAP, validate the use of abdominal actigraphy for monitoring the occurrence of apnea.

Zomer, Peled, Gruen, and Lavie (1989) used wrist actigraphy to measure improvements in sleep efficiency associated with Continuous Positive Air Pressure (CPAP) treatment for sleep apnea syndrome to demonstrate treatment benefits that the patient might not otherwise appreciate.

Primary Insomnia (307.42). This diagnosis is given when the three primary criteria mentioned above for insomnia have been met and cannot be attributed to a mental disorder, organic factor, illness, or substance use.

Bootzin and Engle-Friedman (1981) distinguish among three types of insomnia. Sleep onset insomnia concerns difficulty going to sleep. Sleep maintenance insomnia concerns trouble staying asleep; frequent awakenings. Terminal insomnia refers to early morning awakening with an inability to sleep further.

Hypersomnia Disorder

The three primary criteria for diagnosing Hypersomnia Disorder are "A. The predominant complaint is either (1) or (2): (1) excessive daytime sleepiness or sleep attacks not accounted for by an inadequate amount of sleep; (2) prolonged transition to the fully awake state on awakening (sleep drunkenness). B. The disturbance in A occurs nearly every day for at least one month, or episodically for longer periods of time, and is sufficiently severe to result in impaired occupational functioning or impairment in usual social activities or relationships with others. C. Occurs not exclusively during the course of Sleep–Wake Schedule Disorder." (p. 303)

Criterion A(1) above requires that daytime sleepiness not be accounted for by a lack of sleep. Actigraphy can reveal when the individual went to bed in one of three ways. First, the wearer can be instructed to press the event recording button on the actigraph when they retired for the night to sleep and when they got up in the morning. Second, one can work backward from that portion of the actigraph record unquestionably associated with sleep to the point where activity decreased from typical (for that person) daytime levels to typical "sleep" or "rest" levels to identify sleep onset. Third, computers can be used to implement the sleep scoring algorithms reviewed above to calculate a more exact sleep onset time. The time of awakening can likewise be determined either by event marker, inspection, or computer analysis and thereby determine length of sleep.

Sleep efficiency scores can also be calculated from actigraph records as reviewed above thereby evaluating the extent to which the person slept or was repeatedly awakened during the night.

An interesting combined analysis relevant to criterion A(1) and A(2) above is possible if the person presses the event recorder when they are ready to start sleeping and when they finally feel awake. A latency to fall asleep can be calculated between the time the event recorder was pressed before sleep onset until the time sleep is first scored. Long latencies indicate difficulty initiating sleep. A latency to become fully awake can be calculated between the time the computer scores final awakening and when the wearer presses the event recorder indicating they are fully awake. Difficulty becoming fully awake should be reflected by long latencies.

Actigraphy can assist with the determination that the above disturbances in A occur almost daily for at least one month or less regularly for a longer period of time. Such longitudinal sleep laboratory evaluation is out of the question for economic, personal, and logistic reasons.

The determination that the above symptoms are not part of a Sleep-Wake Schedule Disorder can be facilitated using actigraphy. One would exclude the presence of Sleep–Wake disorder by identifying the individual's actual sleep–wake cycles and showing that they are appropriate to their environmental demands. Criteria for Sleep–Wake disorder presented below require a mismatch between normal actual sleep–wake cycles and environmental demands to diagnose the presence of Sleep–Wake disorder.

Conclusions about the hypersomnias discussed below are all facilitated by actigraphy since one must first determine the presence of hypersomnia before they can relate it to other factors.

Hypersomnia Related to Another Mental Disorder (307.44). Younger persons undergoing the depressive phase of a Bipolar can show hypersomnia. This relationship is usually apparent by age 20.

Hypersomnia Related to a Known Organic Factor (780.50). Prolonged use of sedatives, antihypertensives, and cannabis can produce hypersomnia. Sleep apnea, narcolepsy, sleep-related myoclonus, and "restless legs" syndrome can also produce hypersomnia. Except for narcolepsy, the contribution of actigraphy to the study of these disorders was discussed above regarding Insomnia Related to a Known Organic Factor.

Borbely's (1986) Figures 3 and 4 present 37 days of continuous actigraphy for a person with severe and incapacitating narcolepsy. An hour or longer narcoleptic episode typically followed the first morning activity period with additional narcoleptic episodes distributed throughout the day. Associated nocturnal activity during desired sleep time due to insomnia was clearly in evidence. Both of these behavioral disorders completely fractured this person's normal sleep–wake cycle such that rest and activity were interspersed throughout each 24-hour period, there being no major rest period.

Primary Hypersomnia (780.54). This diagnosis is given when the three primary criteria are satisfied but cannot be attributed to a mental disorder, organic factor, illness, or substance use.

Sleep–Wake Schedule Disorder (307.45)

The primary criteria for Sleep–Wake disorder is "Mismatch between the normal sleep–wake schedule for a person's environment and his or her circadian sleep–wake pattern, resulting in a complaint of either insomnia (criteria A and B of Insomnia Disorder) or hypersomnia (criteria A and B of Hypersomnia Disorder)." (p.307)

Actigraphy can assist in the diagnosis of Sleep-Wake disorder by documenting the person's actual sleep-wake habits so that an independent and objective comparison with environmental demands can be made.

Advanced or Delayed Type. Here sleep onset and offset are advanced or delayed by a specific amount in the absence of environmental demands or sleep disrupting medications. Actigraphy is exceptionally useful in documenting bedtimes within the limitations described above.

Some elderly persons living with their children take afternoon naps out of boredom and consequently go to bed later and later until they have largely switched their sleep–wake cycles relative to other family members. This can interfere with adequate sleep for other family members and occasion placement of the elderly persons in nursing institutions.

Actigraphy can document actual sleep–wake patterns and therefore assist in determining if they have become advanced or delayed as illustrated by the behavioral studies discussed in the next section regarding disorganized sleep–wake cycles. Actigraphy can further document the effects of interventions designed to normalize sleep–wake patterns.

Disorganized Type. No consistent major sleep period is present when Disorganized Type is diagnosed. Actigraphy can readily document the absence of a consistent major sleep period in addition to the return of such a period subsequent to treatment.

Ancoli-Israel, Parker, Sinaee, Fell, and Kripke (1989) estimated sleep behavior from wrist activity in 200 elderly residents (131 females and 69 males; $M = 81.9$ years, $S = 8.6$ years) of a skilled nursing facility using a modified Respitrace-Medilog recording system (Ambulatory Monitoring, Ardsley, NY). About 15% of the patients were bed-bound, 18% were wheel chair-bound, 61% were ambulatory with assistance, and 6% ambulatory without help. The average recording was 15.4 hours per day during which time patients were scored asleep, on average, for 7 hours and 58 minutes and awake for 7 hours and 28 minutes. Hence, they spent approximately half of their day asleep. Moreover, patients averaged no more than 39.5 minutes of sleep during each hour of the night. Hence, patients were awake 20.5 minutes of each night hour. Sometimes this awake time occurred as a single hourly waking episode, but 50% of the patients woke up 2 to 3 times per hour.

A report by Lieberman, Wurtman, and Teicher (1989) indirectly suggests that healthy older adults may have normal activity cycles. Their older group consisted of 17 males aged 65–94 years ($M = 71.4$) and 23 females aged 65–85 years ($M = 74.6$) who were in good health and able to live on their own. Their younger sample consisted of 15 males aged 21–35 years ($M = 27.7$) and 14 females aged 19–31 years ($M = 24.5$). A detailed medical history was obtained and all subjects were given a physical examination and routine laboratory tests. Activity was monitored using an Ambulatory Monitoring, Inc., actigraph programmed for a 15-minute epoch. Data were collected for six days after being admitted to the MIT Clinical Research Center which contained extensive indoor and outdoor exercise facilities plus organized social activities. Subjects were free to create their own schedules. Daytime was defined as 0700 to 2300 hr and nighttime as 2300–0700 hr.

The results indicated that the average daytime activity counts per 15 minutes for the older men ($M = 88.80$, $S = 6.2$) and older women ($M = 83.65$, $S = 5.5$) were significantly ($F(1,65) = 9.77$, $p < .003$) greater than for younger men ($M = 72.64$, $S = 5.8$) and younger women ($M = 69.09$, $S = 4.7$). Likewise, the average nighttime activity counts per 15 minutes for older men ($M = 18.08$, $S = 3.3$) and older women ($M = 13.42$, $S = 1.5$) were significantly ($F(1,65) = 6.05$, $p < .017$) greater than for younger men ($M = 14.03$, $S = 2.0$) and younger women ($M = 8.37$, $S = 1.4$). The average male nighttime activity was significantly greater than for females ($F(1,65) = 7.77$, $p < .007$).

Two comments are important regarding nighttime activity. First, it refers to activity between 2300 and 0700 hours and not specifically to sleep. Persons who go to sleep later than 2300 and rise earlier than 0700 will get higher nighttime readings. This is probably part of the reason why older people were found more active than younger people at night. However, older people remain more active during the day. Perhaps the older sample displayed more of a "cruise effect" where when provided with a rich array of new opportunities, one tries to engage all possible activities.

These data strongly suggest that the elderly did not sleep away large portions of each daytime hour. Their higher nighttime activity was likely due to fewer hours of sleep rather than disturbed sleep though the data do not comment directly upon this possibility. In sum, the disorganized sleep patterns associated with elderly people may be a function of unstimulating environments. Placed in a resort-like setting, this elderly sample were more active than their more youthful counterparts.

Frequently Changing Type. Changing time zones alters the major sleep period and produces "jet lag" as illustrated by Figure 6.7 associated with a 28-day Westerly trip around the world (Gruen, 1987) (cf. Figure 2 in Borbely, 1986, and Lavie and Gruen, 1989). Transmeridian travel places one in the presence of light–dark cycles that are either phase-advanced (West) or -delayed (East) relative to one's home.

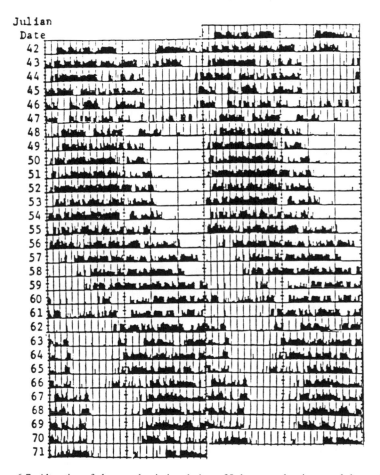

FIGURE 6.7. Alteration of sleep–wake timing during a 28-day westerly trip around the world.

Being phase-advanced means that the traveler will likely go to bed earlier and rise earlier than will local residents. The traveler reaches the end of their day before local residents do. The term "advanced" can be associated with sleeping and rising earlier than local residents. Being phase-delayed means that the traveler will likely go to bed later and get up later than will local residents. The traveler's day is not over when others are going to sleep. The term "delayed" can be associated with sleeping and rising later than local residents.

Dyssomnia Not Otherwise Specified (307.40)

Included here are insomnias, hypersomnias, and sleep–wake schedule disorders that cannot be otherwise diagnosed.

Parasomnias

The primary focus of the parasomnias (308) is upon events occurring during sleep or while semi-asleep. The problem lies in that these events occur at all, not in their interrupting sleep. Actigraphy is relevant to these disorders in that the motor activity associated with them clearly marks when they occur thereby providing an objective index of their frequency and temporal distribution.

Dream Anxiety Disorder (307.47)

"The essential feature is repeated awakenings from sleep with detailed recall of frightening dreams." (p. 308) The time of awakening associated with "Nightmare Disorder" can be determined with actigraphy because of its time base. A one-minute epoch choice would localize awakening to within one minute of its occurrence. Because dreams occur during REM sleep, and because muscle tone dramatically decreases thereby inhibiting activity, a period of inactivity is expected to precede the abrupt awakening. Because REM sleep increases throughout the night, these episodes are more likely to occur near the end than beginning of sleep.

Sleep Terror Disorder (307.46)

"The essential features of this disorder are repeated episodes of abrupt awakening from sleep, usually beginning with a panicky scream. The episode usually occurs during the first third of the major sleep period (the interval of nonrapid eye movement [NREM] sleep . . . and *lasts one to ten minutes*." (emphasis added) (p. 310).

The major distinction between this and the previous disorder is that Dream Anxiety Disorder occurs during REM sleep whereas Sleep Terror Disorder occurs during NREM sleep. Because REM is defined by EEG, EOG, and EMG, only such information can provide a certain distinction. However, because of the profound absence of activity during REM and the fact that Sleep Terror Disorder usually occurs during the first third of sleep, actigraphy can probably distinguish between these conditions quite well. Given the cost and inconvenience of sleep laboratory evaluation, actigraphy may be the preferred initial assessment approach using the more costly alternative only if necessary.

Sleepwalking Disorder (307.46)

During a period of time lasting from 3 to 30 minutes, the person sits up, performs repetitive motor movements such as picking at either their blanket or sheet, and/or walking, dressing, going to the bathroom, opening doors, and eating, all without awareness. The presence of motor control implies the absence of REM state.

Wrist actigraphy will clearly register and time stamp the incidence of the above described movements. Leg actigraphy will also detect the transition from lying to sitting in bed and will clearly respond to walking as will wrist actigraphy. Such information can be used during interview to determine if the person remembers these episodes in order to make a final diagnosis. The person is presumably unaware of these events.

Parasomnia Not Otherwise Specified (307.40)

Sleep disturbances that cannot be otherwise diagnosed are included here. This includes nightmares associated with drug withdrawal. Actigraphy can be used to identify and track such sleep disorders, as described above, despite ignorance of their cause.

Activity, Drugs, and Substance Use

Pharmacologic agents can either increase or decrease daytime or nighttime activity in desired or undesired ways. Carryover effects are possible, wherein medications that reduce nighttime motility may also produce daytime lethargy while drugs that stimulate daytime activity may interfere with sleep. Only some of these issues have been addressed to date.

BARBITURATE HYPNOTICS

Oswald, Berger, Jaramillo, Keddie, Olley, and Plunkett (1963) examined the effects of 200 mg (clinical dose) of heptabarbitone (Medomin) on body movement, eye movement, and EEG in 6 patients over 6 nights. The first night served as adaptation and no data were analyzed. On the subsequent four nights, three patients received medication and the other three received placebo identical in appearance and taste to the real medication. Three of the subjects received two consecutive days of medication at the beginning, middle, and end of the four consecutive nights. One or two placebo nights separated medication nights in the other three patients. Results indicated a significant ($p < .05$) reduction in body movements per minute throughout the entire night. These results were reported as consistent with previous findings by two other investigators regarding the effects of pentabarbitone.

Phase II of the Kast (1964) study began with a three-week activity baseline during which time placebo was administered. Activity was measured from 1500 to 1800 hours daily with a mercury-switch-based forearm-attached activity counter. Twenty-one inpatients were clinically judged to show psychomotor agitation and 21 other inpatients were judged to show psychomotor retardation. Thereafter, 60 mg of phenobarbital was administered three times daily to the agitated patients and 10 mg of dextroamphetamine was administered three times daily to the withdrawn patients. Placebo-treated agitated patients averaged 1433.3 counts per 3 hours, which decreased significantly ($t(41) = 4.13, p < .001$) to 797.0 counts per 3 hours when given phenobarbital. Placebo-treated withdrawn patients averaged 410.0 counts per 3 hours, which increased significantly ($t(41) = 7.11, p < .001$) to 943.3 counts per 3 hours when given dextroamphetamine.

Kast's (1964) third phase examined the behavioral effects of 4× daily placebo, 4× daily 30-mg doses of phenobarbital, 4× daily 50-mg doses of nortryptiline in agitated patients and 4× daily placebo, 4× daily 10-mg doses of amphetamine sulfate, and 4× daily doses of nortryptiline in withdrawn patients. The results were consistent for both groups. Drug was significantly different from placebo for the agitated ($F(1,168) = 57.6, p < .001$) and withdrawn ($F(1,168) = 55.5, p < .001$) patients. However, nortriptyline was not different from phenobarbital ($F(1,168) = 1$, N.S.) for agitated patients and nortriptyline was not different from amphetamine ($F(1,168) = 3.5$, N.S.) for withdrawn patients.

Mattmann, Loepfe, Scheitlin, Schmidlin, Gerne, Strauch, Lehmann, and Borbely (1982) investigated the nighttime and daytime carryover effects of three benzodiazepine hypnotics (triazolam, nitrazepam, and flunitrazepam) in 18 paid volunteer healthy adults aged 20 to 30 years (mean = 24.6 yrs; mean body weight = 63.3 kg: range = 44–90 kg). The drugs were administered according to a double-blind crossover design with placebo. Drug dosage was adjusted to body weight. The following dosages were for 70 kg: triazolam (0.25, 0.5, and 1.0 mg), nitrazepam (10 mg), and flunitrazepam (2.0 mg). Each drug/placebo was given on a different night with 2–3 nights between drugs. Subjects slept at home from 2300–2400 hours until 0700 the next morning when they were awakened with a telephone call. Wrist activity was measured with a modified Colburn et al. (1976) actigraph using a 7.5 min epoch. The dependent variable was the number of 7.5-minute epochs with greater than zero activity counts. Mean differences were expressed as a percentage of placebo values. Hence, placebo levels became zero percent and served as a reference for further comparison.

The nighttime results indicated that activity increased slightly in the placebo condition ($n = 12$) on post-drug night 1 ($M = 3.5\%, S = 3.0\%$), and post-drug night 2 ($M = 3.9\%, S = 6.3\%$). A dose-dependent effect of triazolam with subsequent nighttime carryover was reported. triazolam (0.25 mg; $n = 6$) reduced nighttime activity the first night ($M = -10.4\%, S = 4.37$) but increased it on post-drug nights 1 ($M = 7.7\%, S = 6.1$). These effects were not significant due to small sample size. However, 0.5 mg of triazolam ($n = 11$) produced significant results as indicated next. During the night of administration, activity was significantly ($p < .01$) decreased ($M = -27.8\%, S = 4.9\%$). Some increase was observed on post-drug night 1 ($M = 5.1\%, S = 6.1\%$), but a significant ($p < .05$) activity increase was observed on post-drug night 2 ($M = 14.3\%$, $S = 6.4\%$). Triazolam (1.0 mg; $n = 6$) produced an even greater and still significant ($p < .05$) activity reduction on the administration night ($M = -30.8\%$, $S = 9.9\%$). A slight activity increase was seen on post-drug night 1 ($M = 1.3\%$, $S = 13.0\%$) and a somewhat larger activity increase was seen on post-drug night 2 ($M = 9.4$, $S = 8.6\%$). Nitrazepam (10 mg, $n = 6$) significantly ($p < .05$) reduced activity on the administration night ($M = -18.3\%$, $S = 4.7\%$) and nonsignificantly decreased activity on post-drug night 1 ($M = -3.7\%$, $S = 9.0\%$) and on post-drug night 2 ($M = -5.7\%$, $S = 8.3\%$). Flunitrazepam (2.0 mg; $n = 6$) significantly ($p < .05$) reduced activity on the administration night ($M = -24.7\%$, $S = 6.9\%$), had no discernible effect on post-drug night 1 ($M = 0.0\%$, $S = 7.5\%$), and decreased activity on post-drug night 2 ($M = 0.50\%$, $S = 7.8\%$).

The daytime results indicated that triazolam (0.5 mg) significantly ($p < .05$) reduced activity from 0900 to 1500 the day after drug administration by 10% compared to placebo subjects. Flunitrazepam (2.0 mg) significantly ($p < .05$) reduced daytime activity during the same period by nearly 20%.

The substantial activity reductions during the administration night of all hypnotics at all dosages and the significant activity reductions of all but the lowest dosage of triazolam (0.25 mg) in these very small samples strongly indicates that hypnotics reduce activity during sleep. These effects would all be highly significant in samples of 25 or 50 subjects. The sometimes significant activity increments on post-drug night 2, but not 1, suggest a delayed (48-hour) activity rebound effect. However, a larger sample size might also reveal significant post-drug night 1 decrements plus significant differences between post-drug night 1 and 2 activity decrements. Then we would conclude that hypnotics strongly decreased activity during the administration night, released their grip somewhat during the next night, and reasserted their effect 48 hours later on the second night. This curious oscillatory effect may extend further but would require substantially larger samples for its detection. Conceptually, the effect seems something like displacing a guitar string and letting its vibrations dampen exponentially.

Borbely, Loepfe, Mattmann, and Tobler (1983) studied the effects of midazolam and triazolam on nocturnal and diurnal activity from the perspective of occasional use by healthy young adults. The subjects were 15 paid adults (9 male, 6 female) of mean age = 29.4 years (range = 25–36), and of mean weight = 67.3 kg (range = 55–83) who reported good health including no trouble sleeping. Activity was measured 24 hours each day for five consecutive weeks using a modified Colburn type actigraph with a 7.5-min recording epoch. Subjects were instructed to retire to bed between 2300 and 2400 hours each evening; a 30-minute deviation was permitted. Subjects were further instructed to refrain from napping. Both bedtime and napping could be verified by actigraph records. They were asked to abstain from alcohol and avoid excessive caffeine consumption. Subjects took either medication (7.5 or 15 mg of midazolam, 0.25 or 0.5 mg triazolam) or placebo each

Monday 30 minutes before bedtime according to a 5 × 5 replicated, balanced, double-blind, Latin square design. Nocturnal activity was defined as the number of 7.5-minute epochs containing greater than zero activity counts. The threshold sensitivity of the actigraph was 0.1 g.

Activity data were reported as percent of placebo. The entire nighttime results indicated that both dosages of triazolam significantly ($p < .05$) reduced nighttime activity but did not carry over to either the next day or post-drug nights 1, 2, or 3. The 0.25-mg dose reduced entire nighttime activity to an average of 87.2% ($S = 7.0\%$) of placebo level ($M = 100\%$, $S = 4.4\%$) whereas the 0.5 mg dose reduced entire nighttime activity to an average of 90.0% ($S = 3.7\%$). Activity reductions for the first half of the night were even greater. The 0.25 mg dose reduced first-half nighttime activity to an average of 79.9% ($S = 10.2\%$) of placebo ($M = 100\%$, $S = 6.4\%$) whereas the 0.5 mg dose reduced activity to an average of 82.4% ($S = 6.3\%$). Activity during the second half of the night was nearly normal. Activity for the 0.25 mg dose averaged 93.8% ($S = 6.7\%$) of placebo ($M = 100\%$, $S = 4.4\%$), the 0.5 mg dose average activity being 96.5% ($S = 6.5\%$) of placebo. Post-drug nocturnal activity never came back to 100% of placebo condition through the observed average reductions for 0.25 mg for night 1 ($M = 98.5\%$, $S = 7.6\%$), night 2 ($M = 96.0\%$, $S = 7.3\%$), and night 3 ($M = 93.1\%$, $S = 7.4\%$) and for 0.5 mg for night 1 ($M = 94.8\%$, $S = 5.3\%$), night 2 ($M = 96.2\%$, $S = 6.2\%$), and night 3 ($M = 93.3\%$, $S = 4.5\%$) were not statistically significantly different from placebo night 1 ($M = 100\%$, $S = 5.4\%$), night 2 ($M = 100\%$, $S = 5.7\%$), and night 3 ($M = 100\%$, $S = 4.9\%$) with just 15 subjects but would be significant if these effects held for larger samples.

Midazolam significantly ($p < .05$) reduced entire nighttime activity ($M = 89.4\%$, $S = 5.0\%$) from placebo levels ($M = 100\%$, $S = 4.4\%$) at the 15 mg dose only. Reduction to an average of 97.1% ($S = 5.6\%$) of placebo was not significant in this sample. However, activity during the first half of the night was significantly reduced from placebo for both the 7.5 mg ($M = 85.4\%$, $S = 7.6\%$; $p < .05$) and 15 mg ($M = 75.6\%$, $S = 5.2\%$; $p < .01$) doses. A nonsignificant rebound during the second half of the night for the 7.5 mg dose was observed ($M = 106.9\%$, $S = 6.4\%$) of placebo ($M = 100\%$, $S = 4.4\%$). This effect was much less for the 15 mg dose ($M = 101.1\%$, $S = 5.9\%$). Curious but nonsignificant (in this small sample size) nocturnal oscillations occurred during post-drug night 1 ($M = 98.9\%$, $S = 4.8\%$), night 2 ($M = 101.0$, $S = 5.7\%$), and night 3 ($M = 92.46$, $S = 5.1\%$) for the 7.5 mg dose. The 15 mg dose produced a similar night 1 ($M = 100.9\%$, $S = 5.2\%$), night 2 ($M = 93.3\%$, $S = 4.9\%$), night 3 ($M = 98.6\%$, $S = 5.6\%$) oscillation. Placebo values for these nights are indicated above.

Daytime activity during the first four hours after awakening was examined for carryover effects and none were found. The authors concluded that 15 mg of midazolam and 0.25 mg of triazolam were adequate hypnotic dosages that did not carry over and influence the next day's activity. Results from a random letter, number, symbol typing test of psychomotor performance, corroborate this conclusion. Subjective reports of sleep were consistent with these data in that subjects reported deep and quiet sleep.

Lavie and Gruen (1989) investigated the therapeutic effects of 7.5 mg of midazolam vs placebo on sleep disturbances produced by 11 hour eastward and westward intercontinental flights between New York (westward) and Tel Aviv (eastward) in 18 healthy adults (9 men and 9 women aged 30 to 55 years) who were without sleep complaints. A one-week wrist activity baseline sample was taken in Israel 2–3 weeks before their trip from Tel Aviv using 2-minute epochs. All subjects remained on the Eastern seaboard for 14 days before returning to Israel. Three matched groups of 6 subjects were formed. Group 1 received 7.5 mg of midazolam on the first 4 post-nights in New York and placebo on the first after returning to Israel. Group 2 received reverse treatment; placebo during the first 4 post-nights in New York and 7.5 mg during the first 4 post-nights in Israel. Group 3 received 7.5 mg during the first 4 post-nights after both trips. Medication or placebo were taken 15 minutes before bedtime.

Results for the westward flight to New York showed that the placebo group increased their total sleep time by 6.6% compared to their baseline values during the 4 post-nights whereas the midazolam group slept 16.0% longer. Sleep motility was reduced throughout the night. Diurnal napping was significantly greater in the placebo subjects relative to their baseline.

After the eastward flight back to Israel, the placebo group *decreased* their total sleep time by an average of 11.3% over the 4 post-nights in relation to baseline levels whereas the midazolam subjects *increased* their sleep time by an average of 4%. The drug also decreased nocturnal motility, especially during the first third of the night. These effects would probably have been larger had the 15 mg dose of midazolam been used as recommended by Borbely, Loepfe, Mattmann, and Tobler (1983) above.

Borbely, Mattmann, and Loepfe (1984) measured the behavioral effects of a single bedtime dose (20 or 30 mg) of temazepam (7-chloro-3 hydroxy-1 methyl 5 phenyl-1 H-1,4 benzodiazepine 2(3H) one) short elimination half-life (11.5 hours) benzodiazepine hypnotic in 14 healthy paid adults (6 females, 8 males) ranging in age from 23 to 43 years (mean = 28.9 years) weighing from 45 to 76 kg (mean = 63.4) who did not report either drug usage or sleep disorder. Wrist activity was measured by a the same solid-state device sensitive to 0.1 g recording over 7.5-minute epochs mentioned previously. Activity data were collected 24 hours daily Monday through Friday for 4 weeks. Week 1 was a drug-free baseline week. On the three subsequent Monday nights, subjects took 20 or 30 mg of temazepam or placebo was taken 30 minutes before bedtime according to a double-blind balanced randomized design. Placebo was taken every Tuesday, Wednesday, and Thursday nights.

The dependent variable for nighttime activity was the percentage of 7.5-minute epochs with activity greater than zero expressed as a percentage of all bedtime intervals. For the Monday test night, baseline = 55.7% (SE = 3.2%), placebo =

60.4% ($SE = 3.0$). Activity associated with 20 mg temazepam = 51.3% ($SE = 2.3$) was significantly ($p < .05$) less than placebo. The 30 mg dose of temazepam reduced activity even further ($M = 46.8\%$, $SE = 2.9\%$) which was also significantly ($p < .01$) less than placebo. This effect was entirely explained by the first half of the night where baseline averaged 54.8% ($SE = 3.7\%$), placebo averaged 53.5% ($SE = 4.1\%$); 20 mg temazepam ($M = 42.4\%$, $SE = 3.0\%$) was significantly ($p < .05$) lower than placebo as was 30 mg temazepam ($M = 37.1\%$, $SE = 3.3\%$) ($p < .01$). No significant differences occurred during the second half of the night: baseline ($M = 56.4\%$, $SE = 4.4\%$), placebo ($M = 67.1\%$, $SE = 3.2\%$), 20 mg temazepam ($M = 60.3\%$, $SE = 2.7\%$), 30 mg temazepam ($M = 56.4\%$, $SE = 3.5\%$). Data from Tuesday, Wednesday, and Thursday nights were similar and nonsignificant. Hence, temazepam significantly reduces nocturnal activity during the first half of the first night taken. No evidence of a rebound effect was obtained.

The dependent variable for daytime activity was the mean number of activity counts during the first 8 hours after awakening. No significant differences in either the first four or second four hours of activity were observed across the four experimental conditions. However, self-rated daytime grogginess was significantly elevated over placebo levels in the morning and at noon for the 30 mg temazepam condition but not for the 20 mg condition. The authors concluded that 20 mg was the preferred nighttime dose to be taken 30 minutes before bedtime.

Borbely (1984) represented data from Borbely (1983, 1984) described above. Most notable was their Figure 2 showing decreased nocturnal activity during the first half of the night after taking 30 mg temazepam.

NEUROLEPTICS

Perris and Rapp (1974) used 100,000-capacity step counters (they called them pedometers) to examine the effects of fluspirilene in 10 randomly chosen chronic schizophrenic inpatients. Mean steps taken during 7 baseline days of normal drug treatment were 9079.985. This value increased significantly ($p < .01$) to 9746.185 during the next week when normal chemotherapy was withdrawn. Administration of fluspirilene produced a weekly average of 9089.8 steps, which was not significantly different from baseline. However, their Figure 1 indicates substantial activity reduction on Day 1 compared to the other two conditions followed by a strong linear increase. By Day 7 fluspirilene resulted in slightly more activity than was seen on Day 7 of drug removal.

AKATHESIA

The four major side-effects of neuroleptic medications are: 1) parkinsonism, 2) akathesia, 3) acute dystonic reactions, and 4) chronic tardive dyskinesia (Marsden and Jenner, 1980). Akathesia involves both mental and motor restless resulting in an intense desire to move about to seek relief from these feelings. Munetz and Cornes (1982) cite a 1973 task force report indicating that "Akathesia is a side effect of neuroleptic drugs characterized by a subjective sense of inner restlessness leading to an inability to sit still and a compulsion to move." (p. 345) Different aspects of this definition have been emphasized. Van Putten (1975) reinforces Crane and Naranjo (1971) by specifying that akathesia "refers not to any type of pattern of movement, but rather to a subjective need or desire to move." (p. 43) Stahl (1985) asserts that attempts to distinguish subjective distress from objective movement are controversial. Stahl (1985) indicates that the original observation made by Haskovec (1904) pertained to restless movements that were thought to be hysterical in origin.

Several reasons exist for believing that subjective feelings of restlessness are very often overtly expressed in behavior. Hodge (1959) refers to akathesia as "the syndrome of motor restlessness" and indicates that akathesia may appear as an anxiety state. Hodge (1959) presents akathesia as "a form of rhythmic chorea in which the patient is unable to remain seated." (p. 337) He continues: "Not a few subjects complain paradoxically that they cannot 'sit still' or do so only 'with an effort'; they must get up or move about or shift the position of their limbs, inaction having become unbearable." (p. 337) Raskin (1972) cautioned that akathesia often involves hyperactivity and pacing. Van Putten (1975) concludes by saying that "Even a mild akathesia can preclude sitting through the dinner hour, a movie, a therapy session, or a sedentary job." (p. 46) Raskin (1972) indicates that "Unlike restless legs, akathesia affects the entire body, is present during the day, and does not interfere with sleep to the same extent." (p. 122) These reactions are opposite to the mental and motor quiescence normally expected from neuroleptic medications. Marsden and Jenner (1980) discuss several physiological hypotheses.

While akathesia is often associated with higher dosages and with increasing dosage, Freedman and DeJong (1961) indicate that akathesia can be elicited with low dosages. While usually associated with the beginning of a medication interval during the first three months of treatment, Braude and Barnes (1983) describe a late-onset akathesia associated with the end of each injection interval where drug dose reduction exacerbated akathesia and the appearance of choreiform limb movements which they described as covert dyskinesia.

Stahl (1985) identifies seven types of akathesia. The first three types are unrelated to neuroleptic medication and are: (1) hysterical akathesia (Haskovec's syndrome) associated with neurosis; (2) Bing's akathesia, motor restlessness associated with Parkinson's disease and other basal ganglia disorders; (3) spontaneous akathesia also known as restless legs syndrome and Ekbom's syndrome. The remaining four types of akathesia are neuroleptic dependent; (4) acute akathesia due to medication onset resulting in subjective and motor restlessness; (5) pseudoakathesia where motor restlessness is unaccompanied by subjective restlessness as sometimes occurs in schizophrenic patients with primarily negative symptoms; (6) chronic akathesia type 1 appearing and persisting since the last medication increase and associated with oral and/or limb signs of tardive dyskinesia; (7) chronic akathesia type 2 appearing and persisting in patients whose normal medication dose has been reduced, also known as withdrawal or tardive akathesia. Oral and/or limb symptoms of tardive dyskinesia are also present. An underlying issue concerns how acute forms of akathesia merge into chronic aspects of the disease. Munetz and Cornes (1982) described six patients who initially presented with akathesia, later developed pseudoakathesia, and were finally diagnosed as tardive dyskinesia. They further indicated that 21 of their 45 patients with tardive dyskinesia previously evidenced akathesia sometime during treatment.

Van Putten (1975) estimates that 49 (45%) of the 110 patients they treated with antipsychotic medications developed akathesia. Munetz and Cornes (1982) reported akathesia in 21 of 45 patients (46%). Ayd (1961) reported that 21.2% of 3,775 patients treated with a variety of phenothiazines developed akathesia. Part of the disparity in incidence is undoubtedly due to the extent to which milder cases are included within one's definition of akathesia. Raskin (1972) stated that "Because of its subtle symptoms, a diagnosis of akathesia is often overlooked . . . " (p. 121) Following the research strategy indicated below may augment the percentage of patients developing akathesia well above 45%.

ACTIGRAPHY AND AKATHESIA

The following two research designs are suggested for clinical and research evaluations of akathesia. The first design is based upon a challenge to sit still, while the second draws inferences from a naturalistic activity sample.

Chair-Video Design

This design is based upon the observation that patients with akathesia find it difficult to sit still for an extended period of time, as discussed previously. Baseline activity readings would be taken from both wrists and ankles using a device like the Motionlogger™ or Actillume™ actigraphs (Ambulatory Monitoring, Inc., Ardsley, NY) programmed for a 5- or 10-second epoch for 30 minutes or 1 hour while the patient watches a video of some neutral or calming scenes or while listening to "easy" music prior to receiving neuroleptic medication. Sleeping would not be allowed. Perhaps a simple vigilance task could be assigned where subjects pressed a hand-held event button every time some visual object appeared on the screen or a particular tone was heard including audible instructions to press the button now. The test would be repeated a suitable time after receiving medication and the results compared.

This design has several desirable features. First, perfect performance of zero activity counts is clearly defined. Second, all movements are taken as undesirable since subjects are instructed to move as little as possible after first getting settled. The event recorder buttons on all four actigraphs can be pressed once the subject indicates he or she is ready to remain inactive for the prescribed time period and pressed once again just before terminating the test. Third, changes in daily routine and other extraneous factors that can influence the results of the second design will not affect this test because of its well-defined parameters. Activity data are collected simultaneously from all four limbs because true akathesia is supposed to activate the entire body, not just the legs (cf. Raskin, 1972).

Ambulatory Activity Design

A one-week, 24-hour activity sample from the wrist and/or ankle and/or waist prior to chemotherapy would constitute the baseline data set. The resulting data for each actigraph using a 1-minute epoch (1440 per day × 7 days = 10,080 values) would be presented as a single frequency by activity count distribution describing the statistical properties of ambulatory movement during the week. Medication would be given and after a suitable interval a second week of data would be collected using the same actigraphs at the same locations and a second frequency by activity count distribution calculated and compared to the baseline condition. This procedure assumes that the same daily activities are present to the same degree in both weeks. The resulting distributions should be quite stable and individually descriptive because of the large number of data points over a one-week sampling interval. Post hoc analyses could be done using daily distributions.

A related design is to collect single or multiple limb and/or waist actigraphic measurements daily using 1-minute recording epochs for the first three or four weeks of hospitalization. Daily distributions would be calculated and compared over time. The first few days might be analyzed separately because of habituation to new surroundings and routine. A multiple-day baseline sampling of all relevant activities at least once would precede medication. Daily activity distributions would follow the patient's stay to evaluate responsiveness to medication and other changes in clinical condition.

WITHDRAWAL DYSKINESIA

Gardos, Cole, and Tarsy (1978) indicate that the following symptoms frequently follow abrupt discontinuation of antipsychotic medication: restlessness, insomnia, rhinorrhea, headaches, increased appetite, and giddiness. These symptoms begin to appear within the first few days after discontinuing medication, peak by the end of the first week, and disappear by the end of the second week. Usually only one or two symptoms appear.

ACTIGRAPHY AND WITHDRAWAL DYSKINESIA

Actigraphy offers investigators a quantitative method for following activity during both waking and sleeping hours. By taking such measurements for a week or two prior to discontinuing medication, subsequent restlessness and/or insomnia can be clearly documented for either research or clinical purposes.

It is important to note that both delirium and psychomotor agitation/retardation exist in degrees rather than as qualitative extremes. Actigraphy can contribute to our basic understanding and clinical management of these disorders through better quantification of activity levels including both their intensity and temporal distribution.

MONOAMINE OXIDASE INHIBITOR

Teicher, Cohen, Baldessarini, and Cole (1988) report 8 case studies demonstrating that severe daytime somnolence can occur in patients treated with monoamine oxidase inhibitors (MAOI) in addition to disturbances of sleep already known. The net effect of this combination is to severely disrupt normal circadian sleep–wake cycles. Nondominant wrist actigraphy data was obtained over 15-minute epochs for 40–64 hours in 5 patients to further study the disruptive effects of MAOI. The actigraphic records revealed several times between midday and evening when activity waned dramatically. Multiple nocturnal awakenings were also documented.

Reducing the dosage or substituting isocarboxazid sometimes was beneficial but altering the schedule of drugs and or meals was not. Sedation at bedtime normalized sleep but had little effect on daytime somnolence.

DSM-III-R

Delirium

DSM-III-R defines delirium as the " . . . reduced ability to maintain attention to external stimuli and to appropriately shift attention to new external stimuli, and disorganized thinking as manifested by rambling, irrelevant, or incoherent speech. This syndrome also involves a reduced level of consciousness, sensory misperceptions, *disturbances of the sleep–wake cycle and level of psychomotor activity*, disorientation to time, place, and person, and memory impairment." (emphasis added) (p. 100) Sometimes delirium results in difficulty falling asleep while other times a complete sleep–wake reversal occurs. Nightmares may disrupt sleep. Disordered psychomotor activity can range from stupor to mania.

Alcohol Withdrawal Delirium (291.00) is diagnosed when delirium results after cessation of heavy drinking or within one week of a reduction of habitual alcohol consumption (p. 131). Amphetamine or Similarly Acting Sympathomimetic Delirium (292.81) involves delirium within 24 hours of drug usage (p. 137). Cocaine Delirium (292.81) onsets within 24 hours of drug use (p. 143). Phencyclidine (PCP) or Similarly Acting Arylcyclohexylamine Delirium (292.81) onsets within 24 hours of drug use (p. 156). Sedative, Hypnotic, or Anxiolytic Withdrawal Delirium (292.00) onsets within one week of cessation of heavy use (p. 161).

Other Disorders

Activity disorders during the day and night without delirium are associated with a variety of disorders discussed next.

Uncomplicated Alcohol Withdrawal (291.80) involves insomnia and depressed mood (p. 130). Amphetamine or Similarly Acting Sympathomimetic Intoxication (305.70) involves psychomotor agitation (p. 135). Amphetamine or Similarly Acting Sympathomimetic Withdrawal (292.00) has three inclusion criteria: 1) fatigue, 2) insomnia or hypersomnia, and 3) psychomotor agitation (p. 136). Inclusion criteria for Caffeine Intoxication (305.90) include excitement, insomnia, and psychomotor agitation (p. 139). Group B symptoms of Cocaine Intoxication (305.60) include psychomotor agitation. Group A symptoms of Cocaine Withdrawal (292.00) include insomnia or hypersomnia plus psychomotor agitation. Hallucinogenic Mood Disorder (292.84) is an Organic Mood Syndrome (p. 112) involving symptoms of affective disorders ranging from depression to mania. This includes hypoactivity during the day, insomnia at night through mania. Group C symptoms of Inhalant Intoxication (305.90) include psychomotor retardation ranging to stupor. Group B symptoms for Nicotine withdrawal (292.00) include restlessness. Group B symptoms of Opioid Intoxication (305.50) include psychomotor retardation. Group A symptoms of Opioid Withdrawal (292.00) include insomnia. Group B symptoms for Phencyclidine (PCP) or Similarly Acting Arylcyclohexylamine Intoxication (305.90) include psychomotor agitation. Phencyclidine (PCP) or Similarly Acting Arylcyclohexylamine Mood Disorder (292.84) is an Organic Mood Syndrome (p. 112) involving symptoms of affective disorders ranging from depression to mania. Uncomplicated Sedative, Hypnotic, or Anxiolytic Withdrawal (292.00) involves marked insomnia (p. 160).

8

Activity and Chronic Disease

The decrease in death rates due to advances in medical science and public health have helped more people live longer and thereby increased the prevalence of chronic diseases. The "graying" of America will focus greater attention on geriatric disorders.

NEED FOR AMBULATORY MONITORING

The need for ambulatory monitoring of activity is especially great in connection with chronic disease because of the substantial variability in functional impairment associated with these clinical conditions. Some days patients do much better than others. The degree to which they are more or less able to function normally constitutes important information regarding their clinical management.

Goldstein, Stein, Smolen, and Perlini (1976) described a rapid method for receiving, by telephone, and recording daily self-reported health information in two matched groups ($n = 13$ each) of patients with Laennec's cirrhosis. A more complete description of this study is provided in the cirrhosis section later in this chapter.

Smolen, Stein, Goldstein, and Rosenshein (1978) developed computer software, written in APL, wherein self-measurements, such as those described above, are phoned in to hospital staff who enter them into a data base that reviews all existing data and issues "warnings" when these measurements deviate, by an unspecified amount, from clinically preset criteria. Medical intervention can then be initiated in a timely fashion rather than waiting for a major medical emergency to develop.

SPECIFIC DISORDERS

Arthritis

Osteoarthritis involves cartilage degeneration, usually of the larger weight-bearing joints of the knee, hip, and spine resulting in decreased ambulation as the disease worsens. Rheumatoid arthritis involves a swelling of the lining (synovium) of joints in the hands, wrists, feet, ankles, knees, hips, and shoulders. This destructive process is painful, does not abate with rest, and reduces ambulation.

Goldstein and Stein (1985) report the doctoral dissertation of Perlini (1983) demonstrating pedometer data from 20 chronic stable rheumatic patients sensitive to arthritic inflammatory episodes and hospitalizations. Algozzine, Stein, Doering, Araujo, and Akin (1982) used pedometers to evaluate the therapeutic effects of ten percent trolamine salicylate cream regarding osteoarthritis of the knee. Twenty-six patients received the cream or placebo for one week under double-blind conditions. Subjects on placebo the first week were transferred to cream the second week, and vice versa. Subjects wore their pedometers continuously for all waking hours. The values were read once per week during their clinic visit.

The results did not support the efficacy of the topical cream. The weekly distance walked during cream applications was 12.2 km ($S = 9.1$ km) vs a mean of 14.5 km ($S = 13.0$ km) during placebo. This nonsignificant difference is in the opposite direction of what was predicted; less, not more, activity associated with the cream.

The hypothesis that significantly more activity would be associated with the cream presupposes that the ambulatory activity of the subjects was, at the beginning of the study, below that which they desired on account of arthritis-related pain. It further presupposes that reduction of pain will be met with activity increases. The second assumption may be false on the following grounds. Arthritis is a chronic disease which these subjects undoubtedly had had for several years in advance of this study. Perhaps they had become less active during this time as an adjustment to their disorder. Pain reductions brought about by the cream may have been met by old habits of not being active even though activity would now be less painful or even pain-free. Reinforcement and social support for increased activity may not have followed. Perhaps few occasions on which to be active presented themselves during the two weeks that the test was conducted. No significant difference in activity would therefore be expected; none was observed.

Chronic Obstructive Pulmonary Disease (COPD)

COPD refers to a group of disorders that obstruct air flow on expiration. The most common forms of COPD are: chronic bronchitis, chronic asthma, and pulmonary emphysema. Exacerbating factors are: cigarette smoke (passive and active), allergy, infection, and atmospheric contaminants such as dust and caustic vapors. Symptoms include a combination of cough with sputum, wheezing, and shortness of breath. In advanced cases, oxygen cannot be obtained in adequate quantity and waste carbon dioxide is retained, leading to cardiopulmonary deterioration and heart failure.

Lilker, Karnick, and Lerner (1975) evaluated the effects of portable oxygen treatment on ambulation in 9 COPD men using a double-blind crossover study. A three-week pedometer baseline was obtained prior to the onset of the study. Patients were randomly assigned to five weeks of portable liquid oxygen or liquid air treatment. Each patient was visited at home once each week at which time his pedometer was read.

The subjects walked an average of 1.10 miles per day ($S = 0.94$) during baseline. Miles walked per day under liquid air treatment reduced slightly to 1.03 ($S = 0.66$) but increased somewhat to an average of 1.35 miles ($S = 0.83$) during liquid oxygen. Neither of these differences from the baseline average was significant.

The same reasoning used to explain the null result for arthritis above could be invoked here. Subjects may have adjusted to a more sedentary life and therefore continued with their sedentary ways even though they were more able to move about. For example, young people are often capable of more activity than they show. Documenting low activity levels does not prove reduced capacity for greater movement.

Coronary Heart Disease

Goldstein and Stein (1985) indicate that patients with angina symptoms of ischemic coronary heart disease decrease their activity when they feel pain, which can occur from once a year up to 10 times per day. Patients with congestive heart failure limit their activity because of shortness of breath.

Considerable resources are spent upon the ambulatory monitoring of heart function using the Holter monitor. However, Fentem, Fitton, and Hampton (1976) write that "The analysis of long-term electrocardiogram (ECG) recordings in terms of changes or patterns of change of rate is necessarily incomplete without knowledge of the subject's activity." (p. 163) The output of a pressure-sensitive polyurethane-foam–colloidal-carbon-resistive heel pressure sensor (Barber, Evans, Fentem, and Wilson, 1973) was simultaneously recorded on the same body-borne tape recorder as was the ECG. This allowed the investigators to compare heart rate during active and passive periods for the purpose of evaluating rehabilitation after myocardial infarction and for treatment of ectopic frequency during activity and rest.

Timing of activity and rest can be less invasively accomplished with actigraphs having programmable clocks. Monitoring of wrist and/or ankle activity eliminates the inconvenience associated with the above-mentioned heel sensor and its associated wire connection with the body-borne tape recorder.

The above studies concern treatment of already diseased persons. The studies reviewed next show that activity can be used prophylactically. Unfortunately, none of them directly measured activity. They are reported here in the hope that others will be sufficiently encouraged by their results to conduct more rigorous research on this topic.

Research over more than three decades indicates that inactivity predisposes one to coronary heart disease (Morris, Heady, Raffle, Roberts, and Parks, 1953; Shapiro, Weinblatt, Frank, and Sager, 1965; Paffenbarger, Gima, Laughlin, and Black, 1971; Morris, Chave, Adam, Sirey, Epstein, and Sheehan, 1973; Brunner, Manelis, Modan, and Levin, 1974; Paffenbarger, Wing, and Hyde, 1978; Kannel and Sorlie, 1979; Stallones, 1980; Siscovick, Weiss, Hallstrom, Inui, and Peterson, 1982; Leon, Connett, Jacobs, and Rauramaa, 1987; Paffenbarger, Hyde, Wing, and Hsieh, 1986; Donahue, Abbot, Reed, and Yano, 1988). This relationship is partly because inactivity produces high blood pressure (Olsson, Kaijser, Walldium, Logan, Riemersma, and Oliver, 1979), excessive body weight (Friedlander and Rhoads, 1982), and lower high-density-lipoprotein cholesterol levels (Smith, Mendez, Druckenmiller, and Kris-Etherton, 1982; Haskell, Montoye, and Orenstein, 1985).

The study by Slattery, Jacobs, and Nichaman (1989) is of special interest because it indicates that small amounts of leisure time activity substantially reduce mortality from all causes, including coronary heart disease. Unfortunately, activity was estimated rather than directly measured. This study is being reviewed here in the hope that others will be inspired to conduct more rigorous prospective research. A total of 3043 white male U.S. railroad workers were initially examined from 1957 to 1960, reexamined from 1962 to 1964, and followed until 1977 or death. At first test, 2573 working men were categorized as free of cardiovascular disease (CVD), 465 were categorized as having CVD.

Activity was estimated using items that would later constitute the Minnesota Leisure Time Physical Activity Questionnaire (MLTPA) (Taylor, Jacobs, Schucker, Knudsen, Leon, and DeBacker, 1978). Folsom, Jacobs, Caspersen, Gomez-Marin, and Knudsen (1986) report 1-month test–retest reliability of the MLTPA test to range from 0.79 to 0.88 depending upon the subscale. Test–retest correlations on an unspecified number of men, free of cardiovascular disease at both the first and second (4 to 5 years later) examination, indicated reliability coefficients of 0.25 for light activity, 0.33 for moderate activity, and 0.52 for intense activity. These are unacceptably low reliability coefficients by normal psychometric standards. Hence, interpretation should be restricted to total scores. It appears that habits change over 4 to 5 years' time.

Subjects were divided into four groups on the basis of estimated kilocalories expended per week during leisure time activities. The 635 persons in Group 1 all expended less than 250 kcal/wk with a geometric mean of 40 kcal/wk. Group 2 expended from 251 to 1000 kcal/wk with a geometric mean of 554 kcal/wk. Group 3 expended from 1001 to 1999 kcal/wk with a geometric mean of 1372 kcal/wk. Group 4 expended over 2000 kcal/wk with a geometric mean of 3632 kcal/wk.

Age-adjusted death rates per 100 in the 2562 men free of preexisting cardiovascular disease were calculated. For coronary heart disease, the death rates for coronary heart disease across Groups 1–4 were 12.8, 10.8, 9.5, and 10.2. The greatest single reduction is associated with escaping the most sedentary status. The combined heart disease death rates were 14.7, 12.6, 10.2, and 10.6 across Groups 1–4. Almost the same benefit derived from leaving the most sedentary group was associated with moving up one more activity category. The same is true for combined cardiovascular disease rates of 17.6, 15.4, 12.9, and 13.2 across Groups 1–4. However, the "all-cause" mortality results are more consistent with the coronary heart disease rates presented initially. The age-adjusted death rates for all causes are 29.8, 25.5, 24.7, and 26.2 across Groups 1–4. Hence, the largest single benefit derives from not being sedentary. Further activity increases are not rewarded proportionally with age adjusted all-cause death rate decreases.

Teicher, Lawrence, Barber, Finklestein, Lieberman, and Baldessarini (1986) presented evidence that stroke alters the circadian rhythm of activity. They obtained 48 hours of right wrist activity measurements, using a modified Colburn, Smith and Guarini (1976) actigraph, from a 74-year-old male undergoing rehabilitation 6 weeks after his second stroke. He was reported to be alert and oriented but easily distracted indicating a short attention span. The normal control subject was a 65-year-old recently retired man without significant medical or psychiatric disorder; all evaluations being within normal limits. He wore the actigraph on his left wrist for 48 hours.

A strong activity circadian rhythm was found for the normal man indicating quiet nights and active days. A nonlinear least-squares cosinor analysis revealed a circadian periodicity of 23.5 hours equal to a frequency of 1.02 cycles per day. His peak amplitude was 62 counts per 15 minutes. No discernible circadian rhythm was found for the stroke patient. The closest evidence to a spectral peak was at 3 cycles per day.

Dementia

Teicher, Lawrence, Barber, Finklestein, Lieberman, and Baldessarini (1986) presented a case of a 58-year-old demented alcoholic man with a 6 cycle per day (cpd) ultradian activity cycle that was nearly as prominent as his 0.94 cpd component. Lawrence, Teicher, and Finklestein (1989) reported that nondominant wrist activity on 17 severely demented patients with Alzheimer's disease show increased levels of nocturnal activity both in absolute and percentage terms. They further demonstrate a consistent phase delay; their acrophase (time of peak circadian activity) occurred approximately 1.75 hours later than 9 normal control subjects. A subgroup of 6 "pacers" evidenced a 56% daytime activity increase and a 174% nighttime activity increase.

Meningioma

Teicher, Lawrence, Barber, Finklestein, Lieberman, and Baldessarini (1986) discussed a 24-hour sample of nondominant wrist activity data taken from an 80-year-old woman with a well calcified 3-cm-diameter parasagittal meningioma to the right of the midline. This record contained both a 6- and 11-cpd component in addition to a 0.84-cpd cycle.

Cirrhosis

Goldstein, Stein, Smolen, and Perlini (1976) followed 13 patients with Laennec's cirrhosis and 13 matched controls by telephone, when daily self-reported health information was obtained. The following variables were self-reported daily to hospital staff via the telephone. Morning weight was measured on a home scale at approximately the same time of day. The amount of alcohol consumed was 1 oz of hard liquor = 1, one 12-oz beer = 1, one 4-oz glass of wine = 1. All subjects were mailed blood collection kits monthly. The results were mailed back to the hospital in provided containers and analyzed for ethanol. A list of daily medications and dosages were obtained. Digital pedometers, calibrated according to procedures described by Goldstein and Stein (1985), were worn during all waking hours. Mileage walked was reported daily. The number of hours worked part or full time was reported daily. For patients with questions about fluid retention, they poured an equivalent amount of water into a 64-oz graduated pitcher of all liquids ingested and reported the daily total. The supine abdominal girth at the umbilicus obtained with a tape-measure was reported daily. Perhaps the most important result was the 90% compliance in what is generally considered to be a "difficult" population.

Sickle Cell Crises

Sickle cell anemia is a genetic disorder wherein reduced oxygen causes abnormal hemoglobin S to become distorted into a curved sickle shape causing circulatory blockage in small vessels, called sludging (Rodgers, Noguchi, and Schecter, 1985). The resulting oxygen deprivation causes painful crises experienced as headache, back, chest, limb, and/or abdominal pain and can result in kidney failure, strokes, plus damage to other organs (Rosa, Bierer, and Thomas, 1980; Sheehy and Plumb, 1977). Marked individual variations from mild symptoms to severe disability are found (Bowman, 1975; Conyard, Muthuswamy, and Dosik, 1980). Emotional distress is among the most common precipitants of crisis (Barnhart, Henry, and Lusher, 1979; Kunar, Powers, Allen, and Haywood, 1976).

Dinges, Shapiro, Reilly, Orne, Ohene-Frempong, and Orne (1990) evaluated data from daily diaries kept by 18 children (7 female; 11 male) aged 8 to 17 years ($M = 12.9$) evidencing vaso-occlusive crisis (VOC) greater than once per month and found that they reported their sleep to be "bad" on 43.04% of the nights they experienced VOC-related pain compared to 3.72% of the nights on which such pain was absent. Wrist actigraphy (Ambulatory Monitoring, Ardsley, NY) recorded increased nocturnal activity in response to VOC-related pain thereby disturbing sleep. These crises typically persist for several days and nights. A prolonged period (11 hours) of low-mobility sleep followed VOC-related pain offset in the case of the 14-year-old boy reviewed.

A direct implication of this research is that wrist actigraphy can be used to monitor sleep disturbance caused by VOC-related pain thereby documenting the duration and frequency of these events. Perhaps the length of reduced-mobility sleep following pain offset is a measure of the degree to which the crisis was stressful.

Nocturnal wrist actigraphy may be responsive to other forms of pain than VOC. If so, sleep disturbance due to these clinical conditions could also be monitored with wrist actigraphy as described further in Chapter 6 of this volume.

Colon Cancer

Previous research has emphasized the role of diet in colon cancer risk by reporting that risk is directly proportional to calories consumed (Lyon, Mahoney, West, et al., 1987). Other investigators have indicated that contents other than calories, such as fat, are responsible for increased colon cancer risk (Graham, Dayal, Swanson, et al., 1978; Reedy, 1981). However, Potter and McMichael (1986) demonstrated that the increased risk associated with materials such as fat is due to their greater caloric content.

Exercise has increasingly become the focus of attention in reducing risk of colon cancer because it presumably increases the rate with which food residues pass through the colon thereby reducing the time toxic substances are in contact with tissue (Holdstock, Jisiewicz, Smith, et al., 1970). The studies reported below support this hypothesis. Unfortunately, none of these studies measured physical activity. We review them anyway in the hope that others will be sufficiently encouraged by their results to conduct more definitive research using inexpensive step counters or time-based actigraphy.

Garabrant, Peter, Mack, and Bernstein (1984) selected 2950 male colon cancer patients, aged 20 to 64 years, from the Los Angeles County Cancer Surveillance Program registry of 23,273 persons with cancer between 1972 and 1981. The first two authors rated the primary occupations of these men using a three-category system in accordance with occupational information obtained from the Bureau of the Census 1970 Index. A rating of Highly Active was given if activity was required more than 80% of the time. A rating of Moderately Active was given if activity was required from 20 to 80% of the time. A rating of Sedentary was given if activity was required less than 20% of the time.

The annual age-adjusted incidence rates of colon cancer per 100,000 were: Sedentary = 24.6, Moderate = 21.6, High = 13.4 with a Sedentary/High risk ratio of 1.8. The associated 95% confidence interval of 1.6 to 2.2 excludes 1.0 thereby indicating a statistically significant ($p < .05$) protective activity effect . The annual age-adjusted incidence rates of rectal cancer per 100,000 were: Sedentary = 8.1, Moderate = 9.1, High = 7.9, with a Sedentary/High risk ratio of 1.0. The associated 95% confidence interval of 0.8 to 1.3 includes 1.0 thereby indicating no significant difference in rectal cancer rates as a function of activity.

Vena, Graham, Zielezny, Swanson, Barnes, and Nolan (1985) studied 210 white male patients with colon cancer, 276 white male patients with rectal cancer, and 1431 white male control patients with nonneoplastic nondigestive diseases. All subjects were between the ages of 30 and 79 and were studied between 1957 and 1965. The six jobs each subject held for the longest period of time were rated for activity requirements according to the U.S. Department of Commerce Alphabetical Index of Occupations for the 1960 Census and the Standard Industrial Classification Manual. The categories used were: Sedentary, Light, Medium, Heavy, and Very Heavy work.

The results were presented in terms of age-adjusted odds ratios for developing colon and rectal cancer as determined by logistic regression. The results presented next pertain to developing colon cancer. The first dependent variable was the number of work years in jobs with Sedentary or Light work. The odds ratio for None was 1.0 indicating no risk. The odds ratio for 1–20 years was 1.49 ($p < .05$) indicating a significant risk factor. The odds ratio for more than 20 years was 1.97 ($p < .001$) indicating an even greater risk factor.

The second dependent variable was the proportion of work years in jobs with Sedentary or Light work. The odds ratio for None was 1.0 indicating no risk. The odds ratio for 0.01 to 0.50 was 1.53 ($p < .05$) indicating significant risk. The odds ratio for 0.51 to 0.99 was 1.58 ($p < .05$) indicating a significant and very slightly greater risk. However, the risk factor for having always worked at sedentary jobs or engaged in light work was 2.10 ($p < .001$) indicating a substantially greater risk of colon cancer.

The third dependent variable was the proportion of life in jobs with Sedentary or Light work. Again, None = 1.00 indicating no risk. The odds ratio for 0.01 to 0.40 = 1.66 ($p < .01$) indicating significant risk. The odds ratio for 0.41 to 1.00 = 1.83 ($p < .001$) indicating a somewhat greater risk.

None of the odds ratios were significant regarding the development of rectal cancer. Hence, inactivity appears not to have any effect upon the etiology of rectal cancer like it does for colon cancer.

Slattery, Schumacher, Smith, West, and Abd-Elghany (1988) studied 229 histologically confirmed colon cancer patients (119 females, 110 males) identified from the Utah Cancer Registry and 384 (204 females, 180 males) control subjects obtained by random-digit telephone dialing (Waksberg, 1978). Subjects were interviewed with a precoded inventory regarding their dietary and exercise habits for two years prior to illness for cases and two years prior to the interview for controls. Dietary questions concerned the amount, frequency, and method of preparing specific foods. Exercise questions concerned the time spent per week in specific light-, moderate-, and high-intensity leisure time activities plus open-ended questions about job related activity. Calories expended were calculated using previously published tables (Taylor, Jacobs, Schucker, Knudsen, Leon, and Debacker, 1978).

The results were presented in terms of odds ratios referenced against the lowest activity level after adjusting for body mass index (weight/height squared), age, fiber content, and caloric intake by logistic regression. The odds ratios (90% confidence interval) for men regarding total activity are: Low = 1.0 (referent), Level 2 = 1.19 (0.67–2.13), Level 3 = 0.88 (0.48–1.69), High = 0.70 (0.38–1.29). The odds ratios for men regarding intense activity are: None = 1.0 (referent), Low = 0.83 (0.40–1.75), High = 0.27 (0.11–0.65). The odds ratios for men regarding nonintense activity are: Low = 1.0 (referent), Level 2 = 1.40 (0.76–2.57), Level 3 = 0.93 (0.51–1.72), High = 1.25 (0.68–2.29).

The odds ratios for women regarding total activity after adjusting for body mass index, age, fiber content, and caloric intake by logistic regression are: Low = 1.0 (referent), Level 2 = 0.97 (0.56–1.69), Level 3 = 0.91 (0.52–1.60), High = 0.48 (0.27–0.87). For intense activity the odds ratios are: None = 1.0 (referent) and Any = 0.55 (0.23–1.34). Regarding nonintense activity, the following odds ratios were reported: Low = 1.0 (referent), Level 2 = 1.09 (0.62–1.90), Level 3 = 0.94 (0.53–1.66), High = 0.53 (0.29–0.95).

The results for both men and women regarding total and intense exercise indicate that exercise lowers the odds of getting colon cancer. The odds ratios for men and women are essentially unchanged when corrected for body mass, age, fiber content, but not for caloric intake thereby indicating that the protective effect of exercise does not extend to diet. Total caloric intake was observed to increase colon cancer odds from 1.0 to 2.40 in men and 1.64 in women. Protein intake was observed to increase colon cancer odds from 1.0 to 2.57 in men and 1.49 in women. Fat intake was observed to increase colon cancer odds from 1.0 to 2.18 in men and 2.06 in women. These results are consistent with those of Lyon et al. (1987). Activity does not reduce these odds thereby indicating that the beneficial effects of exercise can be undone by dietary habits. Exercise does not cancel the ill effects of excessive caloric, protein, and fat intake. However, some evidence for an interactive effect was reported. Said otherwise, colon cancer risk is greatest in the most sedentary persons with highest caloric, protein, and fat intake and lowest in the most active persons with lowest caloric, protein, and fat intake. It should be noted that these results do not imply that good nutrition should be neglected in order to minimize caloric intake.

Pain

Patient response to chronic pain can take the form of activity decreases or increases. Withdrawal from normal daily routine, including work and leisure time activities, results in decreased activity. Pacing and other anxiety/distress-related behaviors results in increased activity. Hence, activity measurements are recommended as being clinically informative (Fordyce, 1976; Okeefe, 1982).

Cairns, Thomas, Mooney, and Pace (1976) described an automated "uptime" indicator comprising an electric clock connected to the bedsprings such that being in bed opened a switch and leaving bed closed the switch. The amount of time spent out of bed is therefore automatically recorded.

Sanders (1980) described a device consisting of a miniature calculator connected to a mercury switch. The mercury tilt switch is taped to the thigh with an elastic bandage and is connected to the belt-worn calculator with a small wire where switch changes caused by activity are counted. This device, inexpensive step counters, and sophisticated wrist actigraphs are currently available (cf. Chapter 2).

Morrell and Keefe (1988) reported three studies purporting to evaluate actometers for use with chronic pain patients. The first study reported a correlation of $r(12)$ = .997 ($p < .01$) between one-day (all waking hours) readings of two actometers (Timex Model 101 obtained from Willis and Kaulins, Waterbury, CT) attached to the same place on the patient's dominant ankle. The second study correlated the number of 32-yard laps walked with ankle actometer scores in each of 14 subjects. The resulting 14 correlations ranged from a low of .973 to a high of .999 indicating an extremely strong relationship to distance walked. Actometers have thus far been shown to be highly reliable and valid activity sensors.

In the third study, 15 chronic pain patients were divided into three groups of 5 subjects each. Group 1 walked 32 yards once on each of three consecutive days, Groups 2 and 3 walked a 128- or 224-yard distance once each day. Actometer readings on days 2 and 3 were expressed as a percentage of baseline. Actometer scores were nearly the same across days for some patients and quite different for others. Actometer variability correlated ($r(13) = .47$, $p < .08$) with nurse's ratings of patient walking impairment. No correlation was found between actometer reading and pain and stiffness ratings nor with walking speed. The authors granted the validity of actometers for measuring kinetic energy associated with ambulation but questioned the relevance of such measurements for evaluating chronic pain patients.

They concluded that " . . . actometers may not reliably measure changes in walking in chronic pain patients." (p. 269)

Three comments are pertinent. First, the variability of which the authors complain can be due to inconsistent measurement characteristics of actometers or real behavioral variability over time by chronic pain patients. The results of Studies I and II seem to clearly exclude concerns about actometers as sensing devices yet the authors ignore their own data and conclude that actometers per se are unreliable when it comes to measuring the activity of chronic pain patients. Their studies I and II involved chronic pain patients and the actometers worked well then. The undesired variability seems to be due to the combined condition of placing actometers on chronic pain patients walking a fixed distance on three consecutive days. Perhaps this variance measure reflects an important aspect of their clinical condition. Highly variable uncontrollable behavior is usually a problem.

Second, the authors take "time to traverse a fixed distance" as the gold standard of ambulation. They dismiss their own observations of greater kinetic energy due to limping and less due to guarding or bracing as clinically unimportant. Since such pain behaviors can serve as discriminative stimuli for differential treatment by family, friends, and co-workers, limping and guarding behaviors may well be quite clinically relevant (Fordyce, 1973, 1976).

Third, the time to walk a 32-, 128-, or 224-yard distance under maximally motivating circumstances is probably a good measure of ambulatory capacity; what the patient is maximally capable of. However, it entirely misses the point of what activity level the patient typically chooses to support. Some patients may only use a small fraction of their ambulatory capacity thereby presenting themselves as withdrawn and depressed and consequently setting an occasion for others to intervene on their behalf. Other patients may consistently use most, or all, of their ambulatory capacity by constantly moving about in an agitated fashion thereby setting an occasion for others to attend to their condition. These behavioral features are important to the pain process (Fordyce, 1973, 1976).

In short, the authors have taken an orthopedic rather than behavioral perspective in connection with actometers and their role in comprehensive evaluation of pain behavior.

Infection

Halberg, Fanning, Halberg, Cornelissen, Wilson, Griffiths, and Simpson (1981) report temperature and activity data obtained from an approximately 60-year-old woman before and after hospitalization for a dilatation and curettage. A steady rise in rectal temperature was observed while the subject was at home following the operation. The amplitude of the circadian temperature effect was diminished and more variable after compared to before surgery. Wrist activity data was reported as being more irregular after than before surgery. Acrophase, the period of peak activity, was reported to be variable during the first three post-operative days after which it returned to its presurgery position.

Bedrest is often prescribed for sick children despite indications that early ambulation may be desirable (Bass and Schulman, 1967). The assumption is that children in bed are less active than ambulatory children. To evaluate this conjecture, Bass and Schulman (1967) placed actometers on the dominant wrist and ankle of 32 boys between the ages of 6 and 13 hospitalized on one floor of Chicago's Children's Memorial Hospital. Each week, 2 age-matched boys were placed on complete bedrest for 48 hours between 1100 hours Tuesday to Thursday. One of the two children was randomly selected to remain on bedrest until 1700 hours Friday where-as the other child was permitted full activity.

The results indicated no significant differences in either wrist or ankle activity. This counterintuitive result is not due to extremely low statistical power as they could have detected a correlation of $r = .45$ between group code and activity 80% of the time, $r = .40$ 70% of the time, or $r = .34$ 60% of the time. A possible explanation is that none of these children were especially healthy and therefore may not have been very active despite the opportunity to move about as they pleased. Perhaps being sick reduces ambulation to the point where bedrest does not produce further decrements that can be detected with a sample size of 32. It may be that disease so lowers activity that bedrest would unlikely reduce it further. These questions could be answered by studying the activity of healthy children living on the same ward or in similar surroundings.

References

Achenbach, T. (1980). DSM-III in light of empirical research on the classification of child psychopathology. *Journal of the American Academy of Child Psychiatry, 19,* 395–412.

Achenbach, T., and Edelbrock, C. (1978). The classification of child psychopathology: A review and analysis of empirical efforts. *Psychological Bulletin, 85,* 1275–1301.

Achenbach, B. M., and Edelbrock, C. (1986). *Manual for the Teacher's Report Form and Teacher Version of the Child Behavior Profile.* Burlington, VT: University of Vermont Department of Psychiatry.

Agnew, H. W., and Webb, W. B. (1968). Sleep patterns of 30–39-year-old male subjects. *Psychophysiology, 5,* 228.

Albert, I. B., and Ballas, N. C. (1973). Electroencephalographic and temporal correlates of snoring. *Bulletin of the Psychonomic Society, 1,* 169–170.

Algozzine, G. J., Stein, G. H., Doering, P. L., Araujo, O. E., and Akin, K. C. (1982). Trolamine salicylate cream in osteoarthritis of the knee. *Journal of the American Medical Association, 247,* 1311–1313.

American Psychiatric Association. (1980). *Diagnostic and Statistical Manual of Mental Disorders* (3rd. ed.). Washington D.C.: Author.

American Psychiatric Association (1987). *Diagnostic and statistical manual of mental disorders (3rd ed.—Revised).* Washington, D. C.: Author.

Ancoli-Isreal, S., Kripke, D. F., Mason, W., and Kaplan, O. J. (1985). Sleep apnea and periodic movements in an aging sample. *Journal of Gerontology, 40,* 419–425.

Ancoli-Isreal, S., Parker, L., Sinaee, R., Fell, R. L., and Kripke, D. F. (1989). Sleep fragmentation in patients from a nursing home. *Journal of Gerontology: Medical Sciences, 44,* M18–21.

Antonetti, V. W. (1973). The equations governing weight changes in human beings. *American Journal of Clinical Nutrition, 26,* 64–71.

Andersen, K., Keenan, D. M., and Carson, S. H. (1989). Rest–activity patterns in children: The comparison of retrospective and prospective parental observations compared to objective clinical monitoring. In M. H. Chase, R. Lydic, and C. O'Connor (Eds.) *Sleep Research: 18.* 382. Los Angeles, CA: Brain Information Service/Brain Research Institute.

Aserinsky, E., and Kleitman, N. (1953). Regularly occurring periods of eye motility and concomitant phenomena during sleep. *Science, 118,* 273–274.

Aserinsky, E., and Kleitman, N. (1955). Two types of ocular motility occurring in sleep. *Journal of Applied Physiology, 8,* 1–10.

Ayd, F. J. (1961). A survey of drug-induced extrapyramidal reactions. *Journal of the American Medical Association*, *175*, 1054–1060.

Bakan, D. (1966). The test of significance in psychological research. *Psychological Bulletin*, *66*, 423–437.

Baldridge, B. J., Whitman, R. M., and Kramer, M. (1963). A simplified method for detecting eye movements during dreaming. *Psychosomatic Medicine*, *25*, 78–82

Baldridge, B. J., Whitman, R. M., and Kramer, M. (1965). The concurrence of fine muscle activity and rapid eye movements during sleep. *Psychosomatic Medicine*, *27*, 19–26.

Ball, T. S., Sibbach, L., Jones, R., Steele, B., and Frazier, L. (1975). An accelerometer-activated device to control assaultive and self-destructive behaviors in retardates. *Journal of Behavior Therapy and Experimental Psychiatry*, *6*, 223–228.

Barber, C., Evans, D., Fentem, P. H., and Wilson, M. F. (1973). A simple load transducer suitable for long-term recording activity patterns in human subjects. *Journal of Physiology*, *231*, 94–95.

Barber, N. I., Teicher, M. H., and Baldessarini, R. J. (1989). Effects of selective monoaminergic reuptake blockade on activity rhythms in developing rats. *Psychopharmacology*, *97*, 343–348.

Barkley, R. A. (1977). The effects of methylphenidate on various types of activity level and attention in hyperkinetic children. *Journal of Abnormal Child Psychology*, *5*, 351–369.

Barkley, R. A. (1981). *Hyperactive Children : A handbook for diagnosis and treatment*. New York: Guilford Press.

Barkley, R. A. (1982). Guidelines for defining hyperactivity in children : Attention Deficit Disorder with Hyperactivity. In B. B. Lahey and A. E. Kazdin (Eds.), *Advances in clinical child psychology*, Vol. 5. (pp. 137–180), New York: Plenum Press.

Barkley, R. A., and Cunningham, C. E. (1979a). The effects of methylphenidate on the mother–child interactions of hyperactive children. *Archives of General Psychiatry*, *36*, 201–208.

Barkley, R. A., and Cunningham, C. E. (1979b). Stimulant drugs and activity levels in hyperactive children. *American Journal of Orthopsychiatry*, *49*, 491–499.

Barkley, R. A., and Ullman, D. G. (1975). A comparison of objective measures of activity and distractibility in hyperactive and nonhyperactive children. *Journal of Abnormal Child Psychology*, *3*, 231–244.

Barnhart, M., Henry, R. L., and Lusher, J. (1979). *Sickle cell*. Kalamazoo, Michigan: Upjohn.

Bass, H. N., and Schulman, J. L. (1967). Quantitative assessment of children's activity in and out of bed. *American Journal of Diseases of Children*, *113*, 242–244.

Bell, R. Q. (1968). Adaptation of small wristwatches for mechanical recording of activity in infants and children. *Journal of Experimental Child Psychology*, *6*, 302–305.

Bellack, A. S., and Hersen, M. (Eds.). (1988). Behavioral assessment: A practical handbook (3rd. ed.). New York: Pergamon.

Benoit, O., Royant-Parola, S., Borbely, A. A., Tobler, I., and Widlocher, D. (1985). Circadian aspects of motor activity in depressed patients. *Acta Psychiatricia Belgium*, *85*, 582–592.

Berger, B. G., and Owen, D. R. (1983). Mood alterations with swimming—Swimmers really do "feel better." *Psychosomatic Medicine*, *45*, 425–433.

Birrell, P. C. (1983). Behavioural, subjective, and electroencephalographic indexes of sleep onset latency and sleep duration. *Journal of Behavioral Assessment*, *5*, 179–190.

Blackburn, I. M. (1975). Mental and psychomotor speed in depression and mania. *British Journal of Psychiatry*, *126*, 329–335.

Blake, H., and Gerard, R. W. (1937). Brain potentials during sleep. *American Journal of Physiology*, *119*, 692–703.

Blake, H., Gerard, R. W., and Kleitman, N. (1939). Factors influencing brain potentials during sleep. *Journal of Neurophysiology*, *2*, 48–60.

Blinder, B. J., Freeman, D. M. A., and Stunkard, A. J. (1970). Behavior therapy of anorexia nervosa:

Effectiveness of activity as a reinforcer of weight gain. *American Journal of Psychiatry, 126*, 1093–1098.

Block, J. (1976). Issues, problems, and pitfalls in assessing sex differences: A critical review of the psychology of sex differences. *Merrill-Palmer Quarterly, 22*, 283–308.

Bloom, W. L., and Eidex, M. F. (1967). Inactivity as a major factor in adult obesity. *Metabolism, 16*, 679–684.

Bonato, R. A., and Ogilvie, R. D. (1989). A home evaluation of a behavioral response measure of sleep–wakefulness. *Perceptual and Motor Skills, 68*, 87–96.

Bonnet, M. H., and Johnson, L. C. (1978). Relationship of arousal threshold to sleep stage distribution and subjective estimates of depth and quality of sleep. *Sleep, 1*, 161–168.

Bonnet, M. H., and Moore, S. E. (1982). The threshold of sleep: Perception of sleep as a function of time asleep and auditory threshold. *Sleep, 5*, 267–276.

Bootzin, R. R., and Engle-Friedman, M. (1981). The assessment of insomnia. *Behavioral Assessment, 3*, 107–126.

Borbely, A. A. (1984). Ambulatory motor activity monitoring to study the timecourse of hypnotic action. *British Journal of Clinical Pharmacology, 18*, 83S–86S.

Borbely, A. A. (1986). New techniques for the analysis of the human sleep–wake cycle. *Brain and Development, 8*, 482–488.

Borbely, A. A., Loepfe, M., Mattmann, P., and Tobler, I. (1983). Midazolam and Triazolam: Hypnotic action and residual effects after a single bedtime dose. *Arzneimittel-Forschung/Drug Research, 33*, 1500–1502.

Borberly, A. A., Mattman, P., and Loepfe, M. (1984). Hypnotic action and residual effects of a single bedtime dose of temazepam. *Arzneimittel-Forschung/Drug Research, 34*, 101–103.

Bowman, S. (1975). *Sickle Cell Fundamentals*. Chicago: University of Chicago Press.

Brackbill, Y. (1971). Cumulative effects of continuous stimulation on arousal level in infants. *Child Development, 42*, 17–26.

Bradfield, R. B. (1971). A technique for determination of usual and daily energy expenditure in the field. *American Journal of Clinical Nutrition, 24*, 1148–1154.

Bradfield, R. B., Paulos, J., and Grossman, L. (1971). Energy expenditure and heart rate of obese high school girls. *The American Journal of Clinical Nutrition, 24*, 1482–1488.

Braude, W. M., and Barnes, T. R. E. (1983). Late-onset akathesia—An indicant of covert dyskinesia: Two case reports. *American Journal of Psychiatry, 140*, 611–612.

Bray, G. A. (1976). *The Obese Patient*. Philadelphia: W. B. Saunders.

Bray, G. A. (1978). Definition, measurement, and classification of the syndromes of obesity. *International Journal of Obesity, 2*, 1–14.

Bray, G. A., and Gray, D. S. (1988). Obesity. Part 1—Pathogenesis. *The Western Journal of Medicine, 149*, 429–441.

Brouha, L. *Physiology in industry* (pp. 99–108). NY: Pergamon.

Brown, R. S. (1987). Exercise as an adjunct to the treatment of mental disorders. In W. P. Morgan and S. E. Goldston (Eds.), *Exercise and Mental Health* (pp. 131–137). Washington, DC: Hemisphere.

Brownell, K. D., and Lowney, P. (1986). Obesity: The role of physical activity. In K. D. Brownell and J. Foreyt (Eds.), *Handbook of Eating Disorders: Physiology, Psychology, and Treatment of Obesity, Anorexia and Bulimia* (pp. 146–158). New York: Basic Books.

Brownell, K. D., and Stunkard, A. J. (1980). Physical activity in the development and control of obesity. In A. J. Stunkard (Ed.), *Obesity* (pp. 303–324). Philadelphia, PA: W. B. Saunders Co.

Brownell, K. D., and Wadden, T. A. (1986). Behavior therapy for obesity—Modern approaches and better results. In K. D. Brownell and J. P. Foreyt (Eds.), *Handbook of Eating Disorders: Physiology, Psychology, and Treatment of Obesity, Anorexia, and Bulimia* (pp. 180–197). New York: Basic Books.

Brun, T. (1984). Physiological measurement of activity among adults under free living conditions. In E. Pollitt and P. Amante (Eds.), *Energy Intake and Activity* (pp. 131–156). New York: Alan R. Liss, Inc.

Brunner, D., Manelis, G., Modan, M., and Levin, S. (1974). Physical activity at work and the incidence of myocardial infarction, angina pectoris, and death due to ischemic heart disease: An epidemiological study in Israeli collective settlements (kibbutzim). *Journal of Chronic Disease*, 27, 217–233.

Buss, A. H., and Plomin, R. (1975). *A Temperament Theory of Personality*. New York: Wiley.

Buss, A. H., and Plomin, R. (1984). *Temperament: Early Developing Personality Traits*. Hillsdale, New Jersey: Erlbaum.

Buss, D. M., Block, J. H., and Block J. (1980). Preschool activity level: Personality correlates and developmental implications. *Child Development*, 51, 401–408.

Cairns, D., Thomas, L., Mooney, V., and Pace, J. B. (1976). A comprehensive treatment approach to chronic low back pain. *Pain*, 2, 301–308.

Campbell, D. (1968). Motor activity in a group of newborn babies. *Biology of the Neonate*, 13, 257–270.

Campbell, D., Kuyek, J., Lang, E., and Partington, M. W. (1971). Motor activity in early life. II. Daily motor activity output in the neonatal period. *Biology of the Neonate*, 18, 108–120.

Capella, B., Gentile, J. R., and Juliano, D. B. (1977). Time estimation by hyperactive and normal children. *Perceptual and Motor Skills*, 44, 787–790.

Carskadon, M. A., and Dement, W. C. (1981). Respiration during sleep in the aged human. *Journal of Gerontology*, 36, 420–423.

Carskadon, M. A., Dement, W. C., Mitler, M. M., Guilleminault, C., Zarcone, V. P., and Spiegel, R. (1976). Self-reports versus sleep laboratory findings in 122 drug-free subjects with complaints of chronic insomnia. *American Journal of Psychiatry*, 133, 1382–1383.

Carson, R. C., Butcher, J. N., and Coleman, J. C. (1988). *Abnormal Psychology and Modern Life* (8th ed.). Boston: Scott, Foresman.

Chapman, J. S. (1975). *The Relation between Auditory Stimulation of Short Gestation Infants and Their Gross Motor Limb Activity* (Doctoral dissertation, New York University School of Education). *Dissertation Abstracts International*, 36, 1654B. (University Microfilms No. 75-21, 138)

Chirico, A. M., and Stunkard, A. J. (1960). Physical activity and human obesity. *New England Journal of Medicine*, 263, 935–940.

Christensen, D. E. (1975). Effects of combining methylphenidate and the classroom token system in modifying hyperactive behavior. *American Journal of Mental Deficiency*, 80, 266–276.

Cohen, J. (1977). *Statistical Power Analysis for the Behavioral Sciences* (2nd ed.). New York: Academic Press.

Colburn, T. R., Smith, B. M., Guarini, J. J., and Simmons, N. N. (1976). An ambulatory activity monitor with solid state memory. *Instrument Society of America (ISA) Transactions*, 15, 149–154.

Cole, R. J., Kripke, D. J., and Gruen, W. (1990), Ambulatory monitoring of light exposure: Comparison of forehead and wrist. *Sleep Research*, 19, 364.

Coleman, P. D., Gray, F. E., and Watanabe, K. (1959). EEG amplitude and reaction time during sleep. *Journal of Applied Physiology*, 14, 397–400.

Coleman, R. M. (1982). Periodic movements in sleep (nocturnal myoclonus) and restless legs syndrome. In C. Guilleminault (Ed.), *Sleeping and Waking Disorders: Indications and Techniques* (pp. 265–295). London: Butterworth.

Coleman, R. M. (1986). *Wide Awake at 3:00 A.M.: By Choice or by Chance?* San Francisco: W. H. Freeman.

Coleman, R. M., Pollak, C. P., and Weitzman, E. D. (1979). Periodic movements in sleep (nocturnal myoclonus): Relation to sleep disorders. *Annals of Neurology*, 8, 416–421.

Colvin, R. H., and Olson, S. B. (1983). A descriptive analysis of men and women who have lost significant weight and are highly successful at maintaining the loss. *Addictive Behaviors*, *8*, 287–295.

Conners, C. K. (1969). A Teacher Rating Scale for use in drug studies with children. *American Journal of Psychiatry*, *126*, 884–888.

Conners, C. K. (1973). Rating scales. In *Psychopharmacology Bulletin: Special Issue on Pharmacotherapy of Children*. Washington, D.C.: NIMH, Government Printing Office.

Conners, C. K. (1986). *Hyperkinetic children: A Neuro-Psychosocial Approach*. Beverly Hills, CA: Sage Publications Inc.

Consolazio, C. F. (1971). Energy expenditure studies in military populations using Kofranyi-Michaelis respirometers. *American Journal of Clinical Nutrition*, *24*, 1431–1437.

Consolazio, C. F., Johnson, R. E., and Pecora, L. E. (1963). *Physiological Measurements of Metabolic Functions in Man* (pp. 40–54, and 72–83). New York: McGraw-Hill.

Conyard, S., Muthuswamy, K., and Dosik, H. (1980). Psychosocial aspects of sickle cell anemia in adolescents. *Health and Social Work*, *5*, 20–26.

Cox, G. H., and Marley, E. (1959). The estimation of motility during rest or sleep. *Journal of Neurology, Neurosurgery, and Psychiatry*, *22*, 57–60.

Crane, G. E., and Naranjo, E. R. (1971). Motor disorders induced by neuroleptics. *Archives of General Psychiatry*, *24*, 179–184.

Crawford, M. L. J., and Nicora, B. D. (1964). Measurement of human group activity. *Psychological Reports*, *15*, 227–231.

Cromwell, R. L., Palk, B. E., and Foshee, J. G. (1961). Studies in activity level V. The relationships among eyelid conditioning, intelligence, activity level, and age. *American Journal of Mental Deficiency*, *65*, 744–748.

Cronbach, L. J., and Gleser, G. C. (1965). *Psychological tests and personnel decisions* (2nd ed.). Urbana: University of Illinois Press.

Cunningham, C. E., and Barkley, R. A. (1978). The effects of methylphenidate on the mother–child interactions of hyperactive identical twins. *Developmental Medicine and Child Neurology*, *20*, 634–642.

Cunningham, C. E., and Barkley, R. A. (1979). The interaction of normal and hyperactive children with their mothers in free play and structured tasks. *Child Development*, *50*, 217–224.

Daabs, J. M., Jr., and Clower, B. J. (1973). An ultrasonic motion detector with data on stare, restriction of movement, and startle. *Behavior Research Methods and Instrumentation*, *5*, 475–476.

Daniels, R. J., Katzeff, H. L., Ravussin, E., Garrow, J. S., and Danforth, E., Jr. (1982). Obesity in the Pima indians; Is there a thrifty gene? *Clinical Research*, *30*, 244a (abstract).

Davids, A. (1971). An objective instrument for assessing hyperkinesis in children. *Journal of Learning Disabilities*, *4*, 499–501.

Davidsohn, I., and Henry, J. B. (1974). *Todd–Sanford clinical diagnosis by laboratory methods* (15th ed.). Philadelphia: W. B. Saunders.

Davies, D. R., and Horne, J. A. (1975). Human sleep measurement, characteristics and individual differences. In A. D. Clift (Ed.), *Sleep Disturbance and Hypnotic Drug Dependence* (pp. 43–68). New York: Excerpta Medica.

Dawes, R. M. (1962). A note on base rates and psychometric efficiency. *Journal of Consulting Psychology*, *26*, 422–424.

Decker, M. J., Hoekje, P. L., and Strohl, K. P. (1989). Ambulatory monitoring of arterial oxygen saturation. *Chest*, *95*, 17–22.

Dement, W. C., and Kleitman, N. (1957). The relation of eye movements during sleep to dream activity—An objective method for the study of dreaming. *Journal of Experimental Psychology*, *53*, 339–346.

Detre, T. P., and Jarecki, J. (1971). *Modern Psychiatric Treatment*. Philadelphia: Lippincott.

Dinges, D. F., Shapiro, B. S., Reilly, L. B., Orne, E. C., Ohene-Frempong, K., and Orne, M. T. (1990). Sleep/wake dysfunction in children with sickle cell crisis pain. *Sleep Research, 19,* 323.

Dodd, D. K., Birky, H. J., and Stalling, R. B. (1976). Eating behavior of obese and normal-weight females in a natural setting. *Addictive Behaviors, 1,* 321–325.

Donahue, R. P., Abbot, R. D., Reed, D. M., and Yano, K. (1988). Physical activity and coronary heart disease in middle-aged and elderly men: The Honolulu Heart Program. *American Journal of Public Health, 78,* 683–685.

Dorris, R. J., and Stunkard, A. J. (1957). Physical activity: performance and attitudes of a group of obese women. *American Journal of Medical Science, 233,* 622–628.

Douglas, V. I., Parry, P., Marton, P., and Garson, C. (1976). Assessment of a cognitive training program for hyperactive children. *Journal of Abnormal Child Psychology, 4,* 389–410.

Downey, R., Bonnet, M. H., Lin, P., and Dexter, J. R. (1989). The reliability of leg movements and EEG arousals in patients with Periodic Leg Movements. *Sleep Research, 18,* 170.

Downs, F. S., and Fitzpatrick, J. J. (1976). Preliminary investigation of the reliability and validity of a tool for the assessment of body position and motor activity. *Nursing Research, 25,* 404–408.

Durnin, J. V. G. A. (1984). Some problems in assessing the role of physical activity in the maintenance of energy balance. In E. Pollitt and P. Amante (Eds.), *Energy intake and activity* (pp. 101–113). New York: Alan R. Liss, Inc.

Durnin, J. V. G. A., and Brockway, J. M. (1959). Determination of the total daily energy expenditure in man by indirect calorimetry: Assessment of the accuracy of a modern technique. *British Journal of Nutrition, 13,* 41–57.

Eaton, W. O., and Keats, J. G. (1982). Peer presence, stress, and sex differences in the motor activity levels of preschoolers. *Developmental Psychology, 18,* 534–540.

Eaton, W. O. (1983). Measuring activity level with actometers: Reliability, validity, and arm length. *Child Development, 54,* 720–726.

Eaton, W. O., and Dureski, C. M. (1986). Parent and actometer measures of motor activity level in the young infant. *Infant Behavior and Development, 9,* 383–393.

Eaton, W. O., and Enns, L. R. (1986). Sex differences in human motor activity level. *Psychological Bulletin, 100,* 19–28.

Eaton, W. O., and Yu, A. P. (1989). Are sex differences in child motor activity level a function of sex differences in maturational status? *Child Development, 60,* 1005–1011.

Ebert, M. H., Post, R. M., and Goodwin, F. K. (1972). Effect of physical activity on urinary M.H.P.G. excretion in depressed patients. *Lancet* II, 766.

Edelbrock, C. S., and Achenbach, T. M. (1984). The teacher version of the Child Behavior Profile: I. Boys age 6–11. *Journal of Consulting and Clinical Psychology, 52,* 207–217.

Edelson, R. I., and Sprague, R. L. (1974). Conditioning of activity level in a classroom with institutionalized retarded boys. *American Journal of Mental Deficiency, 78,* 384–388.

Edholm, O. G., (1977). Energy balance in man. *Journal of Human Nutrition, 31,* 413–431.

Ellis, N. R., and Pryer, R. S. (1959). Quantification of gross bodily activity in children with severe neuropathology. *American Journal of Mental Deviance, 63,* 1034–1037.

Elsmore, T. F., and Hursh, S. R. (1982). Circadian rhythms in operant behavior of animals under laboratory conditions In F. M. Brown and R. C. Graeber (Eds.), *Rhythmic aspects of behavior* (pp. 273–310). Hillsdale, New Jersey: Erlbaum.

Epstein, S. (1979). The stability of behavior; I. On predicting most of the people much of the time. *Journal of Personality and Social Psychology, 37,* 1097–1126.

Epstein, S. (1980). The stability of behavior. II. Implications for psychological research. *American Psychologist, 35,* 790–806.

Epstein, L. H., Parker, L., McCoy, J. F., and McGee, G. (1976). Descriptive analysis of eating regulation in obese and non-obese children. *Journal of Applied Behavioral Analysis, 9,* 407–415.

Epstein, L. H., Wing, R. R., and Thompson, J. K. (1978). The relationship between exercise intensity, caloric intake, and weight. *Addictive Behaviors, 3*, 185–190.

Espie, C. A., Lindsay, W. R., and Espie, L. C. (1989). Use of the Sleep Assessment Device (Kelley and Lichstein, 1980) to validate insomniacs' self-report of sleep pattern. *Journal of Psychopathology and Behavioral Assessment, 11*, 71–79.

Falk, J. R., Halmi, K. A., and Tryon, W. W. (1985). Activity measures in anorexia nervosa. *Archives on General Psychiatry, 42*, 811–814.

Feinberg, I., and Carlson, V. R. (1968). Sleep variables as a function of age in man. *Archives of General Psychiatry, 18*, 239–250.

Fentem, P. H., Fitton, D. L., and Hampton, J. R. (1976). Long-term recording of activity patterns. *Postgraduate Medical Journal, 52*, 163–166.

Fisher, C., Gross, J., and Zuch, J. (1965). Cycle of penile erection synchronous with dreaming (REM) sleep—a preliminary report. *Archives of General Psychiatry, 12*, 29–45.

Fitz, D., and Tryon, W. W. (1989). Attrition and augmentation biases in time series analysis: Evaluation of clinical programs. *Evaluation and Program Planning, 12*, 259–270.

Fitzpatrick, J. J., and Donovan, M. (1979). A follow-up study of the reliability and validity of the motor activity rating scale. *Nursing Research, 28*, 179–181.

Folsom, A. J., Jacobs, D. R., Caspersen, C. J., Gomez-Marin, O., and Knudsen, J. (1986). Test–retest reliability of the Minnesota leisure time physical activity questionnaire. *Journal of Chronic Disease, 39*, 505–511.

Fordyce, W. E. (1973). An operant conditioning method for managing chronic pain. *Postgraduate Medicine, 53*, 123–128.

Fordyce, W. E. (1976). *Behavioral Methods for Chronic Pain and Illness*. St. Louis: C. V. Mosby.

Foshee, J. G. (1958). Studies in activity level. I. Simple and complex task performance in defectives. *Journal of Mental Deficiency, 62*, 882–886.

Foster, F. G., and Kupfer, D. J. (1973). Psychomotor activity and serum creatine phosphokinase activity. *Archives of General Psychiatry, 29*, 752–758.

Foster, F. G., and Kupfer, D. J. (1975a). Anorexia nervosa: Telemetric assessment of family interaction and hospital events. *Journal of Psychiatric Research, 12*, 19–35.

Foster, F. G., and Kupfer, D. J. (1975b). Psychomotor activity as a correlate of depression and sleep in acutely disturbed psychiatric inpatients. *American Journal of Psychiatry, 132*, 928–931.

Foster, F. G., Kupfer, D., Weiss, G., Lipponen, V., McPartland, R., and Delgado, J. (1972). Mobility recording and cycle research in neuropsychiatry. *Journal of Interdisciplinary Cycle Research, 3*, 61–72.

Foster, F. G., McPartland, R., and Kupfer, D. J. (1976). Psychotherapy or cycle therapy in affective illness. *Psychosomatic Medicine, 38*, 66–67.

Foster, F. G., McPartland, R. J., and Kupfer, D. J. (1977). Telemetric motor activity in children: A preliminary study. *Biotelemetry, 4*, 1–8.

Foster, F. G., McPartland, R. J., and Kupfer, D. J. (1978a). Motion sensors in medicine, Part I. A report on reliability and validity. *Journal of Inter-American Medicine, 3*, 4–8.

Foster, F. G., McPartland, R., and Kupfer, D. J. (1978b). Motion sensors in medicine, Part II. Application in psychiatry. *Journal of Inter-American Medicine, 3*, 13–17.

Frankel, B. L., Patten, B. M., and Gillin, J. C. (1974). Restless legs syndrome: Sleep-electroencephalographic and neurological findings. *Journal of the American Medical Association, 230*, 1302–1303.

Freedman, D. X., and DeJong, J. (1961). Thresholds for drug-induced akathesia. *American Journal of Psychiatry, 117*, 930–931.

Friedlander, J. S., and Rhoads, J. G. (1982). Patterns of adult weight and fat change in six Solomon Islands societies: A semi-longitudinal study. *Social Science and Medicine, 15*, 205–215.

Garabrant, D. H., Peter, J. M., Mack, T. M., and Bernstein, L. (1984). Job activity and colon cancer risk. *American Journal of Epidemiology, 119*, 1005–1014.

Gardos, G., Cole, J. O., and Tarsy, D. (1978). Withdrawal syndromes associated with antipsychotic drugs. *American Journal of Psychiatry, 135*, 1321–1324.

Garrow, J. S. (1981). *Treat Obesity Seriously: A Clinical Manual*. Edinburgh: Churchill Livingstone.

Garrow, J. S. (1986). Physiological aspects of obesity. In K. D. Brownell and J. P. Foreyt (Eds.), *Handbook of Eating Disorders: Physiology, Psychology, and Treatment of Obesity, Anorexia, and Bulimia.* (pp. 45–52). New York: Basic Books.

Garrow, J. S. (1987a). *Energy Balance and Obesity in Man* (2nd ed.). Amsterdam: Elsevier/North-Holland Biomedical Press.

Garrow, J. S. (1987b). Energy balance in man—an overview. *American Journal of Clinical Nutrition, 45*, 1114–1119.

Garrow, J. S., and Webster, J. (1985). Quetelet's index (W/H^2) as a measure of fatness. *International Journal of Obesity, 9*, 147–153.

Gayle, R, Montoye, H. J. and Philpot, J. (1977). Accuracy of pedometers for measuring distance walked. *Research Quarterly, 48*, 632–636.

Gehardsson, M., Norell, S. E., Kiviranta, H., Pedersen, N. L., and Ahlbom, A. (1986). Sedentary jobs and colon cancer. *American Journal of Epidemiology, 123*, 775–780.

Geissler, C. A., Miller, D. S., and Shah, M. (1987). The daily metabolic rate of the post-obese and the lean. *American Journal of Clinical Nutrition, 45*, 914–920.

Ghali, N., and Durnin, J. V. G. A. (1977). A study of the energy balance of a woman on varying energy intakes during 14 months. *Procedings of the Nutrition Society, 36*, 91a.

Gjessing, R. R. (1976). Motor activity. In L. R. Gjessing and F. A. Jenner (Eds.). *Contribution to the somatology of periodic catatonia* (pp. 129–183). New York: Pergamon.

Gjessing, L. R. (1974). A review of periodic catatonia. *Biological Psychiatry, 8*, 23–45.

Glaros, A. G., and Kline, R. B. (1988). Understanding the accuracy of tests with cutting scores; The sensitivity, specificity, and predictive value model. *Journal of Clinical Psychology, 44*, 1013–1023.

Globus, G. G., Phoebus, E. C., Humphries, J., Boyd, R., and Sharp, R. (1973). Ultraradian rhythms in humans telemetered gross motor activity. *Aerospace Medicine, 44*, 882–887.

Godfrey, H. P. D., and Knight, R. G. (1984). The validity of actometer and speech activity measures in the assessment of depressed patients. *British Journal of Psychiatry, 145*, 159–163.

Goldsmith, R., Miller, D. S., Mumford, P., and Stock, M. J. (1976). The use of long term measurements of heart rate to assess energy expenditure. *Journal of Physiology* (London), *189*, 35 pp.

Goldstein, M. K., Stein, G. H., Smolen, D. M., and Perlini, W. S. (1976). Bio-behavioral monitoring: A method for remote health measurement. *Archives of Physical Medicine and Rehabilitation, 57*, 253–258.

Goode, D. J., Meltzer, H. Y., Moretti, R., Kupfer, D. J., and McPartland, R. J. (1979). The relationship between wrist-monitored motor activity and serum CPK activity in psychiatric in-patients. *British Journal of Psychiatry, 135*, 62–66.

Gottfries, C. G., Gottfries, I., and Olsson, E. (1966). Objective recording of arm and leg activity in normal and clinical samples. *British Journal of Psychiatry, 112*, 1269–1278.

Goyette, C. H., Conners, C. K., and Ulrich, R. F. (1978). Normative data on revised Conners Parent and Teacher Rating Scales. *Journal of Abnormal Child Psychology, 6*, 221–236.

Graham, L. E., II, Taylor, C. B., Hovell, M. F., and Siegel, W. (1983). Five-year follow-up to a behavioral weight-loss program. *Journal of Consulting and Clinical Psychology, 2*, 322–323.

Graham, S., Dayal, J., Swanson, M., Mittelman, A., and Wilkinson, G. (1978). Diet in the epidemiology of cancer of the colon and rectum. *Journal of the National Cancer Institute, 61*, 709–714.

Grande, F., Anderson, J. T., and Keys, A. (1958). Changes of basal metabolic rate in man in semistarvation and refeeding. *Journal of Applied Physiology, 12*, 230–235.

Greist, J. H., Klein, M. H., Eischens, R. R., and Faris, J. T. (1978). Running out of depression. *The Physician and Sportsmedicine*, December, 49–56.

Greist, J. H., Klein, M. H., Eischens, R. R., and Faris, J. T. (1979). Running as a treatment for depression. *Comprehensive Psychiatry*, 20, 41–54.

Griffiths, E., Chapman, N., and Campbell, D. (1967). An apparatus for detecting and monitoring movement. *American Journal of Psychology*, 80, 438–441.

Gruen, W. (1987). Wrist-actigraph measurements of sleep–awake patterns during a 28-day Westerly trip around world. *5th International Congress of Sleep Research* (Poster 490), 691.

Halberg, E., Fanning, R., Halberg, F., Cornelissen, G., Wilson, D., Griffiths, K., and Simpson, H. (1981). Toward a chronopsy: Part III. Automatic monitoring of rectal, axillary and breast surface temperature and of wrist activity: effects of age and of ambulatory surgery followed by nosocomial infection. *Chronobiologia*, 8, 253–271.

Halverson, C. F., Jr., and Waldrop, M. F. (1973). The relations of mechanically recorded activity level to varieties of preschool play behavior. *Child Development*, 44, 678–681.

Halverson, C. F. Jr., and Victor, J. B. (1976). Minor physical anomalies and problem behavior in elementary school children. *Child Development*, 47, 281–285.

Halverson, C. F., Jr., and Post-Gorden, J. C. (1984). Measurement of open-field activity in young children: A critical analysis. In E. Pollitt and P. Amante (Eds.) *Energy Intake and Activity* (pp. 185–203), New York: Alan R. Liss.

Harding, R. M., and Sen, R. N. (1970). Evaluation of total muscular activity by quantification of electromyograms through a summing amplifier. *Medical and Biological Engineering*, 8, 343–356.

Harris, J. A., and Benedict, F. G. (1919). *A Biometric Study of Basal Metabolism in Man* (Publ no 279). Washington, D. C.: Carnegie Institution.

Harris, R. J. (1985). *A Primer of Multivariate Statistics* (2nd ed.). New York: Academic Press, Inc.

Hartman, P. G., and Scrima, L. (1986). Muscle activity in the legs associated with frequent arousals in narcoleptics, nocturnal myoclonus, and abstructive sleep apnea patients. *Clinical Electroencephalography*, 4, 181–186.

Haskell, W. L., Montoye, H. J., and Orenstein, D. (1985). Physical activity and exercise to achieve health-related physical fitness components. *Public Health Report*, 100, 202–211.

Hauri, P. J. (1989). Wrist actigraphy in insomniacs. *Sleep Research*, 18, 239.

Hauri, P. J. (1989). Laboratory sleep and home sleep in insomniacs. *Sleep Research*, 18, 238.

Heiser, J. R., Epstein, L. H., and Wing, R. R. (1981). Technical reliability of pedometers. *The Behavior Therapist*, 4, 21–22.

Hemokinetics, Inc. (1987). *Estimating Activity Level Without the BMR Component (METS); Estimating Basal Metabolic Rate (BMR) Calories.* (Technical Application Note, August 15, 1987). Madison, WI: Author.

Heninger, G. R., and Kirstein, L. (1977). Effects of lithium carbonate on motor activity in mania and depression. *Journal of Nervous and Mental Disease*, 164, 168–175.

Herron, R. E., and Ramsden, R. W. (1967). Continuous monitoring of overt human body movement by radio telemetry: A brief review. *Perceptual and Motor Skills*, 24, 1303–1308.

Hill, S. W., and McCutcheon, N. B. (1975). Eating responses of obese and non-obese humans during dinner meals. *Psychosomatic Medicine*, 37, 395–401.

Hinkle, D. E., Wiersma, W., and Jurs, S. G. (1988). *Applied statistics for the behavioral sciences* (2nd ed.). Chicago: Rand McNally.

Hirsch, J., and Leibel, R. L. (1988). New light on obesity. *The New England Journal of Medicine, 318*, 509–510.

Hobson, J. A., Spagna, T., Malenka, R. (1978). Ethology of sleep studied with time-lapse photography: Postural immobility and sleep-cycle phase in humans. *Science*, 201, 1251–1253.

Hodes, R., and Dement, W. C. (1964). Depression of electrically induced reflexes ("H reflexes") in man during low voltage EEG "sleep". *Electroencephalography and Clinical Neurophysiology, 17*, 617–629.

Hodge, J. R. (1959). Akathesia: The syndrome of motor restlessness. *American Journal of Psychiatry, 116*, 337–338.

Hoiberg, A., Berard, S., Watten, R. H., and Caine, C. (1984). Correlates of weight loss in treatment and at follow-up. *International Journal of Obesity, 8*, 457–465.

Holdstock, D. J., Misiewicz, J. J., Smith, T. and Rowlands, E. N. (1970). Propulsion (mass movement) in the human colon and its relationship to meals and somatic activity. *Gut, 11*, 91–99.

Homatidis, S. and Konstantareas, M. M. (1981). Assessment of Hyperactivity: Isolating Measures of High Discriminant Ability. *Journal of Consulting and Clinical Psychology, 49*, 533–541.

Horton, E. S. (1984). Appropriate methodology for assessing physical activity under laboratory conditions in studies of energy balance in adults. In E. Pollitt and P. Amante (Eds.), *Energy Intake and Activity* (pp. 115–129). New York: Alan R. Liss, Inc.

Hubert, N. C., Wachs, T. D., Peters-Martin, P., and Gandour, M. J. (1982). The study of early temperament: Measurement and conceptual issues. *Child Development, 53*, 571–600.

Huitema, B. E. (1985). Autocorrelation in applied behavior analysis: A myth. *Behavioral Assessment, 7*, 107–118.

Huitema, B. E. (1986). Autocorrelation in behavior modification data: Wherefore art thou? In A. Poling and R. W. Fuqua (Eds.). *Research Methods in Applied Behavior Analysis: Issues and Advances* (pp. 187–208). New York: Plenum Press.

Huitema, B. E. (1988). Autocorrelation: 10 years of confusion. *Behavioral Assessment, 10*, 253–294.

Ingle, D. J. (1949). A simple means of producing obesity in the rat. *Proceedings of the Society of Experimental Biology and Medicine, 72*, 604.

Irwin, O. C. (1932). The distribution of the amount of motility in young infants between two nursing periods. *Journal of Comparative and Physiological Psychology, 14*, 429–445.

Jacobs, D., Ancoli-Israel, S., Parker, L., and Kripke, D. F. (1989). Sleep and wake over 24 hours in a nursing home population. *Sleep Research, 18*, 191.

Jacob, R. G., O'Leary, K. D., and Rosenblad, C. (1978). Formal and Informal Classroom Settings: Effects on Hyperactivity. *Journal of Abnormal Child Psychology, 6*, 47–59.

Jasper, H. H. (1958). Report of the committee on methods of clinical examination in electroencephalography. *Electroencephalography and Clinical Neurophysiology, 10*, 370–375.

Jeffery, R. W., Bjornson-Beson, W. M., Rosenthal, B. S., Kurth, C. L., and Dunn, M. M. (1984). Effectiveness of monetary contracts with two repayment schedules on weight reduction in men and women from self-referred and population samples. *Behavior Therapy, 15*, 273–279.

Jeffrey, D. B., and Katz, R. C. (1977). *Take It Off and Keep It Off: A Behavioral Program for Weight Loss and Healthy Living.* Englewood Cliffs, New York: Prentice-Hall.

Johnson, C. F. (1971). Hyperactivity and the machine: The actometer. *Child Development, 42*, 2105–2110.

Johnson, C. F. (1972). Limits on the measurement of activity level in children using ultrasound and photoelectric cell. *American Journal of Mental Deficiency, 77*, 301–310.

Johnson, M. L., Burke, B. S., and Mayer, J. (1956). Relative importance of inactivity and overeating in the energy balance of obese high school girls. *American Journal of Clinical Nutrition, 4*, 37–44.

Johnsgard, K. W. (1989). *The Exercise Prescription for Depression and Anxiety.* New York: Plenum.

Johnston, J. M., and Pennypacker, H. S. (1980). *Strategies and Tactics of Human Behavioral Research.* Hillsdale, New Jersey: Erlbaum.

Juliano, D. B. (1974). Conceptual tempo activity and concept learning in hyperactive and normal children. *Journal of Abnormal Psychology, 83*, 629–634.

Kagan, J. (1966). Reflection–impulsivity: The generality and dynamics of conceptual tempo. *Journal of Abnormal Psychology, 71*, 17–24.

Kahn, A., Mozin, M. J., Rebuffat, E., Blum, D., Casimir, G., and Duchateau, J. (1991) Chronic insomnia in infants and allergy. (Submitted for publication)

Kannel, W. B., and Sorlie, P. (1979). Some health benefits of physical activity: The Framingham Study. *Archives of Internal Medicine, 139*, 857–861.

Kaspar, J. C., Millichap, J. G., Backus, R., Child, D., and Schulman, J. L. (1971). A study of the relationship between neurological evidence of brain damage in children and activity and distractibility. *Journal of Consulting and Clinical Psychology, 36*, 329–337.

Kast, E. C. (1964). Observations of psychomotor behavior as an index of psychopharmacologic action. *Journal of Neuropsychiatry, 5*, 577–584.

Katahn, M., Pleas, J., Thackrey, M., and Wallston, K. A. (1982). Relationship of eating and activity self-reports to follow-up weight maintenance in the massively obese. *Behavior Therapy, 13*, 521–528.

Katch, F. I., and McArdle, W. D. (1988). *Nutrition, Weight Control, and Exercise*. Philadelphia: Lea and Febiger.

Kavanaugh, T., Shephard, R. J., Tuck, J. A., and Qureshi, S. (1977). Depression following myocardial infarction: The effects of distance running. *Annals of the New York Academy of Science, 301*, 1029–1038.

Keesey, R. E. (1980). A set-point analysis of the regulation of body weight (pp. 144–165). In A. J. Stunkard (Ed.). *Obesity*. Philadelphia: W. B. Saunders.

Kelley, J. E., and Lichstein, K. L. (1980). A sleep assessment device. *Behavioral Assessment, 2*, 135–146.

Kendall, P. C., and Brophy, C. (1981). Activity and attentional correlates of teacher ratings of hyperactivity. *Journal of Pediatric Psychology, 6*, 451–458.

Keys, A. (1970). Coronary heart disease in seven countries. *Circulation, 41*, 1–211.

Keys, A., Brozek, J., Henschel, A., Mickelsen, A., and Taylor, H. L. (1950). *The Biology of Human Starvation*. Minneapolis: University of Minnesota Press.

Khachaturian, Z. S., Kerr, J., Kruger, R., and Schachter, J. (1972). A methodological note: Comparison between period and rate data in studies of cardiac function. *Psychophysiology, 9*, 539–545.

Klein, M. K., Greist, J. H., Gurman, A. S., Neimeyer, R. A., Lesser, D. P., Bushnell, N. J., and Smith, R. E. (1985). A comparative outcome study of group psychotherapy vs. exercise treatments for depression. *International Journal of Mental Health, 13*, 148–177.

Kleitman (1963) *Sleep and Wakefulness*. Chicago: University of Chicago Press (pp. 85–86).

Klesges, R. C., Coates, T. J., Moldenhauer, L. M., Holzer, B., Gustavson, J., and Barnes, J. (1984). The FATS: An observational system for assessing physical activity in children and associated parent behavior. *Behavioral Assessment, 6*, 333–345.

Klesges, L. M., and Klesges, R. C. (1987). The assessment of children's physical activity: a comparison of methods. *Medicine and Science in Sports and Exercise, 19*, 511–517.

Klesges, R. C., Klesges, L. M., Swenson, A. M., and Pheley, A. M. (1985). *American Journal of Epidemiology, 122*, 400–410.

Knapp, T. J., Downs, D. L., and Alperson, J. R. (1976). Behavior therapy for insomnia: A review. *Behavior Therapy, 7*, 614–625.

Kovacevic-Ristanovic, R., Cartwright, R., and Lloyd, S. (1989). Successful non-pharmacologic treatment of periodic leg movements in sleep. *Sleep Research, 18*, 203.

Kraemer, H. C., and Thiemann, S. (1987). *How Many Subjects? Statistical Power Analysis in Research*. Beverly Hills, CA: Sage Publications.

Kripke, D. F., Mullaney, D. J., Atkinson, M., and Wolf, S. (1978). Circadian rhythm disorders in manic-depressives. *Biological Psychiatry, 13*, 335–351.

Kripke, D. F., Mullaney, D. J., Messin, S., and Wyborney, V. G. (1978). Wrist actigraphic measures of sleep and rhythms. *Electroencephalography and Clinical Neurophysiology, 44*, 674–676.

Kunar, S., Powers, D., Allen, J., and Haywood, L. J. (1976). Anxiety, self-concept and personal and social adjustment in children with sickle cell anemia. *Journal of Pediatrics, 88*, 859–863.

Kupfer, D. J., and Detre, T. P. (1971). Development and application of the KDS[tm] 1 in inpatient and outpatient settings. *Psychological Reports, 29*, 607–617.

Kupfer, D. J., Detre, T. P., Foster, F. G., Tucker, G. J., and Delgado, J. (1972). The application of Delgado's telemetric mobility recorder for human studies. *Behavioral Biology*, 7, 585–590.

Kupfer, D. J., and Foster, F. G. (1973). Sleep and activity in a psychotic depression. *Journal of Nervous and Mental Disease*, 156, 341–348.

Kupfer, D. F., Foster, F. G., Detre, T. P., and Himmelhoch, J. (1975). Sleep EEG and motor activity as indicators in affective states. *Neuropsychobiology*, 1, 296–303.

Kupfer, D. J., Sewitch, D. E., Epstein, L. H., Bulik, C., McGowen, C. R., and Robertson, R. J. (1985). Exercise and subsequent sleep in male runners: Failure to support the slow wave sleep-mood-exercise hypothesis. *Neuropsychobiology*, 14, 5–12.

Kupfer, D. J., Weiss, B. L., Foster, F. G., Detre, T. P., Delgado, J., and McPartland, R. (1974). Psychomotor activity in affective states. *Archives of General Psychiatry*, 30, 765–768.

Kupietz, S., Bialer, I., and Winsberg, B. G. (1972). A behavior rating scale for assessing improvement in behaviorally deviant children: A preliminary investigation. *American Journal of Psychiatry*, 128, 116–120.

Lahey, B. B., Green, K. D., and Forehand, R. (1980). On the independence of ratings of hyperactivity. Conduct problems and attention deficits in children: A multiple regression analysis. *Journal of Consulting and Clinical Psychology*, 48, 566–574.

Lahey, B. B., and Piacentini, J. C. (1985). An evaluation of the Quay-Peterson Revised Behavior Problem Checklist. *Journal of School Psychology*, 87, 333–340.

LaPorte, R. E., Cauley, J. A., Kinsey, C. M., Corbett, W., Robertson, R., Black-Sandler, R., Kuller, L. H., and Falkel, J. (1982). The epidemiology of physical activity in children, college students, middle-aged men, menopausal females, and monkeys. *Journal of Chronic Diseases*, 35, 787–795.

LaPorte, R. E., Kuller, L. H., Kupfer, D. J., McPartland, R. J., Matthews, G., and Caspersen, C. (1979). An objective measure of physical activity for epidemiologic research. *American Journal of Epidemiology*, 109, 158–168.

Lavie, P. (1983). Incidence of sleep apnea in a presumably healthy working population: A significant relationship with excessive daytime sleepiness. *Sleep*, 6, 312–318.

Lavie, P., and Gruen, W. (1989). The effects of 7.5 mg midazolam vs placebo on sleep disturbances associated with westward and eastward flights. *Sleep Research*, 18, 386.

Lawrence, J. M., Teicher, M. H., and Finklestein, S. P. (in press). Quantitative assessment of locomotor activity in psychiatry and neurology. In A. B. Joseph and R. Young (Eds.), *Disorders of movement in psychiatry and neurology*. Cambridge, MA: Blackwell Scientific Publications.

Leon, A. S., Connett, J., Jacobs, D. R., Jr., and Rauramaa, R. (1987). Leisure time physical activity levels and risk of coronary heart disease and death: The multiple risk factor intervention trial. *Journal of the American Medical Association*, 258, 2388–2395.

Levine, B., Moyles, T., Roehrs, T., Fortier, J., and Roth, R. (1986). Actigraphic monitoring and polygraphic recording in determination of sleep and wake. *Sleep Research*, 15, 247.

Lewis, M., and Wilson, L. (1970). An infant stabilimeter. *Journal of Experimental Child Psychology*, 10, 52–56.

Lewis, M. (1990). Assessing social intervention: Scientific and social implications. In C. B. Fisher and W. W. Tryon (Eds.). *Ethics in Applied Developmental Psychology* (pp. 81–91). Norwood, New Jersey: Ablex.

Lichstein, K. L., Hoelscher, T. J., Eakin, T. L., and Nickel, R. (1983). Empirical sleep assessment in the home: A convenient inexpensive approach. *Journal of Behavioral Assessment*, 5, 111–118.

Lichstein, K. L., Nickel, R., Hoelscher, T. J., and Kelley, J. E. (1982). Clinical validation of a sleep assessment device. *Behavior Research and Therapy*, 20, 292–298.

Lieberman, H. R., Wurtman, J. J., and Teicher, M. H. (1989). Circadian rhythms of activity in healthy young and elderly humans. *Neurobiology of Aging*, 10, 259–265.

Lilker, E. S., Karnick, A., and Lerner, L. (1975). Portable oxygen in chronic obstructive lung disease with hypoxemia and cor pulmonale: A controlled double-blind crossover study. *Chest*, 68, 236–241.

Lindsley, O. R. (1957). Operant behavior during sleep: A measure of depth of sleep. *Science, 126,* 1290–1291.

Linscheid, T. R., Iwata, B. A., Ricketts, R. W., Williams, D. E., and Griffin, J. C. (1990). Clinical evaluation of the Self-Injurious Behavior Inhibiting System (SIBIS). *Journal of Applied Behavior Analysis, 23,* 53–78.

Lipsey, M. W. (1990). *Design Sensitivity: Statistical Power for Experimental Research.* Beverly Hills, CA: Sage Publications.

Lipsitt, L. P., and DeLucia, C. A. (1960). An apparatus for the measurement of specific response and general activity of the human neonate. *American Journal of Psychology, 73,* 630–632.

Loney, J., Langhorne, J., and Paternite, C. (1978). An empirical basis for subgrouping the hyperkinetic/minimal brain dysfunction syndrome. *Journal of Abnormal Psychology, 87,* 431–441.

Luk, S. L., Thorley, G. and Taylor, E. (1987). Gross overactivity: A study by direct observation. *Journal of Psychopathology and Behavioral Assessment, 9,* 173–183.

Lyon, J. L., Mahoney, A. W., West, D. W., Gardner, J. W., Smith, K. R., Sorenson, A. W. and Stanish, W.: Energy intake: its relationship to colon cancer risk. *Journal of the National Cancer Institute, 78,* 853–861.

Maccoby, E., Dowley, E., Hagen, J., and Dergman, R. (1965). Activity level and intellectual functioning in normal pre-school children. *Child Development, 36,* 761–770.

Maccoby, E. E., and Jacklin, C. N. (1974). *The Psychology of Sex Differences.* Stanford, CA: Stanford University Press.

Marsden, C. D., and Jenner, P. (1980). The pathophysiology of extrapyramidal side-effects of neuroleptic drugs. *Psychological Medicine, 10,* 55–72.

Marston, A. R., and Criss, J. (1984). Maintenance of successful weight loss: Incidence and prediction. *International Journal of Obesity, 8,* 435–439.

McGinty, D. J. (1985). Physiological equilibrium and the control of sleep states. In D. J. McGinty, R. Drucker-Colin, A. Morrison, and P. L. Parmeggiani (Eds.). *Brain Mechanisms of Sleep.* New York: Raven Press.

Mack, R. W., and Kleinhenz, M. E. (1974). Growth, caloric intake, and activity levels in early infancy: A preliminary report. *Human Biology, 46,* 345–354.

Marsden, J. P., and Montgomery, S. R. (1972). A general survey of the walking habits of individuals. *Ergonomics, 15,* 491–504.

Marston, A. R., and Criss, J. (1984). Maintenance of successful weight loss: Incidence and prediction. *International Journal of Obesity, 8,* 435–439.

Martinsen, E. W. (1987). Exercise and medication in the psychiatric patient. In W. P. Morgan and S. E. Goldston (Eds.), *Exercise and Mental Health* (pp. 85–95). Washington, DC: Hemisphere.

Massey, P. S., Lieberman, A., and Batarseh, G. (1971). Measure of activity level in mentally retarded children and adolescents. *American Journal of Mental Deficiency, 76,* 259–261.

Mattmann, P., Loepfe, M., Scheitlin, T., Schmidlin, D., Gerne, M., Strauch, I., Lehmann, D., and Borbely, A. A. (1982). Day-time residual effects and motor activity after three benzodiazepine hypnotics. *Arzneimittel-Forschung/Drug Research, 32,* 461–465.

Matussek, N., Romisch, P., and Ackenheil, M. (1977). MHPG excretion during sleep deprivation in endogenous depression. *Neuropsychobiology, 3,* 23–29.

Mayer, J. (1953). Decreased activity and energy balance in the hereditary obesity diabetes syndrome of mice. *Science, 117,* 504–505.

Mayer, J., and Bullen, B. A. (1974). Nutrition, weight control, and exercise. In W. R. Johnson and E. R. Buskirk (Eds.), *Science and Medicine of Exercise and Sport.* New York: Harper and Row.

Mayer, J., Marshall, N. B., Vitale, J. J., Christensen, J. H., Mashayekhi, M. B., and Stare, F. J. (1954). Exercise food intake and body weight in normal rats and genetically obese adult mice. *American Journal of Physiology, 177,* 544–548.

Mayer, J. E., Roy, P., and Mitra, K. P. (1956). Relation between caloric intake, body weight and physical work: Studies in an industrial male population in West Bengal. *American Journal of Clinical Nutrition, 4*, 169–175.

Mayer, J. E., and Pudel, V. (1972). Experimental studies on food-intake in obese and normal weight subjects. *Journal of Psychosomatic Research, 16*, 305–308.

Maxfield, E., and Knoishi, F. (1966). Patterns of food intake and physical activity in obesity. *Journal of the American Dietetic Association, 49*, 406–408.

McArdle, W. D., Katch, F. I., and Katch, V. L. (1981). *Exercise Physiology*, Philadelphia: Lea and Febiger.

McCann, I. L., and Homes, D. S. (1984). The influence of aerobic exercise on depression. *Journal of Personality and Social Psychology, 46*, 1142–1147.

McConnell, Jr., T. R., Cromwell, R. L., Bialer, I., and Son, C. D. (1964). Studies in activity level: VII. Effects of amphetamine drug administration on the activity level of retarded children. *Journal of Mental Deficiency, 68*, 647–651.

McFarlain, R. A., and Hersen, M. (1974). Continuous measurement of activity level in psychiatric patients. *Journal of Clinical Psychology, 30*, 37–39.

McGowan, C. R., Bulik, C. M., Epstein, L. H., Kupfer, D. J., and Robertson, R. J. (1984). The use of the large-scale integrated sensor (LSI) to estimate energy expenditure. *Journal of Behavioral Assessment, 6*, 51–57.

McGowan, C. R., Epstein, L. H., Kupfer, D. J., Bulik, C. M., and Robertson, R. J. (1986). The effect of exercise on non-restricted caloric intake in male joggers. *Appetite, 7*, 97–105.

McPartland, R. J., Foster, F. G., Kupfer, D. J., and Weiss, B. (1976). Activity sensors for use in psychiatric evaluation. *IEEE Transactions on Biomedical Engineering, 23*, 175–178.

McPartland, R. J., Kupfer, D. J., and Foster, F. G. (1976). The movement activated recording monitor: A third-generation motor activity monitoring system. *Behavior Research Methods and Instrumentation, 8*, 357–360.

Meehl, P. E. (1967). Theory-testing in psychology and physics: A methodological paradox. *Philosophy of Science, 34*, 103–115.

Meehl, P. E. and Rosen, A. (1955). Antecedent probability and the efficiency of psychometric signs, patterns, or cutting scores. *Psychological Bulletin, 52*, 194–216.

Melton, G. B. (1990). Ethical dilemmas in playing by the rules: Applied developmental research and the law. In C. B. Fisher and W. W. Tryon (Eds.). *Ethics in applied developmental psychology* (pp. 145–161). Norwood, NJ: Ablex.

Meltzer, H. Y. (1969a). Creatine kinase and aldolase in serum: Abnormality common to acute psychoses. *Science, 159*, 1368–1370.

Meltzer, H. Y. (1969b). Muscle enzyme release in the acute psychosis. *Archives of General Psychiatry, 21*, 102–112.

Meltzer, H. Y., and Holy, P. A. (1974). Black–white differences in serum creatine phosphokinase (CPK) activity. *Clinica Chimica Acta, 54*, 215–224.

Meltzer, H. Y., and Moline, R. (1970). Plasma enzymatic activity after exercise: Study of psychiatric patients and their relatives. *Archives of General Psychiatry, 22*, 390–407.

Mendelson, W. B. (1987). *Human Sleep: Research and clinical care*. New York: Plenum.

Metropolitan Life Insurance Company. (1983). 1983 Metropolitan Height and Weight Tables. *Statistical Bulletin of the Metropolitan Insurance Company, 64*, 2–9.

Milich, R. (1984). Cross-sectional and longitudinal observations of activity level and sustained attention in a normative sample. *Journal of Abnormal Child Psychology, 12*, 261–276.

Milich, R., and Loney, J. (1979) The role of hyperactive and aggressive symptomatology in predicting adolescent outcome among hyperactive children. *Journal of Pediatric Psychology, 4*, 93–112.

Milich, R., Loney, J., and Landau, S. (1982). Independent dimensions of hyperactivity and aggression: A validation with playroom observation data. *Journal of Abnormal Psychology, 91*, 183–198.

Milich, R. S., Loney, J. and Landau, S. (1982). The independent dimensions of hyperactivity and aggression: A validation with playroom observation data. *Journal of Abnormal Psychology*, *91*, 183–198.

Millichap, J. G. (1974). Neuropharmacology of hyperkinetic behavior: Response to methylphenidate correlated with degree of activity and brain damage. In A. Vernadakis and N. Weiner (Eds.), *Drugs and the Developing Brain* (pp. 475–488). New York: Plenum.

Millichap, J. G., and Boldrey, E. F. (1967). Studies in hyperkinetic behavior II. Laboratory and clinical evaluations of drug treatments. *Neurology*, *17*, 467–471.

Millichap, J., and Johnson, F. (1977). Methylphenidate in hyperkinetic behavior: Relation of response to degree of activity and brain damage. In C. Conners (Ed.), *Clinical Use of Stimulant Drugs in Children*. Amsterdam: Excerpta Medica.

Monroe, L. J. (1967). Psychological and physiological differences between good and poor sleepers. *Journal of Abnormal Psychology*, *72*, 255–264.

Montagu, J. D., and Swarbrick, L. (1975). Effect of amphetamines in hyperkinetic children: Stimulant or sedative? A pilot study. *Developmental Medicine and Child Neurology*, *17*, 293–298.

Montgomery, I., Perkin, G., and Wise, D. (1975). A review of behavioral treatments for insomnia. *Journal of Behavior Therapy and Experimental Psychiatry*, *6*, 93–100.

Montoye, H. J., Washburn, R., Servais, S., Ertl, A., Webster, J. C., and Nagle, F. J. (1983). Estimation of energy expenditure by a portable accelerometer. *Medicine and Science in Sports and Exercise*, *13*, 403–407.

Moore, R. Y. (1978). Central neural control of circadian rhythms. In W. F. Ganong and L. Martine (Eds.). *Frontiers in Neuroendocrinology* (Vol. 5) (pp. 185–206). New York: Raven Press.

Moreland, K. L. (1977). Stimulus control of hyperactivity. *Perceptual and Motor Skills*, *45*, 916.

Morrell, E. M., and Keefe, F. J. (1988). The actometer: An evaluation of instrument applicability for chronic pain patients. *Pain*, *32*, 265–270.

Morris, J. N, Chave, S. P. W., Adam, C., Sirey, C., Epstein, L., and Sheehan, D. J. (1973). Vigorous exercise in leisure-time and the incidence of coronary heart disease. *Lancet*, *1*, 333–339.

Morris, J. N., Heady, J. A., Raffle, P. A. B., Roberts, C. G., and Parks, J. W. (1953). Coronary heart disease and physical activity of work. *Lancet*, *II*, 1111–1120.

Morris, J. R. W. (1973). Accelerometry: A technique for the measurement of human body movements. *Journal of Biomechanics*, *6*, 729–736.

Morrison, D. E., and Henkel, R. E. (1970). *The Significance Test Controversy; A Reader*. Chicago: Aldine.

Morrison, J. R. and Stewart, M. A. (1971). A family study of the hyperactive child syndrome. *Biological Psychiatry*, *3*, 189–195.

Mullaney, D. J., Kripke, D. F., and Messin, S. (1980). Wrist-actigraphic estimation of sleep time. *Sleep*, *3*, 83–92.

Mundel, W. J., and Malmo, H. P. (1979). An accelerometer for recording head movement of laboratory animals. *Physiology and Behavior*, *23*, 391–393.

Munetz, M. R., and Cornes, C. L. (1982). Akathesia, pseudoakathesia, and tardive dyskinesia: Clinical examples. *Comprehensive Psychiatry*, *23*, 345–352.

Naughton, J., Bruhn, J. G., and Lategola, M. T. (1968). Effects of physical training on physiologic and behavioral characteristics of cardiac patients. *Archives of Physical Medicine and Rehabilitation*, *49*, 131–137.

Nazem, S. F. (1988). *Applied Time Series Analysis for Business and Economic Forecasting*. New York: Marcel Dekker, Inc.

Newman, J., Stampi, C., Dunham, D. W., and Broughton, R. (1988). Does wrist-actigraphy approximate traditional polysomnographic detection of sleep and wakefulness in narcolepsy–cataplexy? *Sleep Research*, *17*, 343.

Ogilvie, R. D., and Wilkinson, R. T. (1984). The detection of sleep onset: Behavioural and physiological convergence. *Psychophysiology*, *21*, 510–520.

Ogilvie, R. D., and Wilkinson, R. T. (1988). Behavioral versus EEG-based monitoring of all-night sleep-wake patterns. *Sleep*, *11*, 139–155.

Ogilvie, R. D., Wilkinson, R. T., and Allison, S. (1989). The detection of sleep onset: Behavioral, physiological, and subjective convergence. *Sleep*, *12*, 458–474.

O'Leary, K. D., Pelham, W. W., Rosenbaum, A., and Price, G. H (1976). Behavioral treatment of hyperkinetic children. *Clinical Pediatrics*, *15*, 510–515.

Olsson, A. G, Kaijser, L., Walldium, G., Logan, R. L., Riemersma, R. A., and Oliver, M. F. (1979). Risk factors for ischaemic heart disease with emphasis on nutrition and exercise. *Bibl. Nutr. Dieta*, *27*, 18–24.

Oscai, L. B., Spirakis, C. N., Wolff, C. A., and Beck, R. J. (1972). Effects of exercise and food restriction on adipose tissue cellularity. *Journal of Lipid Research*, *13*, 588–592.

Oswald, I., Berger, R. J., Jamarillo, R. A., Keddie, K. M. G., Olley, P. C., and Plunkett, G. B. (1963). Melancholia and barbiturates—A controlled EEG, body and eye movement study of sleep. *British Journal of Psychiatry*, *109*, 66–78.

Paffenbarger, R. S., Gima, A. S., Laughlin, M. E., and Black, R. A. (1971). Characteristics of longshoremen related to fatal coronary heart disease and stroke. *American Journal of Public Health*, *61*, 1362–1370.

Paffenbarger, R. S., and Hale, W. E. (1975). Work activity and coronary heart mortality. *New England Journal of Medicine*, *292*, 545–550.

Paffenbarger, R. S., Hyde, R. T., Wing, A. L., and Hsieh, C. C. (1986). Physical activity, all-cause mortality and longevity of college alumni. *New England Journal of Medicine*, *314*, 605–613.

Paffenbarger, R. S., Wing. A. L., and Hyde, R. T. (1978). Physical activity as an index of heart attack risk in college alumni. *American Journal of Epidemiology*, *108*, 161–175.

Partington, M. W., Campbell, D., Kuyek, J., and Mehlomakulu, M. (1971). Motor activity in early life III. Premature babies with neonatal tyrosinaemia; a pilot study. *Biology of the Neonate*, *18*, 121–128.

Partington, M. W., Lang, E., and Campbell, D. (1971). Motor activity in early life I. Fries' congenital activity types. *Biology of the Neonate*, *18*, 94–107.

Peacock, L. J., and Williams, M. (1962). An ultrasonic device for recording activity. *American Journal of Psychology*, *75*, 648–652.

Pedersen, F. A., and Bell, R. Q. (1970). Sex differences in preschool children without histories of complications of pregnancy and delivery. *Developmental Psychology*, *3*, 10–15.

Perri, M. G., Shapiro, R. M., Ludwig, W. W, and Twentyman, C. T. (1984). Maintenance strategies for the treatment of obesity: An evaluation of relapse prevention training and posttreatment contact by mail and telephone. *Journal of Consulting and Clinical Psychology*, *52*, 404–413.

Perri, M. G., Shapiro, R. M., Ludwig, W. W., Twentyman, C. T., and McAdoo, W. G. (1984). Maintenance strategies for the treatment of obesity: An evaluation of relapse prevention training and posttreatment cotact by mail and telephone. *Journal of Consulting and Clinical Psychology*, *52*, 404–413.

Perris, C., and Rapp, W. (1974). Ambulatory activity during treatment with Fluspirilene in chronic schizophrenics. *Acta Psychiatrica Scandinavica* (Suppl.), *249*, 117–122.

Pfadt, A., and Tryon, W. W. (1983). Issues in the selection and use of mechanical transducers to directly measure motor activity in clinical settings. *Applied Research in Mental Retardation*, *4*, 251–270.

Pinto, L. P., and Tryon, W. W. (1990a, August). *An Examination of the Situational Specificity Hypothesis in Hyperactive Children*. Paper presented at the American Psychological Association, Boston, Massachusetts.

Pinto, L. P., and Tryon, W. W. (1990b, March). *Construct validity of three hyperactivity rating scales*. Paper presented at the meeting of the Eastern Psychological Association, Philadelphia, Pennsylvania.

Plomin, R., and Foch, T. T. (1980). A twin study of objectively assessed personality in childhood. *Journal of Personality and Social Psychology*, *39*, 680–688.

Poceta, J. S., Hajdukovic, R., Menn, S. J., Ruddy, J. R., and Mitler, M. M. (1989). Periodic leg movements in sleep and obstructive sleep apnea. *Sleep Research, 18,* 233.

Pope, L. (1970). Motor activity in brain injured children. *American Journal of Orthopsychiatry, 40,* 783–794.

Porrino, L. J., Rapoport, J. L., Behar, D., Sceery, W., Ismond, D. R., and Bunney, Jr., W. E. (1983). A naturalistic assessment of the motor activity of hyperactive boys I. Comparison with normal controls. *Archives of General Psychiatry, 40,* 681–687.

Porrino, L. J., Rapoport, J. L., Behar, D., Ismond, D. R., and Bunney, Jr. W. E. (1983). A naturalistic assessment of the motor activity of hyperactive boys II. Stimulant drug effects. *Archives of General Psychiatry, 40,* 688–693.

Post, R. M., Kotin, J., Goodwin, F. K., and Gordon, E. K. (1973). Psychomotor activity and cerebrospinal fluid amine metabolites in affective illness. *American Journal of Psychiatry, 130,* 67–72.

Post, R. M., Stoddard, F. J., Gillin, J. C., Buchsbaum, M. S., Runkle, D. C., Black, K. E., and Bunney, W. E. Jr. (1977). Slow and rapid alterations in motor activity, sleep, and biochemistry in a cycling manic-depressive patient. *Archives of General Psychiatry, 36,* 470–476.

Potter, J. D., and McMichael, A. J. (1986). Diet and cancer of the colon and rectum: A case-control study. *Journal of the National Cancer Institute, 76,* 557–569.

Quay, H. C., and Peterson, D. R. (1987). *Manual for the Revised Behavior Problem Checklist,* Coral Gables, Florida University of Miami.

Rapoport, J. L., Abrahamson, A., Alexander, D., and Lott, I. (1971). Playroom observations of hyperactive children on medication. *Journal of the American Academy of Child Psychiatry, 10,* 524–534.

Rapoport, J. L., Buchsbaum, M. S., Weingartner, H., Zahn, T., Ludlow, C., and Mikkelsen, E. J. (1980). Dextroamphetamine: Its cognitive and behavioral effects in normal and hyperactive boys and normal men. *Archives of General Psychiatry, 37,* 933–943.

Raskin, D. E. (1972). Akathesia: A side effect to be remembered. *American Journal of Psychiatry, 129,* 345–347.

Ravussin, E., and Bogardus, C. (1989). Relationship of genetics, age, and physical fitness to daily energy expenditure and fuel utilization. *American Journal of Clinical Nutrition, 49,* 968–975.

Ray, A. B., Jr., Shotick, A. L., and Peacock, L. J. (1977). Activity level of mentally retarded individuals: Do they reflect the circadian rhythm? *Australian Journal of Mental Retardation, 4,* 18–21.

Reddy, S. (1981). Dietary fat and its relationship to large bowel cancer. *Cancer Research, 41,* 3700–3705.

Redmond, D. P., and Hegge, F. W. (1985). Observations on the design and specification of a wrist-worn human activity monitoring system. *Behavior Research Methods, Instruments and Computers, 17,* 659–669.

Rechtschaffen, A., Hauri, P., and Zeitlin, M. (1966). Auditory awakening thresholds in REM and NREM sleep stages. *Perceptual and Motor Skills, 22,* 927–942.

Reschtschaffen, A., and Kales, A. (1968). *A Manual of Standard Terminology, Techniques and Scoring System for Sleep States of Human Subjects.* NIH Pub #204, Washington, Superintendent of Documents, Book 1-62 or Los Angeles: UCLA, Brain Information Service/Brain Research Institute, University of California at Los Angeles.

Reich, L. H., Kupfer, D. J., Weiss, B L., McPartland, R. J., Foster, F. G., Detre, T., and Delgado, J. (1974). Psychomotor activity as a predictor of sleep efficiency. *Biological Psychiatry, 8,* 253–256.

Reiser, S. J. (1979). The medical influence of the stethoscope. *Scientific American, 240,* 148–155.

Reitman, M., Tryon, W. W., and Gruen, W. (1990). *Detection of obstructive sleep apnea using abdominal actigraphy.* Unpublished Manuscript.

Ribordy, S. C., and Denney, D. R. (1977). The behavioral treatment of insomnia: An alternative to drug therapy. *Behaviour Research and Therapy, 15,* 39–50.

Richardson, J. R. (1971). Heart rate in middle-aged man. *American Journal of Clinical Nutrition, 24,* 1476–1481.

Richter, C. P. (1965). *Biological Clocks in Medicine and Psychiatry.* Springfield, Illinois: C. C. Thomas.

Richter, C. P. (1976). Artifactual seven-day cycles in spontaneous activity in wild rodents and squirrel monkeys. *Journal of Comparative and Physiological Psychology, 90,* 572–582.

Rie, H. E., Rie, E. D., Stewart, S., and Ambuel, J. P. (1976). Effects of methylphenidate on under-achieving children. *Journal of Consulting and Clinical Psychology, 44,* 250–260.

Rimm, D. (1963). Cost efficiency and test prediction. *Journal of Consulting Psychology, 27,* 89–91.

Rodgers, G., Norguchi, C., Schecter, M. (1985). Vaso-occlusive manifestations of sickle cell disease. *American Journal of Pediatric Hematology/Oncology, 7,* 245–253.

Romanczyk, R. G., Crimmins, D. B., Gordon, W. C., and Kashinsky, W. M. (1977). Measuring circadian cycles: A simple temperature recording preparation. *Behavior Research Methods and Instrumentation, 9,* 393–394.

Rorer, l. G., and Dawes, R. M. (1982). A base-rate bootstrap. *Journal of Consulting and Clinical Psychology, 50,* 419–425.

Rorer, L. G., Hoffman, P. J., LaForge, G. E., and Hsieh, K. C. (1966). Optimum cutting scores to discriminate groups of unequal size and variance. *Journal of Applied Psychology, 50,* 153–164.

Rosa, R. M., Bierer, B. E., and Thomas, R. (1980). A study of induced hyponatremia in the prevention and treatment of sickle cell crisis. *New England Journal of Medicine, 303,* 1138–1143.

Rose, H. E., and Mayer, J. (1968). Activity, caloric intake, fat storage, and the energy balance of infants. *Pediatrics, 41,* 18–29.

Rosenbaum, S., Skinner, R. K., Knight, I. B., Garrow, J. S. (1985). A survey of heights and weights of adults in Great Britain, 1980. *Annals of Human Biology, 12,* 115–127.

Rothbart, M. K. (1981). Measurement of temperament in infancy. *Child Development, 52,* 569–578.

Rozeboom, W. W. (1960). The fallacy of the null-hypothesis significance test. *Psychological Bulletin, 57,* 416–428.

Rusak, B., and Zucker, I. (1975). Biological rhythms and animal behavior. *Annual Review of Physiology, 27,* 137–171.

Royant-Parola, S., Borbely, A. A., Tobler, T., Benoit, O., and Widlocher, D. (1986). Long-term activity monitoring in 12 depressed patients. *British Journal of Psychiatry, 149:*288–293.

Rutter, M. (1967). A children's behavior questionnaire for completion by teachers: Preliminary findings. *Journal of Child Psychology and Psychiatry, 8,* 1–11.

Sadeh, A., Alster, J., Urbach, D., and Lavie, P. (1989). Actigraphically based automatic bedtime sleep-wake scoring: Validity and clinical applications. *Journal of Ambulatory Monitoring, 2,* 209–216.

Sander, L. W., and Julia, H. L. (1966). Continuous interactional monitoring in the neonate. *Psychosomatic Medicine, 28,* 822–835.

Sandoval, J. (1977). The measurement of the hyperactive syndrome in children. *Review of Educational Research, 47,* 293–318.

Saris, W. H. M., and Binkhorst, R. A. (1977a). The use of pedometer and actometer in studying daily physical activity in man. Part I: Reliability of pedometer and actometer. *European Journal of Applied Physiology, 37,* 219–228.

Saris, W. H. M., and Binkhorst, R. A. (1977b). The use of pedometer and actometer in studying daily physical activity in man. Part II: Validity of pedometer and actometer measuring the daily physical activity. *European Journal of Applied Physiology, 37,* 229–235.

Saris, W. H. M., Snel, P., and Binkhorst, R. A. (1977). A portable heart rate distribution recorder for studying daily physical activity. *European Journal of Applied Physiology, 37,* 17–25.

Satoh, T., and Haroda, Y. (1973). Electrophysiological study of tooth-grinding during sleep. *Electroencephalography and Clinical Neurophysiology, 35,* 267–275.

Saunders, S. H. (1980). Toward a practical instrument system for the automatic measurement of "up-time" in chronic pain patients. *Pain, 9,* 103–109.

Saunders, K. J., Goldstein, M. K., and Stein, G. H. (1978). Automatic measurement of patient activity on a hospital rehabilitation ward. *Archives of Physical Medicine and Rehabilitation, 59,* 255–257.

Schachar, R., Rutter, M. and Smith, A. (1980). Characteristics of situationally and pervasively hyperactive children: Implications for syndrome definition. *Journal of Child Psychology and Psychiatry*, 22, 375–392.

Schleifer, M., Weiss, G., Cohen, N., Ecman, M., Crejie, H. and Krugar, H. (1975). Hyperactivity in preschools and the effect of methylphenidate. *American Journal of Orthopsychiatry*, 45, 38–50.

Schulman, J. L., Kaspar, J. C., and Throne, F. M. (1965). *Brain Damage and Behavior: A Clinical Experimental Study*. Springfield, Illinois: C. C. Thomas.

Schulman, J. L., and Reisman, J. M. (1959). An objective measure of hyperactivity. *American Journal of Mental Deviance*, 64, 455–456.

Schulman, R. L., Stevens, T. M., and Kupst, M. J. (1977). The biomotometer: A new device for the measurement and remediation of hyperactivity. *Child Development*, 48, 1152–1154.

Schwartz, M., Mandell, A. J., Green, R., and Ferman, R. (1966). Mood, motility, and 17-hydroxycorticoid excretion: A polyvariable case study. *British Journal of Psychiatry*, 112, 149–156.

Scrimshaw, N. S., and Pollitt, E. (1984). In E. Pollitt and P. Amante (Eds.). *Energy intake and activity* (pp. ix–xii): New York: Alan R. Liss, Inc.

Servais, S. B., Webster, J. G., and Montoye, H. J. (1984). Estimating human energy expenditure using an accelerometer device. *Journal of Clinical Engineering*, 9, 159–170.

Shaffer, D., McNamara, N., and Pincus, J. H. (1974). Controlled observations on patterns of activity, attention, and impulsivity in brain damaged and psychiatrically disturbed boys. *Psychological Medicine*, 4, 4–18.

Shaffer, D., and Greenhill, L. A. (1979). A critical note on the predictive validity of the "hyperkinetic syndrome." *Journal of Child Psychology and Psychiatry*, 20, 61–72.

Shapiro, S., Weinblatt, E., Frank, C. W., and Sager, R. V. (1965). The HIP study of incidence and prognosis of coronary heart disease: Preliminary findings on incidence of myocardial infarction and angina. *Journal of Chronic Disease*, 18, 527–558.

Sheehy, T. W., and Plumb, V. J. (1977). Treatment of sickle cell disease. *Archives of Internal Medicine*, 137, 779–792.

Sigel, S. (1956). *Nonparametric Statistics for the Behavioral Sciences*. New York: McGraw-Hill.

Silverman, R. W., Chang, A. S., and Russell, R. W. (1988). Measurement of activity in small animals using a microcomputer-controlled system. *Behavior Research Methods, Instruments, and Computers*, 20, 537–540.

Sime, W. E. (1987). Exercise in the prevention and treatment of depression. In W. P. Morgan and S. E. Goldston (Eds.), *Exercise and Mental Health* (pp. 145–152). Washington, DC: Hemisphere.

Simons, A. D., McGowan, C. R., Epstein, L. H., Kupfer, D. J., and Robertson, R. J. (1985). Exercise as a treatment for depression: An update. *Clinical Psychology Review*, 5, 553–568.

Siscovick, D. S., Weiss, N. S., Hallstrom, A. P., Inui, T. S., and Peterson, D. R. (1982). Physical activity and primary cardiac arrest. *Journal of the American Medical Association*, 248, 3113–3117.

Slattery, M. L., and Jacobs, Jr., D. R. (1987). The interrelationships of physical activity, physical fitness, and body measurements. *Medical Science and Sports Exercise*, 19, 564–569.

Slattery, M. L., Jacobs Jr., D. R., and Nichaman, M. A. (1989). Leisure time physical activity and coronary heart disease death: The U.S. Railroad study. *Circulation*, 79, 304–311.

Slattery, M. L., Schumacher, M. C., Smith, K. R., West, D. W., and Abd-Elghany, N. (1988). Physical activity, diet, and risk of colon cancer in Utah. *American Journal of Epidemiology*, 128, 989–999.

Smith, R. C. (1985). Relationship of periodic movements in sleep (nocturnal myoclonus) and the Babinski sign. *Sleep*, 8, 239–243.

Smith, M. P., Mendez, J., Druckenmiller, M., and Kris-Etherton, P. M. (1982). Exercise intensity, dietary intake, and high-density lipoprotein cholesterol in young female competitive swimmers. *American Journal of Clinical Nutrition*, 36, 251–255.

Smolen, D. M., Stein, G. H., Goldstein, M. K., and Rosenshein, J. S. (1978). NEW: An interactive data management system for monitoring ambulatory patients. *Computer Programs in Biomedicine*, 8, 71–76.

Snyder, F., and Scott, J. (1972). The psychology of sleep. In N. S. Greenfield and R. A. Sternback (Eds.). *Handbook of Psychophysiology* (pp. 645–708). Toronto: Holt, Rinehart and Winston.

Sopko, G., Jacobs, D. R. Jr., and Taylor, H. L. (1984). Dietary measures of physical activity. *American Journal of Epidemiology*, *120*, 900–911.

Sprague, R. L., Barnes, K. R., and Werry, J. S. (1970). Methylphenidate and Thioridazine: Learning, reaction time, activity, and classroom behavior in disturbed children. *American Journal of Orthopsychiatry*, *40*, 615–628.

Sprague, R. L., Christensen, D. E., and Werry, J. S. (1974). Experimental psychology and stimulant drugs. In C. K. Conners (Ed.) *Clinical Use of Stimulant Drugs in Children* (pp. 141–163). The Hague: Excerpta Medica.

Sprague, R. L., and Sleator, E. K. (1973). Effects of psychopharmacologic agents on learning disorders. *Pediatric Clinics of North America*, *20*, 719–735.

Sprague, R. L., and Toppe, L. K. (1966). Relationship between activity level and delay of reinforcement in the retarded. *Journal of Experimental Child Psychology*, *3*, 390–397.

Stahl, S. M. (1985). Akathesia and tardive dyskinesia. *Archives of General Psychiatry*, *42*, 915–917.

Stallones, R. A. (1980). The rise and fall of ischemic heart disease. *Scientific American*, *243*, 53–59.

Stampi, C., and Broughton, R. (1989). Ultrashort sleep-wake schedule: Detection of sleep state through wrist actigraph measures. *Sleep Research*, *18*, 100

Stefanik, P. A., Heald, F. P., and Mayer, J. (1959). Caloric intake in relation to energy output of obese and non-obese adolescent boys. *American Journal of Clinical Nutrition*, *7*, 55–62.

Stern, M. J., and Cleary, P. (1982). The national exercise and heart disease project: Long-term psychosocial outcome. *Archives of Internal Medicine*, *142*, 1093–1097.

Stern, J. S., and Lowney, P. (1986). Obesity: The role of physical activity (pp. 145–158). In K. D. Brownell and J. P. Foreyt (Eds.). *Handbook of Eating Disorders: Physiology, Psychology, and Treatment of Obesity, Anorexia, and Bulimia*. New York: Basic Books.

Stevens, E. A. (1971). Some effects of tempo changes on stereotyped rocking movements of low-level mentally retarded subjects. *American Journal of Mental Deficiency*, *76*, 76–81.

Stevens, T. M., Kupst, M., Suran, B. G. and Schulman, J. L. (1978). Activity level: A comparison between actometer scores and observer ratings. *Journal of Abnormal Child Psychology*, *6*, 163–173.

Stewart, A. L., and Brook, R. H. (1983). Effects of being overweight. *American Journal of Public Health*, *73*, 171–178.

Stoddard, F. J., Post, R. M., and Bunney, W. E., Jr. (1977). Slow and rapid psychobiological alterations in a manic-depressive patient: Clinical phenomenology. *British Journal of Psychiatry*, *130*, 72–78.

Stoff, D. M., Stauderman, K., and Wyatt, R. J. (1983). The time and space machine: Continuous measurement of drug-induced behavior patterns in the rat. *Psychopharmacology*, *80*, 319–324.

Stonehill, E., and Crisp, A. H. (1971). Problems in the measurement of sleep with particular reference to the development of a motility bed. *Journal of Psychosomatic Research*, *15*, 495–499.

Stott, F. D. (1977). Ambulatory monitoring. *British Journal of Clinical Equipment*, *2*, 61–68.

Stradling, J., Warley, A., and Sharpley, A. (1987). Wrist actigraphic assessment of sleep. *5th International Congress of Sleep Research Abstracts*, (Poster 521) 672.

Straw, M. K., and Rogers, T. (1985). Obesity assessment. In W. W. Tryon (Ed.), *Behavioral Assessment in Behavioral Medicine* (pp. 19–65). New York: Springer.

Stunkard, A. E. (1958). Physical activity, emotions, and human obesity. *Psychosomatic Medicine*, *20*, 366–372.

Stunkard, A. J., and McLaren-Hume, M. (1958). The results of treatment for obesity. *Archives of Internal Medicine*, *103*, 80–85.

Stunkard, A. J. (1960). A method of studying physical activity in man. *American Journal of Clinical Nutrition*, *8*, 595–601.

Stunkard, A., and Pestka, J. (1962). The physical activity of obese girls. *American Journal of Diseases of Children, 103*, 812–817.

Sykes, D. H., Douglas, V. I., Weiss, G., and Minde, K. K. (1971). Attention in hyperactive children and the effect of methylphenidate (Ritalin). *Journal of Child Psychology and Psychiatry, 12*, 129–139.

Taylor, C. B., Kraemer, H. C., Bragg, D. A., Miles, L. E., Rule, B., Savin, W. M., and Debusk, R. F. (1982). A new system for long-term recording and processing of heart rate and physical activity in outpatients. *Computers and Biomedical Research, 15*, 7–17.

Taylor, H. L., Jacobs, D. R., Schucker, B., Knudsen, J, Leon, A. S., and DeBacker, G. (1978). A questionnaire for the assessment of leisure time physical activities. *Journal of Chronic Disease, 31*, 741–755.

Teicher, M. H., Barber, N. I., Baldessarini, R. J., and Shaywitz, B. A. (1988). Amphetamine accelerates and attenuates ultradian activity rhythms in preweanling rats. *Pharmacology Biochemistry and Behavior, 29*, 517–523.

Teicher, M. H., Barber, N. I., Lawrence, J. M., and Baldessarini, R. J. (1989). Motor activity and antidepressant drugs: A proposed approach to categorizing depression syndromes and their animal models. In D. Kupfer, G. Koobs, and C. Ehlers (Eds.) (1980). *Animal Models of Depression* (pp. 135–161). Boston: Birkhauser Press.

Teicher, M. H., Cohen, B. M., Baldessarini, R. J., and Cole, J. O. (1988). Severe daytime somnolence in patients treated with an MAOI. *American Journal of Psychiatry, 145*, 1552–1556.

Teicher, M. H., Lawrence, J. M., Barber, N. I., Finklestein, S. P., Lieberman, H., and Baldessarini, R. J. (1986). Altered locomotor activity in neuropsychiatric patients. *Progress in Neuro-Psychopharmacology and Biological Psychiatry, 10*, 755–761.

Teicher, M. H., Lawrence, J. M., Barber, N. I., Finklestein, S. P., Lieberman, H. R., and Baldessarini, R. J. (1988). Increased activity and phase delay in circadian motility rhythms in geriatric depression: Preliminary observations. *Archives of General Psychiatry, 45*, 913–917.

Terman, M. (1983). Behavioral analysis and circadian rhythms. In M. D. Zeiler and P. Harzem (Eds.), *Advances in Analysis of Behaviour* (Vol. 3) (pp. 103–141). New York: Wiley.

Terman, M., and Terman, J. S. (1970). Circadian rhythm of brain self-stimulation behavior. *Science, 168*, 1242–1244.

Terman, M., and Terman, J. S. (1975). Control of the rat's circadian self-stimulation rhythm by light–dark cycles. *Physiology and Behavior, 14*, 781–789.

Thomas, A., and Chess, S. (1977). *Temperament and Development*. New York: Brunner/Mazel.

Thompson, J. K., Jarvie, G. J., Lahey, B. B., and Cureton, K. J. (1982). Exercise and obesity: Etiology, physiology, and intervention. *Psychological Bulletin, 91*, 55–79.

Tizard, B. (1968b). Observations of over-active imbecile children in controlled and uncontrolled environment. II: Classroom studies. *American Journal of Mental Deficiency, 72*, 548–553.

Trites, R. L., Blouin, A. G. A., Ferguson, H. B., and Lynch, G. (1981). The Conners Teacher Rating Scale: An epidemiologic, interrater reliability and follow-up investigation. In K. D. Gadow and J. Loney (Eds.), *Psychological Aspects of Drug Treatment for Hyperactivity*. Boulder, Colorado: Westview Press.

Tryon , W. W. (1984a), Principles and methods of mechanically measuring motor activity. *Behavioral Assessment, 6*, 129–139.

Tryon, W. W. (1984b). Measuring activity using actometers: A methodological study. *Journal of Behavioral Assessment, 6*, 147–153.

Tryon, W. W. (1985a). Measurement of human activity. In W. W. Tryon (Ed.) *Behavioral Assessment in Behavioral Medicine* (pp. 200–256). New York: Springer.

Tryon, W. W. (1986). Motor activity measurements and DSM-III. *Progress in Behavior Modification, 20*, 36–66.

Tryon, W. W. (1987). Activity as a function of body weight. *American Journal of Clinical Nutrition, 46*, 451–455.

Tryon, W. W. (1989a). Behavioral assessment and psychiatric diagnosis. In H. Hersen (Ed.). *Innovations in Child Behavior Therapy* (pp. 35–56). New York: Springer.

Tryon, W. W. (1989b). Motor activity and DSM-III-R. In M. Hersen and S. M. Turner (Eds.). *Adult Psychopathology and Diagnosis*. New York: Wiley.

Tryon, W. W. (1989c). Behavioral measurement of activity: Obtaining stable clinical measurements. (Submitted for publication.)

Tryon, W. W., Pinto, L. P. and Morrison, D. F. (in press). Reliability assessment of pedometer activity measurements. *Journal of Psychopathology and Behavioral Assessment*.

Tryon, W. W. (1990). Predictive parallels between clinical and applied developmental psychology. In C. B. Fisher and W. W. Tryon (Eds.). *Ethics in Applied Developmental Psychology* (pp. 203–214). Norwood, New Jersey: Ablex.

Tzischinsky, O., Epstein, R., Zomer, J., Barak, S., and Lavie, P. (1987). Pre- and post-puberty changes in motility in sleep: An actigraphic study. *5th International Congress of Sleep Research Abstracts* (Poster 541), 692.

Ullman, D. G., Barkley, R. A., and Brown, H. W. (1978). The behavioral symptoms of hyperkinetic children who successfully responded to stimulant drug treatment. *American Journal of Orthopsychiatry, 48*, 425–437.

Urbach, D., Lavie, P., and Alster, J. (1989). Screening for sleep disorders by actigraphic recordings. *Sleep Research, 18*, 357.

Van Itallie, T. B. (1985). Health implications of overweight and obesity in the United States. *Annals of Internal Medicine, 103*, 983–988.

Van Praag, H. M., and Korf, J. (1971). Retarded depression and the dopamine metabolism. *Psychopharmacologia, 19*, 199–203.

Van Putten, T. (1975). The many faces of akathesia. *Comprehensive Psychiatry, 16*, 43–47.

Vena, J. E., Graham, S., Zielezny, M., Swanson, M K., Barnes, R. E., and Nolan, J. (1985). Lifetime occupational exercise and colon cancer. *American Journal of Epidomiology, 122*, 357–365.

Waksberg, J. (1978). Sampling methods for random-digit-dialing. *Journal of American Statistical Association, 73*, 40–46.

Waldrop, M. F., and Halverson, C. F., Jr. (1971). Minor physical anomalies and hyperactive behavior in young children. In J. Hellmuth (Ed.). *Exceptional Infant: Studies in Abnormalities*. Vol. 2. New York: Brunner/Mazel.

Warnold, I., and Arvidsson-Lenner, R. (1977). Evaluation of the heart rate method to determine the daily energy expenditure in disease. A study in juvenile diabetics. *American Journal of Clinical Nutrition, 30*, 304–315.

Washburn, R., Chin, M. K., and Montoye, H. J. (1980). Accuracy of pedometer in walking and running. *Research Quarterly for Exercise and Sport, 51*, 695–702.

Waxman, M., and Stunkard, A. J. (1980). Caloric intake and expenditure of obese boys. *Journal of Pediatrics, 96*, 187–193.

Webb, P., and Annis, J. F. (1983). Adaptation to overeating in lean and overweight women. *Human Nutrition and Clinical Nutrition, 37C*, 117–131.

Webster, J. B., Kripke, D. F., Messin, S., Mullaney, D. J., and Wyborney, G. (1982). An activity-based sleep monitor system for ambulatory use. *Sleep, 5*, 389–399.

Webster, J. B., Messin, S., Mullaney, D. J., and Kripke, D. F. (1982). Transducer design and placement for activity recording. *Medical and Biological Engineering and Computing, 20*, 741–744.

Wehr, T. A., and Goodwin, F. K. (1979). Rapid cycling in manic-depressives induced by tricyclic antidepressants. *Archives of General Psychiatry, 36*, 555–559.

Wehr, T. A., and Goodwin, F. K. (1980). Desynchronization of circadian rhythms as a possible source of manic-depressive cycles. *Seventh Annual Meeting of the ACNP—Abridged Proceedings, 15*, 19–20.

Wehr, T. A., and Goodwin, F. K. (1980). Desynchronization of circadian rhythms as a possible source of manic-depressive cycles. *Psychopharmacology Bulletin, 16,* 19–20.

Wehr, T. A., Goodwin, F. K., Wirz-Justice, A., Breitmaier, J., and Craig, C. (1982). 48-hour sleep-wake cycles in manic-depressive illness: Naturalistic observations and sleep-deprivation experiments. *Archives of General Psychiatry, 39,* 559–565.

Wehr, T. A., Muscettola, G., and Goodwin, F. K. (1980). Urinary 3-methoxy-4-hydroxyphenylglycol circadian rhythm: Early timing (phase-advance in manic depressives compared with normal subjects). *Archives of General Psychiatry, 37,* 257–263.

Wehr, T. A., Wirz-Justice, A., Goodwin, F. K., Duncan, W., and Gillin, J. C. (1979). Phase advance of the sleep–wake cycle as an antidepressant. *Science, 206,* 710–713.

Weiss, B. L., Foster, F. G., Reynolds, C. F. III, and Kupfer, D. J. (1974). Psychomotor activity in mania. *Archives of General Psychiatry, 31,* 379–383.

Weiss, B. L., Kupfer, D. J., Foster, F. G., and Delgado, J. (1974). Psychomotor activity, sleep, and biogenic amine metabolites in depression. *Biological Psychiatry, 9,* 45–54.

Werry, J., and Aman, M. (1975). Methylphenidate and halperidol in children: Effects on attention, memory, and activity. *Archives of General Psychiatry, 32,* 790–795.

Werry, J. S., and Sprague, R. L. (1970). Hyperactivity. In C. G. Costello (Ed.), *Symptoms of Psychopathology.* New York: Wiley.

Westover, S. A., and Lanyon, R. I. The maintenance of weight loss after behavioral treatment. *Behavior Modification, 14,* 123–137.

Whalen, C. K., and Henker, B. (1980). The social ecology of psychostimulant treatment: A model for conceptual and empirical analysis. In C. K. Whalen and B. Henker (Eds.), *Hyperactive Children, Social Ecology of Identification and Treatment.* New York: Academic Press.

Whalen, C. K., Henker, B., Collins, B. E., Finck, D. and Dotemoto, S. A. (1979). A social ecology of hyperactive boys: Medication effects in systematically structured classroom environments. *Journal of Applied Behavioral Analysis, 12,* 65–81.

Wilkinson, P. W., Parkin, J. M., Pearlson, G., Strong, H., and Sykes, P. (1977). Energy intake and physical activity in obese children. *British Medical Journal, 1,* 756.

Wilkinson, R. T. (1968). Sleep deprivation: Performance tests for partial and selective sleep deprivation. In B. F. Fiess and L. A. Abt (Eds.). *Progress in Clinical Psychology* (pp. 28–43). New York: Grune and Stratton.

Wilkinson, R. T. (1970). Methods for research on sleep deprivation and sleep function. In Hartmann, E. (Ed.), *Sleep and Dreaming* (pp. 369–382). Boston: Little and Brown.

Willett, W., and Stampfer, M. J. (1986). Total energy intake: Implications for epidemiologic analyses. *American Journal of Epidemiology, 124,* 17–27.

Williams, H. L., Hammack, J. T., Daly, R. L., Dement, W. C., and Lubin, A. (1964). Responses to auditory stimulation, sleep loss and the EEG stages of sleep. *Electroencephalography and Clinical Neurophysiology, 16,* 269–279.

Williams, R. L., and Karacan, I. (1976). *Pharmacology of Sleep.* New York: Wiley.

Williamson, D. A., Calpin, J. P., DiLorenzo, T. M., Garris, R. P., and Petti, T. A. (1981). Treating hyperactivity with dexedrine and activity feedback. *Behavior Modification, 5,* 399–416.

Winchell, C. A. (1981). *The Hyperkinetic Child: An Annotated Bibliography, 1974–1979.* Westport, Connecticut: Greenwood Press.

Winer, B. J. (1971). *Statistical Principles in Experimental Design* (2nd ed.). New York: Wiley.

Wing, R. R., Epstein, L. H., Marcus, M. D., and Koeske, R. (1984). Intermittent low-calorie regimen and booster sessions in the treatment of obesity. *Behaviour Research and Therapy, 22,* 445–449.

Woggon, B., Angst, J., Curtius, H. Ch., Niederwieser, A., Levine, R. A., Borbely, A. A., and Tobler, I. (1985). Tetrahydrobiopterin (BH$_4$) in endogenous depression. *Pharmacopsychiatry, 18,* 98–99.

Wolff, E. A., III, Putnam, F. W., and Post, R. M. (1985). Motor activity and affective illness: The relationship of amplitude and temporal distribution to changes in affective state. *Archives of General Psychiatry, 42,* 288–294.

Wolpert, E. (1960). Studies in psychophysiology of dreams II. An electromyographic study of dreaming. *Archives of General Psychiatry, 2,* 231–241.

Wong, T. C., Webster, J. G., Montoye, H. J., and Washburn, R. (1981). Portable accelerometer device for measuring human energy expenditure. *IEEE Transactions on Biomedical Engineering, BME-28,* 467–471.

Woo, R., Garrow, J. S., and Pi-Sunyer, F. X. (1982a) Effect of exercise on spontaneous calorie intake in obesity. *American Journal of Clinical Nutrition, 36,* 470–477.

Woo, R., Garrow, J. S., and Pi-Sunyer, F. X. (1982b). Voluntary food intake during prolonged exercise in obese women. *American Journal of Clinical Nutrition, 36,* 478–484.

Word, T., and Stern, J. A. (1958). A simple stabilimeter. *Journal of the Experimental Analysis of Behavior, 1,* 199–203.

Wren, F. J., Teicher, M. H., Baldessarini, R. J., and Lieberman, H. (1988). Locomotor activity patterns and stimulant response in children with attention deficit hyperactivity disorder. *American Academy of Child Adolescent Psychiatry Abstracts, 4,* 65.

Zentall, S. S. (1980). Behavioral comparisons of hyperactive and normally active children in natural settings. *Journal of Abnormal Child Psychology, 8,* 93–109.

Zentall, S. S., and Zentall, T. R. (1976). Activity and task performance of hyperactive children as a function of environmental stimulation. *Journal of Consulting and Clinical Psychology, 44,* 693–697.

Zomer, J., Peled, R., Gruen, W., and Lavie, P. (1989). Actigraphic monitoring to encourage CPAP treatment. *Sleep Research, 18,* 406.

Zomer, J., Pollack, I., Tzischinsky, O., Epstein, R., Alster, J., and Lavie, P. (1987). Computerized assessment of sleep time by wrist actigraph. *5th International Congress of Sleep Research* (Poster 528), 528.

Index